T0275450

Population Politics in the Tropics

Population Politics in the Tropics explores colonial population policies in Angola between 1890 and 1945 from a transimperial perspective. Using a wide array of previously unused sources and multilingual archival research from Angola, Portugal and beyond, Samuël Coghe sheds new light on the history of colonial Angola, showing how population policies were conceived, implemented and contested. He analyses why and how doctors, administrators, missionaries and other colonial actors tried to grasp and quantify demographic change and 'improve' the health conditions, reproductive regimes and migration patterns of Angola's 'native' population. Coghe argues that these interventions were inextricably linked to pervasive fears of depopulation and underpopulation, but that their implementation was often hampered by weak state structures, internal conflicts and multiple forms of African agency. Coghe's fresh analysis of demography, health and migration in colonial Angola challenges common ideas of Portuguese colonial exceptionalism.

SAMUËL COGHE is Postdoctoral Research Fellow in Global History at the Freie Universität Berlin.

Global Health Histories

Series editor:

Sanjoy Bhattacharya, *University of York*

Global Health Histories aims to publish outstanding and innovative scholarship on the history of public health, medicine and science worldwide. By studying the many ways in which the impact of ideas of health and well-being on society were measured and described in different global, international, regional, national and local contexts, books in the series reconceptualise the nature of empire, the nation state, extra-state actors and different forms of globalisation. The series showcases new approaches to writing about the connected histories of health and medicine, humanitarianism and global economic and social development.

Population Politics in the Tropics

Demography, Health and Transimperialism in Colonial Angola

Samuël Coghe

Freie Universität Berlin

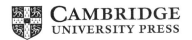

CAMBRIDGE
UNIVERSITY PRESS

CAMBRIDGE
UNIVERSITY PRESS

University Printing House, Cambridge CB2 8BS, United Kingdom

One Liberty Plaza, 20th Floor, New York, NY 10006, USA

477 Williamstown Road, Port Melbourne, VIC 3207, Australia

314–321, 3rd Floor, Plot 3, Splendor Forum, Jasola District Centre,
New Delhi – 110025, India

103 Penang Road, #05-06/07, Visioncrest Commercial, Singapore 238467

Cambridge University Press is part of the University of Cambridge.

It furthers the University's mission by disseminating knowledge in the pursuit of
education, learning, and research at the highest international levels of excellence.

www.cambridge.org
Information on this title: www.cambridge.org/9781108837866
DOI: 10.1017/9781108943307

First published 2022

A catalogue record for this publication is available from the British Library.

Library of Congress Cataloging-in-Publication Data
Names: Coghe, Samuël, author.
Title: Population politics in the tropics : demography, health, and transimperialism in
   colonial Angola / Samuël Coghe, Freie Universitat Berlin.
Description: Cambridge, United Kingdom ; New York, NY : Cambridge
University Press, 2022. | Series: Global health histories | Originally presented as the
   author's thesis (doctoral)–European University Institute (EUI) in Florence, 2014. |
   Includes bibliographical references and index.
Identifiers: LCCN 2021039264 | ISBN 9781108837866 (hardback) | ISBN
   9781108932103 (paperback) | ISBN 9781108943307 (epub)
Subjects: LCSH: Angola–Population policy. | Angola–Population–Histoy. |
   Portugal–Colonies–Angola–History. | Angola–Politics and
   government–1855-1961. | Public health–Angola–History. |
   BISAC: MEDICAL / History
Classification: LCC HB3664.4.A3 C64 2022 | DDC 967.3/03–dc23
LC record available at https://lccn.loc.gov/2021039264

ISBN 978-1-108-83786-6 Hardback

For Laura and Nora

Contents

Maps

Figures

Tables

x

Acknowledgements

This book grew out of my PhD thesis defended at the European University Institute (EUI) in Florence in 2014. Over the years, it has greatly benefited from discussions with colleagues at the project's various intellectual homes. I wish to thank first my supervisor Sebastian Conrad, who has given this project his continuous intellectual and moral support, at the EUI and later at the Freie Universität Berlin. The EUI provided a most stimulating scholarly environment in which to embark on a transimperial project on colonial Africa. Formative for this book were also my long stays at the Max Planck Institute for the History of Science (MPIWG), where I had the chance to be part of Veronika Lipphardt's vibrant research group. Here I also met Alexandra Widmer, with whom I happened to share a common interest in colonial population politics and whose feedback, encouragement and friendship have accompanied me ever since. The workshops of the research network on Demography and Population (funded by the German Research Foundation) greatly enlarged my vision on population and demography, for which I thank fellow network members Regula Argast, Maria Dörnemann, Ursula Ferdinand, Heinrich Hartmann, Axel Hüntelmann, Teresa Huhle, Morgane Labbé, Jesse Olszynko-Gryn, Petra Overath, Christiane Reinecke, Thomas Robertson, Corinna Unger and, again, Alexandra Widmer. In Berlin, Andreas Eckert and Baz Lecocq have opened the doors to the world of African history for me. Further, the informal reading group on African history provided me with crucial feedback and collegial support during the last periods of revision. Many sincere thanks to Sarah Bellows-Blakely, Marie Huber, Stephanie Lämmert, Dörte Lerp, Christoph Kalter, Marcia Schenck and Daniel Tödt. I would also like to thank my other (former) Berlin colleagues Catherine Davies, Franziska Exeler, Sebastian Gottschalk, Minu Haschemi Yekani, and Christoph Kamissek, as well as Teresa Huhle for reading chapters at various stages of this project.

This book has been supported by pre- and postdoctoral scholarships provided by the Belgian Ministry of Foreign Affairs, the EUI and the MPIWG. I am also indebted to the staff of numerous archives and libraries. I want to express my special gratitude to all employees at the National Library in Lisbon and the library of the Ibero-American Institute in Berlin, the main libraries I consulted for this book and places where I felt very much at home; to Ruth Gbikpi at the EUI and Ellen Garske and Ruth Kessentini at the MPIWG for providing me innumerable books and articles through their fabulous interlibrary loan systems; to Jacques Oberson at the League of Nations Archives in Geneva; to Emily Burgoyne at the Baptist Missionary Society Archives in Oxford and to Fathers Gérard Vieira and Martin Dejonge at the Archives de la Congrégation du Saint-Esprit in Chevilly-Larue near Paris. Not the least I want to thank the entire staff of the Arquivo Histórico Ultramarino in Lisbon, who endured my insatiable demands for more sources and brought me, over the years, hundreds of boxes and bundles of (often still unsorted) documents. My sincere gratitude also goes to Alexandra Aparício and Seu Mateus for facilitating and guiding my archival research at the Arquivo Nacional de Angola and to Luiz Damas Mora for sharing private letters from his great-uncle with me. Finally, I am also indebted to Márcia Gonçalves and Léo Péria-Peigné who retrieved some additional sources for me in Lisbon and Chevilly-Larue at a time when the COVID-19 pandemic made travelling impossible.

Portions of Chapter 3 appeared in earlier versions in 'Inter-imperial Learning and African Health Care in Portuguese Angola in the Interwar Period', *Social History of Medicine* 28.1 (2015), 134–54 and 'Sleeping Sickness Control and the Transnational Politics of Mass Chemoprophylaxis in Portuguese Colonial Africa', *Portuguese Studies Review* 25.1 (2017), 57–89. Chapter 4 is a substantially revised and enlarged version of 'Medical Demography in Interwar Angola. Measuring and Negotiating Health, Reproduction and Difference', in: Alexandra Widmer and Veronika Lipphardt, (eds.), *Health and Difference. Rendering Human Variation in Colonial Engagements*, New York/Oxford: Berghahn Books, 2016, 178–204. It also contains a few reworked paragraphs published earlier in 'Tensions of Colonial Demography. Depopulation Anxieties and Population Statistics in Interwar Angola', *Contemporanea. Rivista di Storia dell'800 e del '900* 18.3 (2015), 472–8. I would like to thank Oxford University Press, Baywolf Press, Berghahn and il Mulino for their kind permission to re-use this material.

During archival stays and conferences in Portugal, Angola and Brazil, I had the chance to discuss parts of this book project with many eminent colleagues working on Portuguese colonial history and the lusophone world, most notably Eric Allina, Warwick Anderson, Cristiana Bastos, Mariana Candido, Cláudia Castelo, José Curto, Rita Garnel, Ana Carolina Vimieiro-Gomes, João Pedro Gomes, Márcia Gonçalves, Philip Havik, Miguel Bandeira Jerónimo, Alexander Keese, Paulo Teodoro de Matos, Maria da Conceição Neto, Inês Queiroz, Eugénia Rodrigues, Ricardo Roque, Ricardo Boaventura Santos,

Ana Cristina Nogueira da Silva, Jorge Varanda and Jelmer Vos. I am very grateful for their active support and the convivial discussions. I also gratefully recognise the comments received during many other workshops, most notably those in Florence, Berlin, Rostock and London organised by Moritz von Brescius, Daniel Hedinger, Nadin Heé, Christoph Kamissek, Jonas Kreienbaum and Valeska Huber, and not the least the incomparable 'platform' workshops staged by Sebastian Conrad in exquisite places in and around Berlin. Finally, I also want to thank Shane Doyle, Sarah Ehlers, Guillaume Lachenal and Myriam Mertens for sharing their thoughts on colonial demography and medicine with me.

During the final stages of this project, I greatly benefited from the generous, detailed and constructive feedback from the anonymous reviewers, which helped me in rethinking and revising the manuscript. I am also indebted to Rachel Blaifeder, Lucy Rhymer, Emily Sharp and Natasha Whelan for skilfully guiding me through the publication process at Cambridge University Press; Maria João Lourenço Pereira for drawing the maps; Natasha Klimenko for taking care of the other maps and pictures; and Jess Farr-Cox for making the index and, together with Margot Wylie at an earlier point, correcting and improving the English of this manuscript. Of course, any errors and imperfections that may remain are mine.

This book would have been much more difficult in the making without the hospitality and conviviality of my friends in Lisbon. To Ana, Bernadette, Emiliana, Inês, João, Márcia, Rui and Teresa, Sofia, Susana and Xico: *muito obrigado*! I am immensely grateful to my family in Belgium and Bremen, and to my closest friends, most notably Carl and Olivier, for their enduring support, love and friendship. Finally, my greatest debt is to Laura Stielike and our daughter Nora, to whom I dedicate this book. From the beginning, Laura has accompanied this project, engaging in countless discussions, reading and commenting on chapters, and enduring my late nights, absences and preoccupations. Her love and support, as well as Nora's affection and humour, have sustained me through the many vicissitudes of this project.

Note on the Spelling of Proper Names

Geographical names are spelt according to the current official norms in Angola. Orthography has changed at various times in the twentieth and twenty-first centuries and is now close to the orthography used in the 1920s and 1930s (e.g. Luanda, Cuanza river, Quiçama). Many places in Angola and neighbouring countries have changed names during and after the colonial period. I have retained the names most commonly used by the Portuguese during the period under study (e.g. São Salvador do Congo, Nova Lisboa, Léopoldville, Northern Rhodesia). At the time, Portuguese names were often interchangeably used with African names (e.g. Nova Lisboa = Huambo). Names of African peoples are spelt according to international Bantu standards (e.g. Kuvale, Kwanyama).

Introduction

In 1918, former colonial administrator Luiz de Mello e Athayde published an article in the influential Bulletin of the Geographical Society of Lisbon, warning about the ongoing depopulation of Angola, Portugal's long-standing colony in West Central Africa. While old calculations, he argued, had assumed a total population of 10–12 million, or a density of nine inhabitants per square km, newer ones suggested a density of six, or even as low as 3.3, confirming his intuition that Angola's once abundant population had been and was still diminishing markedly. For the causes, Athayde pointed at the old emigration of slaves to the Americas, new emigration flows to Angola's neighbouring colonies and various factors that diminished fertility and augmented mortality. For the Ganguela population in southern Angola that he had administrated and studied, these were constant raids by the neighbouring Kwanyama, who enslaved Ganguela people and destroyed their livelihoods; diseases such as smallpox and the lesser-known local scourges of *michila* and *lindunda*; alcoholism; and birth-spacing practices. Athayde's rationales were less humanitarian than political and economic. If depopulation continued, he argued, Angola would soon face the same labour problem as other colonies, since only 'natives' could provide the necessary labour force needed for the colonial economy.[1]

Athayde was neither the first nor the last Portuguese colonial official to warn about Angola's demographic decline. From the late nineteenth century until the aftermath of the Second World War, a steady flow of alarming reports expressed, provoked and cemented great concern about the 'quantity and quality' of Angola's 'native' population. Many of them made a similarly uncritical use of available demographic data and expressed rationales and solutions similar to those of Athayde, who urged the complete pacification

---

[1] Athayde, 'Perigo do despovoamento'. I use 'native' *(indígena)* as an actor's term. Contemporary Europeans used the terms interchangeably, either to designate the vast majority of Angolans still considered 'uncivilised' and hence subject to a specific political and civil status *(indigenato)* or, in a broader 'racial' sense, to designate all 'black', 'African' people in Angola. See also footnote 4.

and 'civilisation' of the colony, the spread of modern medicine, protection of infants and reduction of emigration. Fears among the colonisers that the African population, so crucial to the colonial project, was declining and degenerating dovetailed with broader (and shifting) ideological and political, economic and scientific concerns and interests and gave rise to a wide range of medical and administrative interventions.

These population discourses and policies are the subject of this book. It examines fears around depopulation and how these were entangled with a broad array of policies aimed at preserving, increasing and physically improving the 'native' population in Portuguese Angola. It argues that discourses and practices of population improvement affected Angola's African population in multiple ways, even if they were often underfunded, half-hearted, inconsistent and contested, as they involved a wide array of actors with sometimes converging, but often also conflicting, interests. It therefore analyses the agency and mutual interactions of ministers and governors, local administrators and imperial inspectors, doctors and missionaries, journalists and scientists, national and international organisations and networks, as well as Africans in their role as patients and nurses, mothers and midwives, labourers and chiefs, migrants and peasants. It also argues that depopulation anxieties and population politics in Angola were inextricably linked to similar discourses and practices in other parts of the (colonial) world. By exploring transnational and transimperial connections, I show that Portuguese colonialism was firmly embedded in a larger European context and thus make a broader argument against reductionist views of Portuguese exceptionalism so common in the literature.

The narrative is picked up in the 1890s, when colonial expansion, ideological shifts and epidemic sleeping sickness challenged conventional views on the 'native' population and triggered unprecedented concern among doctors, administrators and missionaries in Angola. The book follows this depopulation discourse through the first half of the twentieth century, showing how it was constantly reiterated by alarming reports about deadly diseases, low fertility, high infant mortality, endemic labour scarcity and rampant emigration, until it gradually faded away after the Second World War. I thereby explore the ambiguous role of demographic knowledge, arguing that anxieties about the size and evolution of the 'native' population were partly based on demographic data that colonial actors did not hesitate to instrumentalise for their purposes, even though these data were (often ostensibly) incomplete, flawed and contested.

Simultaneously, this volume shows how depopulation fears gave rise to a broad array of policies aiming to increase both the 'quantity and quality' of the population. It attends to the colonial response to sleeping sickness from the late nineteenth century onwards and the emergence of an ambitious programme of African healthcare after the First World War. This *Assistência Médica aos*

Indígenas (Native Medical Assistance) attempted to combat epidemic and endemic diseases, but also included new approaches to reduce infant mortality and improve maternal fertility and health. Finally, I underline the importance of colonial attempts to curb cross-border emigration via prohibiting most forms of labour migration and providing incentives for border populations to stay in Angola.

The book transcends major political caesuras. In October 1910, the revolutionary overthrow of the old constitutional monarchy (1822–1910), which had been dominated by landed elites, led to a republican form of parliamentary democracy in Portugal, commonly called the First Portuguese Republic (1910–26). It had its power base in 'progressive' urban bourgeois and intellectual milieus and was marked by huge social tensions, anti-clerical laws and endemic political instability, with 45 governments in 16 years. While these shifts had repercussions for colonial policies, the most fundamental change was the decentralisation of the Empire. New organic laws granted greater autonomy to the colonies, a change that reached its apogee in the 1920s, when Angola and Mozambique were governed by high commissioners with far-reaching prerogatives.[2]

In May 1926, the Republic was overthrown and replaced by a military dictatorship, during which royalists, conservative republicans and radical nationalists struggled for power, until, around 1930, the Minister of Finance (and from 1932 Prime Minister) António de Oliveira Salazar consolidated his position and began to construct the *Estado Novo*, resulting in a new constitution in 1933. The conservative, authoritarian and corporatist policies of the *Estado Novo*, which also included financial austerity and an increasingly pro-clerical stance, were gradually applied to the colonies. Perhaps the most defining moments were the reaffirmation of the unity of Empire and its political recentralisation in Lisbon, with the Colonial Ministry receiving strong powers of oversight, through the Colonial Act (*Acto Colonial*) of 1930 and the Organic Law of the Portuguese Colonial Empire (*Carta Orgânica do Império Colonial Português*) and the Overseas Administrative Reform (*Reforma Administrativa Ultramarina – RAU*), both in 1933.[3]

This volume attends to the impact of these regime changes on the colonies, as they entailed ideological changes, the renewal of political elites and the reform of governmental and administrative structures. However, it is critical of the extent to which they determined important shifts in demographic discourses and 'native' population policies. The long time-span of this book allows it to show that such changes were often gradual and that some milestone events, such as setting up the *Assistência Médica aos Indígenas* at the

---

[2] Proença, 'Questão colonial'. See also Rosas and Rollo (eds.), *História*.
[3] Meneses, *Salazar*; Oliveira, 'Ciclo africano', 479–86.

beginning of the military dictatorship in 1926, resulted from plans that had been conceived under earlier regimes. This is not surprising given the fundamental continuities in colonial policies between political regimes. All of them were strongly nationalist, pro-colonialist and anxious about Portugal's colonial prestige. Moreover, throughout the late nineteenth and first half of the twentieth century, deeply entrenched racism pervaded their paternalistic 'civilising missions' and discriminatory policies towards the 'native' population in Angola. The *indigenato* system, gradually established after the official abolition of European-controlled slavery in the 1870s and frequently (re)codified in the first half of the twentieth century, was only legally abolished in 1961. During that period, the vast majority of 'black' Angolans were considered 'uncivilised' *indígenas* and, much like in the French colonies, subject to a specific political, civil and judicial regime that excluded them from citizenship and key political rights and imposed specific labour duties and sanctions unless they had gained the status of 'civilised' *assimilados*.[4] Certainly in some cases regime changes clearly mattered, but the continuities in population policies across political regimes underline the fact that the prisms of political, metropolitan and national history are not sufficient to understand changes in demographic and medical discourses and practices in Angola. A key argument made herein is that these were also – and sometimes primarily – provoked by international disruptions such as the two World Wars and the world economic crisis of the early 1930s and driven by broader changes in ideas, perceptions and practices that circulated among colonial powers through processes of inter-imperial learning and competition.

This book also acknowledges the particular position of Angola within the larger framework of the Portuguese Empire and hence the situatedness of Portuguese population politics in Angola. Angola was not just any Portuguese colony. With about 1.25 million square kilometres and presumably about 3–4 million inhabitants in the early twentieth century, it was by far the largest in area and the second largest in population (after Mozambique) of the eight remaining colonies in what had arguably once been Europe's first global maritime empire.[5] Moreover, by the late nineteenth century, Portuguese colonial influence in Angola was already four centuries old. 'Discovered' (from a European perspective) by Diogo Cão in the 1480s, Angola's coastal regions were, in the sixteenth and seventeenth century, gradually brought under formal Portuguese control.[6] They played a major role in the transatlantic slave trade.

---

[4] See Cruz, *Estatuto do indigenato*; Silva, *Constitucionalismo e Império*; Silva, 'Natives'. See also Jerónimo, *Civilising Mission*, 26–30, 38–41. Compare with Mann, 'What Was the Indigénat?'.

[5] See, for instance, Bethencourt and Curto (eds.), *Portuguese Oceanic Expansion*.

[6] Birmingham, *Trade and Conflict*; Thornton, 'Early Kongo-Portuguese Relations'; Heintze, *Studien*.

Between 1500 and 1867, an estimated 5.6 million Africans were shipped as slaves from West Central Africa to the Americas, about two-thirds of them from the Portuguese-controlled port cities of Luanda and Benguela alone.[7] Most were brought to Brazil and, over the centuries, cross-Atlantic exchanges forged an almost symbiotic relationship between both Portuguese colonies, to the extent that historians such as Luiz Felipe de Alencastro have characterised Angola as a sub-colony of Brazil.[8] With Brazilian independence in 1822 and the end of the Portuguese slave trade from Angola in the mid-nineteenth century, Angola's position within the Empire changed dramatically. Driven by a widespread belief in the colony's immeasurable resources and economic opportunities and (compared to Mozambique) greater geographic proximity to Portugal, many colonialists came to see Angola as the new cornerstone of the reconfigured 'Third' Portuguese Empire (1822–1975).[9] Angola's particular status, I suggest, exacerbated depopulation anxieties and, alongside local factors, shaped how population policies were conceived and implemented.

Reframing Portuguese Colonialism

By examining population discourses and policies, this book not only moves beyond existing scholarship on colonial Angola and the 'Third' Portuguese Empire in general; it also inevitably challenges how Portuguese colonialism in the late nineteenth and twentieth centuries has usually been framed and interpreted. Over recent decades, historians have mainly focused on explaining three issues: the particularities and contradictions of Portuguese imperial and racial ideologies;[10] the persistence of forms of unfree labour well into the twentieth century;[11] and the belated and violent decolonisation process, with its protracted colonial wars (1961–74), late developmental policies and African nationalist movements.[12] Looking through these specific lenses has often

---

[7] Eltis and Richardson, 'New Assessment'; Silva, *Atlantic Slave Trade*. On the social history of the transatlantic slave trade in Angola, see Miller, *Way of Death*; Candido, *African Slaving Port*.

[8] See particularly Alencastro, *Trato dos Viventes*; Curto, *Enslaving Spirits*; Ferreira, *Cross-Cultural Exchange*.

[9] See Chapter 1. The first (maritime) empire was organised around the Portuguese trading posts in India, the second (territorial) empire around the Brazilian economy and the third centred on Portugal's African colonies. For an overview, see Costa, Rodrigues and Oliveira (eds.), *História da Expansão*. See also Clarence-Smith, *Third Portuguese Empire*.

[10] See Castelo, *Modo português*; Alexandre, *Velho Brasil, novas Áfricas*; Matos, *Côres do Império*; Bethencourt and Pearce (eds.), *Racism and Ethnic Relations*; Jerónimo, *Civilising Mission*.

[11] See Higgs, *Chocolate Islands*; Allina, *Slavery*; Ball, *Angola's Colossal Lie*; Cleveland, *Diamonds in the Rough*; Jerónimo, *Civilising Mission* and Monteiro, *Portugal*.

[12] Messiant, *Angola colonial*; Morier-Genoud (ed.), *Sure Road?*; Jerónimo and Pinto (eds.), *Portugal e o fim do colonialismo*; Jerónimo and Pinto (eds.), *Ends of European Colonial Empires*; Péclard, *Incertitudes*; Jerónimo, 'Battle'; Alexandre, *Contra o vento*.

induced historians to – implicitly or explicitly – characterise Portuguese colonialism as distinctly brutal and backward compared to other European colonialist projects. Tying in with some newer studies that challenge this idea of Portuguese colonial exceptionalism, this book contributes to rethinking and reappraising Portuguese colonialism in two ways. First, by focusing on the important but understudied domains of demography, medicine and 'native' policy, it contributes to a more complex and nuanced picture of Portuguese colonialism, especially since there are few studies on colonial policies 'on the ground' in Angola for the period between 1890 and 1945. Second, by adopting comparative, transnational and transimperial perspectives, I show that population politics in Angola were firmly embedded in broader European discourses and practices and, in many regards, not so 'different', let alone exceptional.

Population Politics and the Colonial State

Portuguese colonialism in Angola cannot be understood by looking at ideological formations, forced labour regimes and late-imperial intransigence alone, however real and afflicting they were for many Angolans. Portuguese colonialism in Angola was also (often in contradictory ways) underwritten by discourses, logics and practices that, following Michel Foucault, can be described as the 'biopolitics of the population'.[13]

When Foucault coined the terms 'biopower' and 'biopolitics' in the mid-1970s, he referred to a set of technologies that emerged in seventeenth- and eighteenth-century Europe, used to know (*savoir*) and optimise the life of both the individual and the collective body.[14] According to Foucault, the individual body was addressed through disciplinary institutions like the clinic, the prison and the army in order to 'produce human beings whose bodies are at once useful and docile', while the collective body required a different 'series of interventions and regulatory controls: a biopolitics of the population'. Made possible by medicine and the emergence of statistics as a new scientific discipline, these interventions targeted the biological basis of the population, aiming to monitor and improve both its quantity and 'quality'.[15] My use of the term 'population politics' refers to this latter part of Foucault's biopower/biopolitics paradigm. As summarised by Philipp Sarasin, this involved

the registration and regulation of the population 'movements' in a given society, ranging from the statistical registration of births and deaths, the state's efforts to increase the birth rate and the most diverse forms of public hygiene and healthcare to

---

[13] Foucault, *Volonté de savoir*, 183.

[14] Foucault, 'Cours du 17 mars 1976'; Foucault, *Volonté de savoir*, 177–91.

[15] Inda, 'Analytics of the Modern', 6 (first quote); Foucault, *Volonté de savoir*, 183 (second quote).

the actual regulation of the population from a 'qualitative' point of view, in the end to the eugenically motivated extirpation of life deemed 'unworthy of living'.[16]

Historians of colonialism have criticised Foucault's biopower/biopolitics paradigm for two main reasons. On the one hand, some have rightly condemned the Eurocentrism of his account, which can be said to be both empirical and epistemological: Foucault neither used non-European (con)texts to support his claims nor does the rise of 'biopower' seem to have been influenced by events or thought from outside Western Europe. Thus, Ann Laura Stoler has asked what Foucault's analysis and chronologies would look like if one included colonial settings.[17] On the other hand, scholars like Frederick Cooper and Megan Vaughan have downplayed the relevance of 'biopower' in the context of colonial rule in Africa, arguing that in most colonial settings power was 'repressive' rather than 'productive', more 'arterial' than 'capillary'.[18] Against the latter critique, however, Nancy Rose Hunt has argued that 'Foucault's notion of biopower needs to be taken seriously for colonial Africa', since 'these were not just extractive economies, but ones that wilfully, if ambivalently, promoted life'.[19]

This book refrains from adopting Foucault's general epistemological and analytical framework, with his contested concepts of (bio)power and governmentality, or from entering theoretical discussions about the validity of his chronologies. Rather, it follows Nancy Rose Hunt's intuition and uses Foucault's concept of 'population politics' as an analytical lens through which to examine 'native policy' in colonial Angola. This unites the variegated discourses and policies targeting the biological basis of Angola's African population, allowing them to be considered holistically. This study even broadens the scope of the concept. Beyond policies geared towards reducing mortality and increasing natality, which have usually been the focus of historical studies on colonial biopolitics,[20] it also analyses policies aimed at curbing African emigration, as these related directly to the size of Angola's 'native' population. Most fundamentally, this book explores how population politics played out in a colonial context where power asymmetries were arguably larger than in Europe and, due to claims of racial difference, differently shaped. Simultaneously, it examines how Portuguese population politics were influenced by the fact that Angola was part of the tropics.

---

[16] Sarasin, *Michel Foucault*, 167.
[17] Stoler, *Race*, 1–18. On epistemological Eurocentrism, see Mudimbe, *Invention of Africa*, 19–20.
[18] Vaughan, *Curing Their Ills*, 8–12 (quotes 10); Cooper, *Colonialism in Question*, 48–9 (quotes 48).
[19] Hunt, 'Fertility's Fires', 429 (quote). See also Hunt, *Nervous State*, 7–8.
[20] See, for instance, Hunt, *Colonial Lexicon*; Thomas, *Politics of the Womb*; Bashford, *Imperial Hygiene*.

Tropics was not merely a geographical term, designating the area between the Tropics of Cancer and Capricorn, 23°26′ north and south respectively of the equator, and hence including the Portuguese colony of Angola that stretches from latitude 4° to 18° S. It was also a powerful discursive term and social construct: the tropics were imagined as fundamentally different from temperate zones like Europe in climate and vegetation, diseases and human life.[21] Unlike much of the historiography linking colonialism and the tropics, however, this book does not focus on the protracted scientific and political debates about the possibilities of white settlement and acclimatisation,[22] but on how tropical visions and conditions shaped European politics towards indigenous populations. I claim that the indigenous populations in Angola were the object of overlapping processes of Othering, conceived and governed as a racial, colonial and climatic Other. Considered inferior and incapable of self-government and self-improvement, they had to be protected from the particular dangers of tropical nature – or to be torn out of their 'innate laziness' in order to take advantage of the immense possibilities tropical fertility apparently offered for agriculture.[23] As Warwick Anderson has argued, the domestication of the tropics, which became conceivable in the early twentieth century, justified colonial rule and 'technoscientific' interventions.[24]

Of course, population politics in Angola were neither monolithic nor all-encompassing. Although most colonisers viewed a growing and healthy African population as a precondition for the colony's *mise en valeur*, colonial rule in practice often ran counter to this logic, due to the conflicting interests and priorities of different colonial actors. On the one hand, competing rationales such as the search for short-term economic gains or the desire for comprehensive political and military control explain why colonial rule in twentieth-century Angola was never about population improvement alone, but continued to be marked also by exploitation and oppression, and in some cases outspoken indifference or extreme violence. Moreover, although colonial population discourse usually spoke of 'natives' in a generalising and totalising manner, policies sometimes differentiated between population groups. Largely based on the theories and categorisations of colonial anthropology, certain ethnic groups were deemed less important for – or even detrimental to – the future of the colony and 'excluded' from 'positive' population politics. Cases in point are the 'Bushmen' in Southern Angola, who were conceptualised as a

---

[21] Stepan, *Picturing Tropical Nature*; Arnold, *Tropics*, 110–4; Anderson, 'Natures of Culture'.
[22] For a brief analysis, see Chapter 1.
[23] On the 'climatic Other' and tropical laziness, see Duncan, *In the Shadows*, 8, 12, 182–4.
[24] Anderson, 'Natures of Culture'.

'primitive and dying race' and largely neglected by the Portuguese colonial state until the 1950s, or the 'unruly' pastoralist Kuvale, who suffered genocidal violence and forced relocation in the late 1930s and early 1940s.[25] On the other hand, the outcome of population policies was often more modest than, or simply different from, what had been planned or expected, because their implementation was hampered by practical problems and internal conflicts in the colonial administration and/or undermined by the attitudes and actions of the Angolan population. Angolans not only resisted but also actively (re)shaped policies intended to govern them.

This argument about the tensions and boundaries of population politics links to a broader shift in the conceptualisation of the colonial state in Africa. Counter to earlier visions of a powerful and autonomous colonial state, historians have in the last two decades increasingly highlighted its weakness and internal contradictions. Especially before 1945, that is before the 'second colonial occupation' and the rise of the 'developmental state' with increased funding and expanding bureaucratic apparatuses,[26] colonial states were almost permanently underfinanced and understaffed, and hence unable to completely fulfil their own far-reaching claims of controlling and transforming colonial territories and populations that were often larger than those of their metropoles. According to this revisionist view, the power of colonial states was also limited insofar as they relied heavily on African and European intermediaries and operated with little expert knowledge. Thus, their impact on African societies and cultures was often fragmentary.[27]

Various studies have shown that African intermediaries such as 'traditional' or newly appointed authorities, clerks, interpreters, soldiers, policemen, nurses and catechists were crucial for the functioning of the colonial state but were also difficult to control as they often followed their own agenda.[28] Some scholars, such as the sociologist Trutz von Trotha, have emphasised that the colonial state not only depended on African intermediaries ('external inter- mediarity'), but also on local European administrators ('internal intermediar- ity'), who in practice had significant discretionary powers. Until well into the twentieth century, these 'men on the spot', sometimes called 'the real chiefs of the empire', often acted independently from – and even contrary to the policies

---

[25] On the 'Bushmen', see Coghe, 'Reassessing Portuguese Exceptionalism'; on the Kuvale, see Pélissier, *História das campanhas*, vol. 2, 267–75 and Campos, *Ocupação*.

[26] See Cooper, 'Modernizing Bureaucrats' and Eckert, 'We Are All Planners Now'.

[27] Compare Young, *African Colonial State* with Berman, 'Perils'; Eckert, 'Vom Segen der (Staats-) Gewalt?' and Conrad and Stange, 'Governance and Colonial Rule'.

[28] See particularly the essays in Lawrance, Osborn and Roberts (eds.), *Intermediaries* and Glasman, 'Penser les intermédiaires'. On medical intermediaries, see also footnote 82.

devised by – the central administrations in the colonial capitals. Bringing them under more continuous and tight control was a long and difficult process.[29] Moreover, before 1945, and certainly before the 1920s, colonial rule in Africa was based on much less, and less systematic and stable, scientific knowledge than many colonial governments wished for, as the number of scientific institutions and experts remained low until the 'second colonial occupation' after the Second World War.[30]

This book further teases out the implications of this paradigm shift for Angola, drawing on recent work by Alexander Keese and Philip Havik.[31] It looks at the internal conflicts within and limitations of the colonial state that conditioned medical, demographic and administrative population policies. Attentive to the tension between colonial discourse and the 'contested, fragmentary and often ineffective nature of colonial practices', it sees failure as inherent to colonial rule.[32] It also attends to the 'epistemological worries' of colonial officials and the feelings of vulnerability and helplessness they often experienced in the colonial situation – topics that have received increased historiographical attention in recent years and further bolstered the notion of a 'weak' colonial state.[33] Portuguese colonial officials not only worried about the size and the health of Angola's 'native' population, but many of them also feared that Portugal was not as effective as other colonial powers in ruling and 'developing' them – or, at least, was perceived in this way by other colonial nations and Angolans alike. These deep-seated and multi-layered anxieties about Portugal's comparative position as an imperial power played out at various levels of the colonial administration and gave way to variegated 'politics of comparison': comparing and emulating practices from colonial competitors in some cases; avoiding being compared in others; and struggling for international recognition of important 'firsts' or particularly 'benevolent' practices. Following Ann Laura Stoler on the 'politics of imperial comparison', this study examines why, how and to what effect colonial actors constantly engaged in comparisons with other colonial powers.[34]

---

[29] Trotha, 'Was war Kolonialismus?', 63–4. See also, in greater detail, Spittler, *Verwaltung* and Trotha, *Koloniale Herrschaft*.

[30] See Tilley, *Africa* and, for the Portuguese empire, Castelo, 'Investigação científica'.

[31] See most notably Keese, *Living with Ambiguity*; Keese, 'Searching'; Havik, '"Direct" or "indirect" rule?' and Havik, Keese and Santos (eds.), *Administration and Taxation*.

[32] Duncan, *In the Shadows*, 2 (quote).

[33] See Stoler, *Carnal Knowledge*, 10; Stoler, *Along the Archival Grain*, 3 (quote). See also Reinkowski and Thum (eds.), *Helpless Imperialists*; Fischer-Tiné (ed.), *Anxieties, Fear and Panic*. For Portuguese Angola, see Roque, 'Razor's Edge'.

[34] Stoler and McGranahan, 'Introduction', 13–5.

Challenging Exceptionalism

This study challenges ideas of Portuguese colonial exceptionalism that under-write much of the historiography.[35] The notion that Portuguese colonial rule in the late nineteenth and twentieth century was different from that of other European powers was already actively promoted by the colonial state itself. In the 1930s and 1940s, the *Estado Novo* revived and exalted an imperial ideology, already prominent in the late nineteenth century, according to which Portuguese 'overseas expansion' and colonialism was not only particularly benevolent, pious and assimilationist, but also an historical and essential mission of the Portuguese nation.[36] In the 1950s, the *Estado Novo* adopted 'lusotropicalism', a concept that had been nurtured by the Brazilian sociologist Gilberto Freyre since the 1930s, as its legitimising ideology. Including many of the aforementioned ideas, its main claim was that Portuguese colonialism was uniquely benign due to the absence of racial discrimination and a positive stance on miscegenation.[37] Arguably, claiming imperial exceptionalism was not exceptional for colonial empires, but it was, as Stoler has convincingly argued, 'part of the discursive apparatus of empires'. Virtually all of them adopted self-images and imperial ideologies that set them apart and legitimised their 'civilising mission'.[38]

It is partly in reaction to such overly positive, lusotropicalist views, which continued to pervade debates on Portugal's colonial past until long after decolonisation (and sometimes still do), that recent historians of Portuguese colonialism have focused on debunking the contradictions of its racial ideologies, the violence of its labour regimes, the mismanagement of its developmental policies and the belatedness of its decolonisation.[39] By doing so, however, they have contributed to an opposite form of exceptionalism, describing a particularly unfit, backward and cruel empire. This notion was already present in international critique during colonial times, and positive self-images promulgated by *Estado Novo* colonialists were partly directed at this. Negative exceptionalism has also been fed by the writings of the influential Portuguese sociologist Boaventura de Sousa Santos, who posited that, due to Portugal's semiperipheric position in the capitalist world-system, its colonial rule was particularly weak and subaltern, marked by the 'incapacity to colonize efficiently' and a strong dependency on Great Britain.[40]

---

[35] For a critique of Portuguese colonial exceptionalism that addresses some of the same points, see Havik, Keese and Santos (eds.), *Administration and Taxation*, x–xi, 18–23.

[36] Polanah, 'Imperial Mystique'.

[37] See Castelo, *Modo português* and Anderson, Roque and Santos (eds.), *Luso-Tropicalism.*

[38] Stoler and McGranahan, 'Introduction', 10–13 (quote 10).   [39] See footnotes 10, 11 and 12.

[40] Santos, 'Between Prospero and Caliban', 9 (quote).

Arguably, this negative form of exceptionalism has, for a long time, also thrived on the lack of in-depth empirical studies on many other aspects of twentieth-century colonial rule in the Portuguese Empire, not least Angola, and the lack of comparative and transimperial studies that include the Portuguese colonies. In many domains (such as colonial medicine), Portuguese colonies have been ignored or at best been covered in a cursory way, thus leaving room for the assumption that 'the Portuguese' did things differently, or did not do anything. Portugal's absence is, for instance, very striking in the newer and often explicitly transimperial historiography on sleeping sickness, one of the major themes of this book.[41] This situation is now slowly changing, due to the work of a new generation of scholars probing deeper into the local practices and tensions of Portuguese colonial rule before 1945 and adopting comparative and transimperial perspectives.[42]

While the main difference might ultimately have been the protracted and violent decolonisation process in the 1960s and 1970s, this does not, of course, mean that there are no specificities of Portuguese colonial rule prior to 1945.[43] Nevertheless, this volume challenges Portuguese colonial exceptionalism in three intertwined ways. First, it questions the analytical value of generalisations that, as Boaventura Santos and lusotropicalist ideology did, conflate discourses and practices over vast spaces and time periods into a single theorem about the exceptional characteristics of Portuguese colonialism. It proposes to look beyond ideology and to acknowledge the situatedness, internal contradictions and shifting character of colonial discourses and practices 'on the ground'. Second, it questions the idealised norms of British (allegedly successful, peaceful and developmental) colonialism against which Portuguese colonial rule often seems to have been pitted. As Havik, Santos and Keese have argued, economic exploitation, repression and crude violence were 'common features' of European colonialism in late nineteenth- and early twentieth-century Africa. Although Portuguese administrations might often (though not always) have been comparatively underfunded and understaffed, this did not entail fundamental differences in policies, although, as I will show, such differences sometimes haunted Portuguese colonial officials.[44] Alongside Keese, this study advocates a shift in perspective to see Portuguese colonial rule not as 'different', but rather as a variation that was 'in its own ways representative of European colonial practices'.[45] Third and most directly, it shows that Portuguese population discourses, anxieties and policies in Angola

---

[41] See Chapters 1 and 2.   [42] See footnote 31.
[43] Havik, Keese and Santos (eds.), *Administration and Taxation*, 21. See also Jerónimo and Pinto (eds.), *Ends of European Colonial Empires*.
[44] Havik, Keese and Santos (eds.), *Administration and Taxation*, 21–3.
[45] Keese, 'Searching', 241 (quote).

were in many regards connected and similar to those in other colonial spaces, particularly in (Central) Africa.

To substantiate this claim, this study adopts a double, that is comparative and transimperial, approach. On the one hand, it compares colonial debates, policies and practices regarding Angola's 'native' population with those of other colonial powers, thus embedding them in the broader history of colonialism in Africa and beyond. Therefore, it draws on existing historiography as well as primary sources from these other empires. On the other, it examines how colonial actors, ideas and practices circulated across colonial and imperial borders.[46] By using these transcolonial and transimperial lenses, this study demonstrates that Angola was not exclusively tied to its metropole, Portugal, but also connected in multiple ways with actors, debates and policies in other parts of the (colonial) world, including other parts of the Portuguese Empire. This book argues that neither depopulation anxieties nor the policies attempting to address them were unique to Angola, but in large part the result of multiple intra- and inter-imperial exchanges of ideas, fears and practices. It thereby shows that such exchanges were conditioned by changing situations and power relations. Some ideas and practices did not circulate widely, due to ignorance, indifference or outright rejection by colonial actors; others underwent important changes while circulating and being (re-)adapted to different local circumstances; and still others were applied with a time lag or in a different situation.[47]

Simultaneously, this study also questions the 'Portugueseness' of population politics in Angola by attending to intra-imperial differences. Empires were not homogenous entities: not only did their parts have different levels of sovereignty, as Stoler has argued, but these were often also ruled in different manners, as George Steinmetz has masterfully shown by comparing 'German' native policy in South West Africa, Samoa and Qingdao.[48] The Portuguese Empire was also highly heterogeneous, with colonies that were all situated within the tropics, but as different in size, population, economics and geopolitics as the Cape Verde Islands, Macau and Angola. Rather than being the sole product of 'national' character, traditions or styles of thought, population discourses and policies varied considerably within the Portuguese Empire, due to differences in demographic conditions and disease environments, economic importance and geographical position, ethnographic representations and legal status of the populations they were targeting.

---

[46] On the chances and challenges of transimperial history, see Hedinger and Heé, 'Transimperial History'.

[47] See Raj, 'Beyond Postcolonialism', 343–4. On the non-circulation of knowledge and cultural production of ignorance, see Proctor and Schiebinger (eds.), *Agnotology*.

[48] Stoler, 'Degrees of Imperial Sovereignty'; Steinmetz, *Devil's Handwriting*.

A striking example can be found in the migration policies discussed in Chapter 6. Whereas, from the late nineteenth century, the colonial government in Lourenço Marques (now Maputo) allowed tens of thousands of Mozambican labourers to work in the mines and farms of neighbouring South Africa and Southern Rhodesia every year and organised a monitoring system for this massive labour migration, the Colonial Ministry in Lisbon did not allow the government in Luanda to copy this model when corresponding foreign demands for Angolan labourers arose in the interwar years. Fears of labour scarcity might have been stronger in Angola, but the main reason for this differential treatment was arguably the different position Angola held in the imperial imagination: the heart of the Portuguese Empire and exclusively national terrain.

Rethinking Population History in the Twentieth Century

By analysing population politics in colonial Africa before 1945, this book also departs from, and simultaneously speaks to, both main strands in the historiography on twentieth-century population politics, thus challenging some of the main narratives in population history.[49] The first major strand of research has analysed the decline of fertility that was first diagnosed for France in the mid-nineteenth century and began to affect many other European countries around the turn of the century. Initially, this topic interested mainly historical demographers, who sought to statistically reconstruct and explain falling birth rates in Europe.[50] From the 1980s onwards, however, historians shifted attention to the political, social and cultural dimensions of this demographic phenomenon.[51] They have shown how, in the late nineteenth and early twentieth centuries, declining birth rates triggered anxieties of both quantitative and qualitative population decline, the former threatening the external power of the nation-state, the latter the power balance within it. In the era of nationalism, both the size and composition of the population mattered for the future of the nation. Declining birth rates strengthened discourses of degeneration, as many contemporaries believed that this decline was greater among the 'educated classes' than among the 'lower and dangerous classes', and that this in turn would result in a growing dominance of 'undesirable elements'. Historians have argued that, although intertwined, fears over the size and the differential fertility of the population gave rise to the divergent intellectual answers and

---

[49] For an overview of these analytical strands, see Bashford, 'Nation, Empire, Globe', 170–1.
[50] For an authoritative analysis, see the contributions in Coale (ed.), *Decline of Fertility*.
[51] For the political history of population, see Rosental, 'Histoire politique'.

political programmes of pronatalism and eugenicism.[52] Pronatalist and eugenicist debates and policies have received much scholarly attention, also with regard to Portugal.[53] Colonial populations, however, are generally absent in this analytical framework, except for the anxieties of non-adaptation, degeneration and miscegenation regarding white Europeans in the colonies.[54]

The second major strand, which has gained momentum over the past 15 years, explores the global dimensions of the population problem and puts non-Europeans centre-stage. It has, however, a strong focus on the problem of overpopulation and, concomitantly, the global population control movement after the Second World War. Scholars like Matthew Connelly and Marc Frey have shown how, between the late 1940s and early 1980s, neo-Malthusian concerns regarding rapid population growth in Asia and parts of Africa and Latin America gripped international 'experts' and national policy-makers. Partly due to the support of a small but powerful transnational epistemic community of 'population experts', these concerns triggered numerous programmes aimed at monitoring and limiting population growth in what had begun to be referred to as the 'Third World'.[55] A growing number of case studies have analysed how such 'family planning' programmes functioned in national contexts, in other words, how they were enmeshed with imperatives of modernisation and development or implemented through contraceptives and sterilisation procedures.[56]

This book addresses the 'blind spots' of both strands of research. By studying pre-1945 Angola and showing that it was in many regards typical of large parts of tropical Africa and the Pacific, it makes the broader argument that discourses and policies with regard to colonial, non-European populations in the twentieth century were not only about overpopulation.[57] As such, this book also serves as a counterpoint to the work of Alison Bashford, who has retraced the genealogy of the global overpopulation discourse back into the

---

[52] Teitelbaum and Winter, *Fear of Population Decline*; Schneider, *Quality and Quantity*; Soloway, *Demography and Degeneration*; Cole, *Power*.

[53] From the vast literature, and in addition to the previous footnote, see, on pronatalist policies, Thébaud, 'Mouvement nataliste'; Pedersen, *Family*; Cova, 'Histoire de la maternité' and, on eugenics, Adams (ed.), *Wellborn Science*; Stepan, *Hour of Eugenics* and Turda and Gillette, *Latin Eugenics*. For Portugal, see, on pronatalist policies, Pimentel, *História das organizações femininas*; on eugenics, Pereira, 'Eugenia'; Matos, 'Aperfeiçoar a "raça"' and Cleminson, *Catholicism, Race and Empire*.

[54] See, for instance, Campbell, *Race and Empire*; Saada, *Empire's Children*. For the Portuguese Empire, see Williams, 'Migration and Miscegenation'; Bastos, 'Migrants, Settlers and Colonists'; Cleminson, *Catholicism, Race and Empire*, 203–45.

[55] See especially Connelly, *Fatal Misconception* and Frey, 'Neo-Malthusianism'.

[56] See, for instance, Briggs, *Reproducing Empire*; Huhle, *Bevölkerung*; Dörnemann, *Plan Your Family* and various contributions in Hartmann and Unger (eds.), *World of Populations*.

[57] For this broader argument, see also Coghe and Widmer, 'Colonial Demography'.

interwar period.[58] It does not question that the – mostly Anglophone – experts at the centre of Bashford's argument were indeed beginning to view overpopulation, already apparent in some Asian countries, as a global challenge, in (geo) political, economic and environmental terms, in the 1920s and 1930s. Rather, it demonstrates that there was another, simultaneous, population discourse. Parallel to fears of fertility and population decline in Europe, Portuguese, French, Belgian and British colonial 'experts' in tropical Africa and the Pacific were still predominantly concerned with the intertwined problems of de- and underpopulation. In many of these colonies, including Angola, fears of rapid population growth and overpopulation only emerged after 1945, and often even much later still, after decolonisation.

These depopulation anxieties and corresponding population policies have not gone completely unheeded in the historiography on tropical Africa and the Pacific, but they have thus far been analysed in a fragmentary and unsystematic way. One strand of studies has focused on discourse, discussing how European observers attributed de- and underpopulation in a particular colony or empire to a variety of causes, most notably deadly diseases, low fertility, high infant mortality, the persistence of 'native' customs, emigration and the nefarious influence of colonial rule.[59] Another body of literature has analysed particular colonial policies aimed at countering depopulation, such as medical campaigns against epidemic diseases[60] or interventions in indigenous women's reproduction.[61]

This book goes beyond this insightful literature, broadening the scope of analysis in three main ways. First, analysing both discourses and policies, it provides the first book-length analysis of how depopulation discourses and population politics in colonial Africa were interwoven, and how the latter played out locally. Second, it does not focus on a single cause of depopulation but examines a broad variety of causes and policies. Looking at all three basic demographic movements (natality, mortality and migration), it connects various fields of study rarely analysed together, such as demography, health, reproduction, migration and border policies. Third, this book transcends the national framework that usually limits the scope of analysis in the aforementioned studies. It shows how (de)population discourses and policies crossed

---

[58] Bashford, 'Nation, Empire, Globe' and especially Bashford, *Global Population*.

[59] For colonial Africa, see particularly van Beusekom, 'From Underpopulation to Overpopulation'; Sanderson, 'Congo belge'; Hunt, 'Colonial Medical Anthropology' and Ittmann, *Problem of Great Importance*, 48–82. On depopulation anxieties in the Pacific, see Brantlinger, *Dark Vanishings*, 141–63 and the work of Alexandra Widmer, in particular Widmer, 'Of Field Encounters'.

[60] See further in this chapter.

[61] See, for instance, Summers, 'Intimate Colonialism'; Hunt, *Colonial Lexicon*; Thomas, *Politics of the Womb*; Widmer, 'Imbalanced Sex Ratio'.

colonial and imperial boundaries and, without ignoring dissimilarities, argues that, in many regards, their actuation in Angola was typical of large parts of tropical Africa and the Pacific.

The Tensions of Colonial Demography

Population Politics in the Tropics also takes a closer look at the role of demographic knowledge in colonial population discourses and policies. Although population figures and indices figured prominently in debates about colonial populations, it is striking that how they were used has barely been examined in historiography, certainly with regard to Africa. Instead, much of the literature has been written from the vantage point of historical demography and/or social history. The main thrust of such studies has been to gather and 'correct' the scanty demographic data produced by colonial bureaucracies and religious actors to reconstruct demographic 'realities' and assess the influence of colonialism on African demographic regimes (fertility, mortality and migration).[62] Since the late 1980s, historians have also looked at colonial demography from the perspectives of cultural and postcolonial history. However, many of these studies have, perhaps excessively, focused on the classificatory logics of the colonial census, thereby turning the idea that census categories reinforced or even created ethnic identities and differences, with all the social consequences, into a historiographical commonplace.[63]

This book explores a different path of analysis. It does not pay much attention to the role of census categories in the production of Angola's ethnic landscape, nor does it aim to reconstruct its demographic past. It is not unlikely that the Angolan population effectively declined in the late nineteenth and early twentieth century, due to the long-term effects of the transatlantic slave trade, colonial wars of conquest, epidemic diseases, famine, and other disruptions caused or reinforced by colonial encroachment. Jan Vansina, for instance, in a nuanced case study on the Kuba in the neighbouring Belgian Congo, estimated population decline between 1880 and 1920 at 15–19 per cent.[64] Yet whether and to what extent such a decline occurred in Angola is a question that this book cannot and does not want to answer. There are no

---

[62] See the studies in Cordell and Gregory (eds.), *African Population and Capitalism* and Fetter (ed.), *Demography from Scanty Evidence* as well as Cordell, Gregory and Piché, *Hoe and Wage* and Walters, 'Counting Souls'. For Angola, see Heisel, 'Indigenous Populations'; Heisel, 'Demography'; Heywood and Thornton, 'Demography'; Heywood and Thornton, 'African Fiscal Systems'.

[63] Classic texts are Cohn, 'Census' and Anderson, *Imagined Communities*, 164–70. See also the critique in Appadurai, 'Number in the Colonial Imagination', 316. For Africa, examples include Christopher, 'To Define the Indefinable'; Uvin, 'Counting' and, though embedded in a broader analysis, also van den Bersselaar, 'Establishing the Facts'.

[64] Vansina, *Being Colonized*, 127–49.

detailed case studies like Vansina's for Angola and, in recent macro-studies, historical demographers and economic historians have not reached a consensus on whether the population in Angola, and (West) Central Africa as a whole, effectively declined. Using back-projections of late-colonial censuses, usually of 1950 and/or 1960, to cope with the lack of reliable data from earlier periods, they have come to different conclusions. While Patrick Manning has suggested a very low, but continuous population growth in Angola between 1850 and 1920, which then accelerated from the 1920s onwards, Ewout Frankema and Morten Jerven have posited a net population loss of 15 per cent between 1890 and 1920 for the whole of Central Africa, without providing any detail on Angola.[65] The differences between these studies reveal the basic tension of back-projections: they are always estimates that hinge on how authors determine 'standard' growth rates and quantify the impact of colonial 'disruptions' such as wars, famines, and epidemics.[66] Exemplary of the epistemological problems of reconstructing early colonial African demography is the infamous case of the Belgian Congo. Whereas some historians, followed by elements of public opinion, have assumed a net population loss of up to 50 per cent between the onset of colonial conquest in 1885 and 1930, much more than the 15–19 per cent calculated for the Kuba by Jan Vansina, others remain sceptical as to whether decline exceeded 10 per cent or even occurred at all.[67]

Rather than trying to reconstruct Angola's demographic evolution, this volume approaches demographic knowledge from a constructivist perspective. It examines why, how and by whom demographic data in Angola were produced, and how these numbers, percentages and indices subsequently circulated and were interpreted, debated and used by a broad array of colonial actors. In line with recent historiography on other colonies, it shows that the production of demographic data on Angola's 'native' population met many obstacles and that hence data were relatively scarce and inaccurate, certainly before the first 'scientific' census of 1940.[68] It also draws attention to the contradictions that arose from the fact that these data were produced by various departments in the colony, each with their own rationale and method of data gathering. It thereby foregrounds the role of medical doctors in colonial

---

[65] Manning, 'African Population' and the appendices (esp. B15) available as spreadsheet at www.dataverse.pitt.edu/archive/users.php (last accessed 10 December 2020); Frankema and Jerven, 'Writing History Backwards', 925–7.

[66] For a critique of population estimates and back-projections, see Caldwell and Schindlmayr, 'Historical Population Estimates', 192–202.

[67] See the discussion in Sanderson, *Démographie coloniale congolaise*. Compare with Vansina, *Being Colonized*, 127–49 and Manning, 'African Population', appendix B15, who attests population stagnation and even slow growth for this period.

[68] See, for instance, Fetter, 'Demography in the Reconstruction'; van den Bersselaar, 'Establishing the Facts'; Gervais and Mandé, 'Comment compter'; Barbieri, 'Utilité des statistiques'.

demography, which has been almost completely overlooked by historians (see Chapter 4).

Moreover, by analysing the circulation and consumption of colonial demographic intelligence, this study also draws attention to a crucial, though thus far unexplored tension of colonial demography, at which the eminent demographer Robert René Kuczynski hinted in 1937 when he bemoaned the 'appalling' extent to which colonial officials were 'tempted to draw far-reaching conclusions from the scanty population data at their disposal'.[69] Indeed, although colonial officials were mostly aware of the deficiencies of their demographic data, they continued to circulate and interpret these data, either because they perceived this as their bureaucratic duty or because particular numbers, percentages or indices suited their agenda. The fiction of the numbers not only promoted the 'illusion of bureaucratic control', as Arjun Appadurai has stated with regard to British India;[70] numbers also served to fuel or appease depopulation anxieties and to legitimise particular population policies.[71]

Colonial Medicine

Most of the population policies studied in this book relate to medicine. While demography was about measuring change within a population, medicine promised to increase its 'quantity and quality'. Following Foucault's idea of population politics, this book attends to the multiple and varied efforts to reduce the mortality, increase the natality and improve the overall health of Angola's 'native' population. Somewhat surprisingly, this story has hardly been told. Although colonial medicine is a burgeoning historiographical field, with a vast and growing number of articles and book-length studies on British, French, Belgian or German colonies in Africa,[72] twentieth-century Angola has thus far received very little scholarly attention. Notable exceptions are Martin Shapiro's pioneering, though rather broad PhD thesis and Jorge Varanda's work on the health policies of Diamang, a major diamond company in northeastern Angola.[73] Scholars of the Portuguese Empire have mostly

[69] Kuczynski, *Colonial Population*, xii–iii.
[70] Appadurai, 'Number in the Colonial Imagination', 316–20 (quote 317).
[71] For this instrumental use, see also Dörnemann, Overath and Reinecke, 'Competing Numbers'.
[72] See particularly Vaughan, *Curing Their Ills*; Lyons, *Colonial Disease*; Headrick, *Colonialism, Health and Illness*; Bado, *Médecine coloniale*; Hunt, *Colonial Lexicon*; Bell, *Frontiers of Medicine*; Neill, *Networks*; Webel, *Politics of Disease Control*.
[73] Shapiro, *Medicine*; Varanda, *A Bem da Nação*; Varanda, 'Crossing Colonies and Empires'; Varanda, 'Cuidados biomédicos'.

focused on earlier time periods[74] or other colonies, most notably Goa and Guinea.[75]

While exploring this virtually uncharted empirical terrain, this volume draws upon and contributes to major turns in the historiography of colonial medicine that have, over the past four decades, vanquished the 'humanitarian' master narrative, reframed the interactions between colonial health officials and indigenous populations and embedded them in broader transnational and global contexts. The first, and perhaps most fundamental, of these turns started in the 1970s–1980s, when the often heroic narrative of medical progress, which focused on the conquest of particular tropical diseases and the achievements of 'great European men', began to give way to a more critical view of the connection between medicine and imperialism that paid greater attention to the social, political, cultural and economic contexts of health, disease and medicine.[76] Drawing upon Daniel Headrick's influential work on the role of technology and infrastructure in nineteenth-century European imperialism, many have questioned the disinterested, humanitarian and benevolent character of colonial medicine. Some reframed it as a 'tool of empire', used by colonial powers to penetrate, control and exploit the territories under their rule.[77] Others, particularly scholars working on urban sanitation measures or large-scale disease campaigns, stressed the violence, racism and disruptive effects of colonial medicine in practice.[78] Still others have focused on the confrontation between Western medicine and African healing practices, refuting the assumption that Western epistemes and practices simply eclipsed African 'therapeutic practices' often dubbed 'traditions'. Instead, they claim that this encounter often led to medical pluralism, that is the co-existence of beliefs and practices from different healing systems.[79]

In concert with such critical perspectives, this book shows that colonial medicine in late nineteenth- and twentieth-century Angola indeed served as a 'tool of empire'. Beyond facilitating the survival of European settlers, state officials and missionaries in tropical environments, the introduction of Western

---

[74] See, for instance, Walker, 'Acquisition and Circulation'; Kananoja, *Healing Knowledge*.

[75] See in particular the work of Cristiana Bastos and Philip Havik, most notably Bastos, 'Doctors for the Empire'; Bastos, 'Medical Hybridisms'; Havik, 'Public Health and Tropical Modernity' and Havik, 'Public Health, Social Medicine'. See also Silva, *Land of Flies* and Williams, *Healthy Colonial State*.

[76] For this shift, see MacLeod, 'Introduction', 4–6. Paradigmatic works are Arnold (ed.), *Imperial Medicine*; MacLeod (ed.), *Disease, Medicine, and Empire*; Feierman and Janzen (eds.), *Social Basis*.

[77] Headrick, *Tools of Empire*, 3–14, 58–79. See also Curtin, *Disease and Empire*.

[78] See Swanson, 'Sanitation Syndrome'; Lyons, *Colonial Disease* and Lachenal, *Médicament*.

[79] See the groundbreaking Janzen, *Quest for Therapy*. On the concept of medical pluralism, see also Vaughan, 'Healing and Curing', 290–2; Bruchhausen, 'Medical Pluralism'. I have borrowed the term 'therapeutic practices' from Janzen and Feierman, 'Preface', xvi, who reject the term 'traditional' for being (or suggesting to be) antithetical to 'modern'.

biomedicine increasingly aimed to improve the health of Africans needed as labourers for the economic *mise en valeur*, extend social control over them and, by framing healthcare as part of Europe's civilising mission, increase the international legitimacy of colonialism.[80] Using a broad range of previously unexplored sources, the demographic, political and economic rationales of colonial medicine are analysed in this volume. Yet, as various historians have pointed out, the 'tool of empire' concept does not fully render the complexities of medical interactions in the colonial situation.[81] In the first half of the twentieth century, biomedical interventions in Angola, as in most parts of colonial Africa, were still limited in scope and efficiency, due to internal shortcomings and conflicts, and the resilience of competing indigenous beliefs and practices. Local beliefs about disease causation often persisted and many Africans continued to prefer local remedies over biomedical treatment, or combined elements of each in local forms of medical pluralism. Further, Western biomedical practices were often brutal and disruptive. During the vast anti-sleeping sickness campaigns extensively analysed in Chapters 2 and 3, colonial health services forcibly relocated, incarcerated and treated a large number of people.

Despite this violence, this book rejects a binary opposition between (passive) African patients and European health workers. In line with a growing body of literature on other (African) colonies inspired by subaltern studies and the postcolonial turn, it shows that medical interventions depended on the collaboration of Africans. The agency of African 'patients' could take multiple forms, ranging from avoidance and outright resistance (for instance through hiding, evasion or non-compliance) to the (partial) acceptance of, and even demand for, new biomedical interventions. Often, their views and actions forced colonial health officials to rethink and reshape their programmes and practices. Moreover, African agency was not limited to 'the sick'. The spread and acceptance of new biomedical practices largely hinged on the collaboration of African intermediaries, such as local chiefs, nurses and midwives. Trained by both state and missionary doctors, medical auxiliaries played an important role in colonial health campaigns, but often followed their own agenda.[82]

The fault lines of colonial medicine not only ran between Africans and Europeans. While leading European doctors in Angola championed the organisation and expansion of medical campaigns and basic African healthcare for the sake of demographic improvement and international legitimacy, parts of

---

[80] See also Shapiro, *Medicine*.
[81] See, for instance, Arnold, *Colonizing the Body*, 15, 292–3; Au, *Mixed Medicines*, 6–7.
[82] See, for instance, Lyons, 'Power to Heal'; Turrittin, 'Colonial Midwives'; Kalusa, 'Language' and Webel, 'Medical Auxiliaries'.

the colony's administration and public opinion criticised the costs, the modalities and sometimes even the very utility of such population politics. Hence, ambitious health plans were recurrently thwarted by reluctant governors-general and austerity-led colonial ministers, or eroded by the passive resistance of local administrators anxious about their authority and on whose collaboration medical officers largely depended. Although personnel and budget were significantly expanded in the 1920s, the colonial health services in Angola (as in virtually all colonies) were almost permanently underfinanced and understaffed. Moreover, conflicts over goals, methods and individual career paths also arose within the health services themselves or between doctors in Angola and experts in tropical medicine in Lisbon – a new medical specialty based on parasitology that was institutionalised in Europe's imperial metropoles in the early twentieth century to deal with the major diseases in the (tropical) colonies.[83] Colonial medicine, hence, was not simply a 'tool of empire', but the result of continuous and complex negotiation processes between a multitude of colonial actors.

These negotiations did not only take place within Angola or between Angola and Portugal. Tying in with the recent transnational and global turns in medical history, this book emphasises that, as for colonialism in general, medical knowledge and practices circulated across colonial and imperial boundaries, furthered by the intra-imperial mobility of doctors, international conferences and journals and transimperial collaborations.[84] The transnational and global perspectives adopted throughout this study reveal the multiple, varied and changing connections between medical ideologies, programmes and practices in Angola and other parts of the (colonial) world. Thus, this study not only provides a first book-length transimperial history of colonial medicine in Angola: it also serves as an addition and corrective to various recent and explicitly transimperial histories of colonial medicine in Africa that have, for epistemological or practical reasons, 'forgotten' the Portuguese colonies.[85]

Angola's transnational connections not only included state actors, but also international organisations and private philanthropies, such as the League of Nations Health Organisation (LNHO) and the Rockefeller Foundation, whose global involvement in health campaigns has received much scholarly attention

---

[83] See Chapter 1.

[84] While first programmatic calls were published in the late 1990s, major transnational and transimperial studies appeared only in the 2010s. Compare Arnold, 'Introduction', 11 and Anderson, 'Postcolonial History' with Digby, Ernst and Muhkarji (eds.), *Crossing Colonial Historiographies*; Neill, *Networks*; Mertens, *Chemical Compounds* and Lachenal, *Médicament*. For the Portuguese empire, see Varanda, 'Crossing Colonies and Empires'; Bastos and Barreto (eds.), *Circulação do conhecimento*.

[85] See Chapters 1 and 2.

recently.[86] Missionary societies intervened in the health of Angola's 'native' population as well: by hiring professional doctors and nurses and training African nurses and midwives, foreign Protestant missions provided basic healthcare and targeted specific diseases and health problems.[87] Examining their involvement in fighting sleeping sickness and medicalising childbirth, this book also reveals the ambivalent attitudes of Portuguese state doctors and the colonial administration towards them.

Sources and Archives

Population Politics in the Tropics draws upon a large number and variety of primary sources, many of which have hardly, if at all, been used in historical research. These were unearthed during extensive research stays in libraries and archives in Angola, Portugal and various other European countries.

The published sources used in this study range from official government documents such as administrative reports, law texts and statistical publications to more personal considerations such as memoirs and travelogues. Within this range are also numerous scientific, medical and more generalist colonialist pieces, presented at national and international conferences or published as journal articles or monographs. Angolan newspapers, a large collection of which is held in the National Library in Lisbon, also conveyed valuable insights. Beyond providing information on local events and institutions, they were also the sites where high-ranking colonial officials aired ideas, policies and results. It is necessary to remember, however, that virtually all documents published in Portugal and its colonies during the military dictatorship (1926–33) and the *Estado Novo* (1933–74) underwent state censorship.[88] Sensitive issues and voices particularly critical of state policies were hence largely filtered out.

In order to analyse the inner life of the colonial state, archival sources were crucial. The present study is based on extensive research in the collections of the Portuguese Colonial Ministry, stored in the *Arquivo Histórico Ultramarino* (AHU) in Lisbon, and of the central government (*Governo Geral*) of Angola, preserved in the *Arquivo Nacional de Angola* (ANA) in Luanda. In these official, though still much under-used, repositories of Portuguese colonial rule in Angola, I have consulted a wide array of sources produced by agents of the

---

[86] On the LNHO, see Weindling, 'Philanthropy'; Borowy, *Coming to Terms*; Sealey, *League of Nations Health Organisation* and Tworek, 'Communicable Disease'. On the medical work of the Rockefeller Foundation, see Farley, *To Cast Out Disease* and Stepan, *Eradication*.

[87] On missionary medicine in colonial Africa, see Ranger, 'Godly Medicine'; Landau, 'Explaining Surgical Evangelism'; Jennings, 'Healing of Bodies' and the contributions in Hardiman (ed.), *Healing Bodies*.

[88] See, for instance, Barreto, 'Censura' and Gomes, *Militares*.

colonial state such as colonial doctors, administrators, governors and inspectors. While these sources offer valuable insights into the depopulation anxieties
that haunted colonial officials and the related population policies, they also
present two basic problems.

The first is that the sources available in the aforementioned archives only
constitute a small part of the documents produced by the Portuguese Colonial
Ministry and the central government in Angola between 1890 and 1945.
Whole collections are missing or, due to the lack of personnel, have not yet
been processed by archivists, so that they are (still) inaccessible to the scholarly community.[89] In Portugal, this not only concerns the AHU: the incorpor-
ation and processing of archival collections on Portugal's national and colonial
history of the twentieth century has long not been given priority, since the
undertaking of twentieth-century history was hampered by censorship and
taboos.[90] In Angola, many local archives were destroyed during the colonial
and civil wars, or are almost inaccessible to (foreign) researchers.[91]
A particular setback for this study was that the records of the Angolan health
services for the time period under consideration here have never entered the
ANA or AHU, and that I was unable to locate them elsewhere. I have found
(copies of) reports and correspondence in other collections in the same
archives, but, overall, my analysis of health policies relied on printed sources
to a greater extent than I would have wished. Further, it is important to note
that both AHU and ANA only possess rudimentary catalogues, making
research a time-consuming, haphazard and often frustrating experience.

Using sources from the AHU also raises a second issue. Most of these
documents were written or compiled either by officials of the Colonial
Ministry in Lisbon or high-ranking colonial authorities in Angola, such as
governors-general, provincial governors and directors of services. These were
the documents considered important enough to be sent from Luanda to Lisbon,
whereas reports from and correspondence with the lower echelons of the
colonial administration in Angola were usually not forwarded. It is important
to acknowledge the biases this creates. High-level documents tend to be more
polished and programmatic and contain less information on the local practical-
ities and everyday complexities of colonial population policies, not to speak of
African attitudes and actions. Fortunately, some local reports and correspondence did end up in the AHU, often as part of larger files, conveying a more
actor-oriented and nuanced picture of colonial rule. Even so, the main

---

[89] On the situation in the AHU, see also Castelo, *Passagens para África*, 34–5; Ball, *Angola's Colossal Lie*, 14–5; Keese, 'Why Stay?', 80–1; Havik, 'Public Health and Tropical Modernity', 642.

[90] Domingos and Pereira, 'Introdução', 15.

[91] Pacheco, 'Arquivos queimados', 33–7; Thompson, 'Taking the Graduate Students'.

consequence is that this study tells more about the thoughts and actions of Portuguese colonial officials in Angola than about African views and actions, and is hence much less Africanist than originally conceived.

To attenuate the gaps and biases of the sources in the AHU and ANA, and to introduce transnational perspectives, these are complemented with archival material from over a dozen other archives located in Portugal, Belgium, France, Germany, Great Britain and Switzerland. In Portugal, I found important reports on the 1930s and 1940s in the personal archives of António de Oliveira Salazar and his successor Marcello Caetano, who was Minister of Colonies from 1944 to 1947, stored in the National Archives in Lisbon, the *Arquivo National da Torre do Tombo* (ANTT). To grasp Angola's connections with other colonies and international organisations, such as the League of Nations, I consulted the Foreign Ministry's *Arquivo Histórico-Diplomático* (AHD-MNE). For some more specific questions, I have drawn on documents from the *Arquivo Histórico Parlamentar* (AHP) and a small collection of letters from a leading medical doctor in Angola, held by his great-nephew Luiz Damas Mora.[92] Visits to public archives in Brussels, London and Berlin and to the archives of the League of Nations in Geneva served to further explore the international and transimperial connections of Portuguese population policies in Angola. Finally, I consulted the archives of the Protestant Baptist Missionary Society (BMS) in Oxford and of the Catholic Congregation of the Holy Spirit in Chevilly-Larue (AGCSSp) near Paris, two of the most important missionary societies present in colonial Angola, to elucidate the role of missionaries in healthcare and other population policies.

Structure of the Book

The book is organised both chronologically and thematically. Following the unfolding of the depopulation discourse and the policies adopted to turn the tide, it gradually advances from the late nineteenth to the mid-twentieth century, when depopulation fears slowly faded. Each chapter focuses on different aspects of Portuguese population politics.

Chapter 1 charts the emergence of depopulation anxieties and population politics in Angola around the turn of the twentieth century. It argues that a new epidemic of sleeping sickness in the 1890s played a key role in this process, as it served as a catalyst for various shifts in the configuration of Portuguese colonialism in Africa. Raging in the historical heartland of colonial Angola, sleeping sickness was thought to cause tremendous population loss and, hence, seen as a threat to the economic future and legitimacy of Portuguese

---

[92] These are now published in Mora, *António Damas Mora*, 91–106.

colonialism. Medical intervention became a demographic and economic necessity, a national and international imperative and a scientific opportunity. Moving beyond demographic discourse and broader shifts in colonialism, Chapter 2 analyses the multi-faceted practical efforts to check sleeping sickness in Angola until the end of the First World War. It argues that Portuguese doctors actively contributed to the transimperial efforts to understand and cure this deadly disease, but that the implementation of new biomedical knowledge and practices 'on the ground' was seriously hampered by various factors, most notably the distrust and resistance of many Angolans, difficult ecological conditions and a chronic lack of resources.

The next three chapters move forward into the interwar period, showing how the scope of medical and demographic intervention broadened with the establishment of a more comprehensive and better funded programme of African healthcare, the so-called *Assistência Médica aos Indígenas* (AMI), in the 1920s and its orientation towards social (i.e. collective and preventive) medicine. Chapter 3 examines the debates leading up to the establishment of this AMI programme in 1926, the programme's general structures and objectives as well as the structural constraints that eventually limited its expansion in the 1930s. It shows that, aside from demographic, medical and economic considerations, a decisive rationale for the AMI programme was Portugal's desire to defend its legitimacy as a colonial power against growing international critique after the First World War, most notably from within the newly established League of Nations. The chapter also looks at how the anti-sleeping sickness campaign became an essential part of this new health scheme. The main argument of the chapter is that, in the interwar years, the history of both the AMI scheme and anti-sleeping sickness measures were profoundly shaped by processes of inter-imperial comparison and exchange. These could take the form of (explicit or implicit) inter-imperial borrowing, collaboration, but also competition.

Chapters 4 and 5 concentrate on further aspects of the AMI programme and the dynamics of practical implementation. Chapter 4 attends to the barely studied role of doctors as 'field demographers' and population experts in tropical Africa. As depopulation anxieties grew even stronger after the First World War due to new statistical data, doctors used the structures of the AMI programme to collect and analyse demographic data in a far more systematic manner. The chapter explores the rationales, methods and tensions of this 'medical demography' in interwar Angola, attending to the transnational circulation of practices and the agency of the African population. It argues that, despite the multiple difficulties in gathering accurate data, doctors often drew far-reaching conclusions. By suggesting that the population had begun growing again and that the major problem was no longer excessive mortality from diseases nor low fertility, but rather rampant infant mortality, they used their demographic data to legitimise the AMI programme and to shift attention towards infant healthcare.

Chapter 5 discusses how this shift played out in practice. It looks more closely at three kinds of interventions aimed at curbing maternal and infant mortality in Angola in the 1920s–1940s and connects them with debates and policies in Portugal and other African colonies: the establishment of state maternity hospitals and concomitant education of Angolan midwives; philanthropic initiatives such as infant welfare dispensaries promoted by high-ranking Portuguese women in urban areas; and the Protestant mission maternities and midwife training schemes. The chapter argues that all three schemes were underwritten by a strongly negative image of African mothers, whom they wanted to instil with the 'art of motherhood', but that passive resistance and selective appropriation by African mothers changed their orientation.

Finally, Chapter 6 goes beyond medical interventions and highlights the spatial dimensions of population politics in the first half of the twentieth century. It focuses on the anxieties and counter-policies that the emigration of Angolans to neighbouring colonies provoked among colonial officials. Presumably, Angolans emigrated, temporarily or permanently, to work in foreign mines, plantations or infrastructure, to avoid taxes and forced labour, or to improve their standard of living. Although demographic knowledge about these migration movements was partial and unstable, they reinforced existing fears of population decline and about Portugal's prestige as a colonial power. In turn, they led to administrative and religious policies in border regions, such as tax reductions, the settlement of Catholic missions and the improvement of administrative control. The chapter also reveals conflicting views between the Colonial Ministry in Lisbon and the central government in Luanda about the advantages of prohibiting intra- and transimperial labour migration.

The Conclusion summarises the findings of the book and wraps up its key arguments. It is followed by an Epilogue on posterior developments, showing that after the Second World War depopulation fears gradually faded away, but that, unlike what happened with regard to many other parts of Africa and the emerging 'Third World', indications of sustained natural population growth did not readily spark fears of overpopulation. Densities were still considered low and the massive influx of white settlers was justified with Angola's allegedly tremendous potential to absorb population growth.

1   Sleeping Sickness, Depopulation Anxieties and the Emergence of Population Politics

From the mid-1890s, an epidemic of sleeping sickness in the eastern hinterland of Luanda generated increasingly dramatic accounts. Observers reported staggering mortality rates and empty villages where agriculture and commerce had once thrived. The missionary pro-colonial journal *Portugal em África* wrote the following in 1896: 'The majority of the *concelhos* [administrative areas] are depopulating. Mortality is high. Sleeping disease has victimised the indigenous population in the *concelhos* of Zenza do Golungo, Muxima, Massangano and Icolo Bongo [*sic*]: this disease is a crying shame'.[1] Doctors in the region, like the medical officers (*delegados de saúde*) stationed in Dondo and the naval doctor and naturalist José Pereira do Nascimento, were equally appalled by the devastation of the disease.[2] And the British consuls for Angola reported that 'the margins of the River Coanza, which a few years ago were thickly populated, may now be traversed for hours without encountering a single native hut' and warned that 'if European medicine cannot find a remedy, entire districts of South-West Africa [*sic*] will be either stripped of their present inhabitants or kept in a perpetual state of underpopulation'.[3]

The sleeping sickness epidemic in late nineteenth-century Angola was not the first Portuguese (let alone European) encounter with the disease, which had most probably existed in various spots on the African continent for many centuries.[4] Throughout the nineteenth century and sporadically even earlier, European doctors had repeatedly signalled its deadly presence among Africans living along the West Coast of Africa, from the Gulf of Guinea to the Congo basin and Central Angola.[5] In European languages, the disease had come to be

---

[1] *Portugal em África* 3 (1896), 420. Icolo Bongo should read Icolo e Bengo.
[2] Luis Fernando Collaço, 'Relatório do serviço de saúde da villa do Dondo (1896)', 31 December 1896, AHU, SEMU, DGU 942 and the alarming reports from his successor, Alfredo Lopes, referred to in Junta de Saúde (Luanda), Session 25 August 1900, ANA, Cód. 1867, fls. 107r–108r. For Nascimento, see 'Relatório duma viagem de Ndalla-Tando (Cazengo) ao Rio Zaire, 1899', summarised in AHU, CCart001104 and extensively cited in Leitão, *Relatório da visita sanitária*, 116–9.
[3] Nightingale, *Report*, 8 and Casement, *Report*, 10.   [4] Steverding, 'History'.
[5] See Lyons, *Colonial Disease*, 64–6; Bado, *Médecine coloniale*, 38–9. See also Bettencourt, Kopke, Rezende and Mendes, *Maladie du sommeil*, 1–4.

known under such names as 'lethargus/lethargy', 'hypnosis' and 'sleeping sickness' (Port. *doença do so(m)no*), insofar as its main clinical symptom was 'an irresistible urge to sleep', which grew stronger over time and invariably led to death.[6] In Portuguese medical circles, the symptoms and possible causes and cures of the disease were already being extensively discussed in 1871, after colonial physician Manuel Ferreira Ribeiro informed the Society of Medical Sciences in Lisbon *Sociedade das Sciências Médicas de Lisboa* of several cases of this still obscure disease on the islands of São Tomé and Príncipe.[7]

Nor was it the first time that sleeping sickness was observed in northern Angola. Called *hoxa* by the Mbundu population in Luanda's hinterland and *lalangolo* or *láála-negoulo* ('sleep-force') in Kikongo further north in the Lower Congo basin, the disease might have been known to them for many decades, as Portuguese doctors later suggested.[8] Certainly, from the 1870s, the disease attracted the attention of colonial administrators and doctors, merchants and travellers, as it caused epidemics in various commercial and agricultural centres along the Cuanza and Bengo rivers east of Luanda, such as Dondo and Massangano, and even further north (in Musserra) and east (in Malanje) (see Map 1.1).[9] The medical officer in Dondo, for instance, reported 232 victims between 1872 and 1877.[10] Later, Portuguese sleeping sickness experts speculated that the disease had probably originated in the Quiçama region south of the Cuanza river.[11] Though scarce and limited in scope, medical reports and statistics suggest that the disease abated somewhat thereafter in the region, only to manifest in a new major epidemic starting in the mid-1890s.[12] Meanwhile, however, the disease had become 'endemic' in Luanda's hinterland, 'with more or less frequent upsurges', as the director of the Angolan health services wrote in 1887.[13] In the 1880s and early 1890s, the disease was also reported to be widespread in the area around São Salvador do

---

[6] Sociedade das Sciências Medicas, 'Relatório da comissão', 251 (quote). For the different designations, see Bado, *Médecine coloniale*, 40–1 and Leitão, *Relatório da visita sanitária*, 97.

[7] Ribeiro, 'Molestia'; Sociedade das Sciências Medicas, 'Relatório da Comissão'; Sociedade das Sciências Medicas, 'Acta da Sessão 15 July 1871'.

[8] Leitão, *Relatório da visita sanitária*, 97–9; Silva, 'Doença do somno'.

[9] See Dias, 'Famine and Disease', 371 and, additionally, Monteiro, *Angola and the River Congo*, vol. I, 143–4. See also Bettencourt, Kopke, Rezende and Mendes, *Maladie du sommeil*, 5.

[10] Collaço, 'Relatório Dondo (1877)', 100.

[11] Bettencourt, Kopke, Rezende and Mendes, *Maladie du sommeil*, 5.

[12] Correia, 'Doença do sono', 159–62.

[13] Curto, 'Relatório do Chefe do Serviço de Saúde de Angola', 333–4. See also Ribeiro, *Estudos medico-tropicaes*, 191.

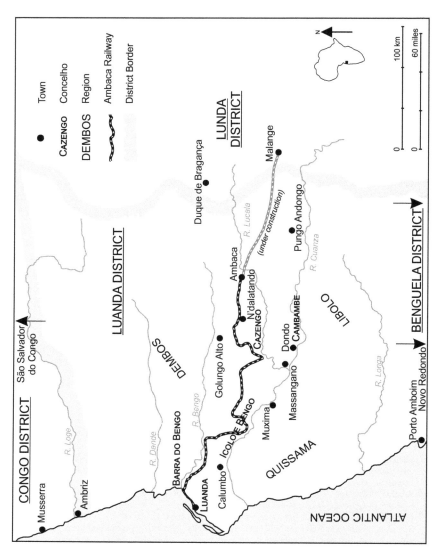

Map 1.1 The hinterland of Luanda around 1900.

30

Congo (now Mbanza Kongo) and in the Cabinda enclave, regions close to the Congo river.[14]

Certainly, European doctors had not remained completely inactive between the 1870s and mid-1890s. They proposed and discussed various theories about the cause of the disease. Many believed sleeping sickness to be a 'racial disease', since it seemed to only affect Africans. Accordingly, most of their theories blamed the supposedly unhealthy African habits, such as abuse of alcohol and hashish, sun exposure, sexual excess, toxic or adulterated food, or even Africans' alleged propensity to strong forms of 'nostalgia', as the disease had also been observed among newly arrived African slaves in the Americas in the 1860s. However, there was no unanimity about the racial character of the disease and some doctors related sleeping sickness to other tropical diseases such as malaria or helminthiasis.[15] In search for a cure, some doctors had also tried out a wide range of medications. However, attempts at understanding and curing the disease (discussed in greater detail in Chapter 2) were piecemeal, often individual initiatives without much institutional support and not widely publicised. Most importantly, they failed to reveal the cause of the disease and to provide an effective cure before the 1900s.

The relative neglect of sleeping sickness in the 1870s and 1880s stood in stark contrast to the strong official and public reactions to the epidemic in the late 1890s. Epidemic sleeping sickness now triggered massive depopulation fears and jolted medical and political authorities in Luanda and Lisbon into action. In August 1900, in the face of terrifying accounts from Angola's interior, the Health Council (*Junta de Saúde*) in Luanda, the colony's highest ranked medical board composed of the director of the health services and two senior health officials, appointed a medical officer to investigate the matter.[16] Between November 1900 and February 1901, Alberto de Souza Maia Leitão travelled through Luanda's hinterland and recorded information on numerous sleeping sickness cases.[17] Even before his report was published, the Portuguese Overseas Ministry in Lisbon also took action. In February 1901, minister António Teixeira de Sousa, a medical doctor himself, appointed a scientific commission to elucidate the aetiology and epidemiology of this

---

[14] For São Salvador do Congo, see Barroso, 'Relatório', 447, 455 and Mense, *Rapport sur l'état sanitaire*, 46–7. For Cabinda, see Silva, *Contribuição*, 394–5.

[15] See the controversial discussions at the Society of Medical Sciences in Lisbon in 1871 (Sociedade das Sciências Medicas, 'Relatório da Comissão'; Sociedade das Sciências Medicas, 'Acta da Sessão 15.07.1871') and the critical overviews in Corre, 'Recherches', 347–55; Azevedo, *Algumas palavras*, 33–6; Manson, 'Clinical Lecture', 125–6; Leitão, *Relatório da visita sanitária*, 111–20. On nostalgia, see also Kananoja, *Healing Knowledge*, 179.

[16] Junta de Saúde (Luanda), Session 25 August 1900, ANA, Cód. 1867, fls. 107r–108r.

[17] Leitão, *Relatório da visita sanitária*.

deadly disease.[18] The commission comprised some of Portugal's foremost bacteriologists: the director of the Royal Bacteriological Institute in Lisbon Annibal Bettencourt, one of his collaborators Gomes de Rezende, the naval doctor Ayres Kopke and the director of the Bacteriological Laboratory in Luanda Annibal Correia Mendes. Between May and December 1901, the commission conducted extensive research in Angola and on the island of Príncipe, a Portuguese colony in the Gulf of Guinea, where the disease had also taken on epidemic forms in the late 1890s.[19]

The first European mission of its kind, the Portuguese sleeping sickness commission was soon followed by a host of similar endeavours in what Kirk Hoppe has termed the 'scientific scramble for sleeping sickness'.[20] Indeed, in the late nineteenth and early twentieth centuries, sleeping sickness epidemics were also signalled in many other tropical African territories, most famously British Uganda in 1901, and all colonial powers – even Spain in its tiny possessions in the Gulf of Guinea – organised medical missions to investigate causes of, and possible remedies for, the disease.[21] After it was discovered in 1903–4 that sleeping sickness was caused by parasitic trypanosomes transmitted to humans through the bite of the tsetse fly, colonial governments and their medical services, including the Portuguese, set up unprecedented campaigns to map, control and eradicate the disease.[22]

While embedding Angola in this larger transimperial context, this chapter argues that epidemic sleeping sickness or Human African Trypanosomiasis (HAT), as the disease came to be officially called,[23] played a crucial role in the emergence of both depopulation anxieties and population politics at the turn of the twentieth century. First, it examines the socio-economic impact of sleeping sickness in Angola, particularly in the supposed epicentre of the epidemic, the eastern hinterland of Luanda, which was also the historical heartland of Portuguese colonisation. Here, it also argues that ongoing colonisation processes might not only have heightened awareness and anxieties about the epidemic, but also contributed to the spread of the disease. Second, the chapter shows that, even for Luanda's hinterland, let alone for the whole colony, it was

---

[18] 'Portaria nomeando uma commissão para estudar na provincia de Angola a doença do somno', *COLP* (1901), 41.

[19] See their final report Bettencourt, Kopke, Rezende and Mendes, *Maladie du sommeil* and Chapter 2.

[20] Hoppe, *Lords of the Fly*, 28.

[21] For an overview, see ibid., 11–5. Helen Tilley lists 17 research commissions, but omits the Spanish one in 1909 and three Portuguese sleeping sickness missions, to Angola (1904), Mozambique (1910–11) and Príncipe (1911–14). Compare Tilley, *Africa*, 174–6 with Amaral, 'Emergence', 313 and Corral-Corral and Quereda Rodriguez-Navarro, 'Gustavo Pittaluga'.

[22] See Chapter 2.

[23] www.who.int/mediacentre/factsheets/fs259/en/ (last accessed 13 March 2021).

and is impossible to measure the demographic impact of the epidemic, as mortality statistics revealed only a fraction of the casualties and census figures did not specify the causes of registered population decline. More than on precise numbers, depopulation anxieties thrived on estimates and eyewitness information about deserted villages and empty districts. Moreover, various contemporaries identified further major causes of depopulation. While this makes it even more difficult to disentangle the demographic impact of sleeping sickness, it also shows that a broader (crisis) discourse of population decline was emerging, in which sleeping sickness was only one, but probably the noisiest, element. Finally, the chapter examines the underlying reasons as to why, around 1900, epidemic sleeping sickness and assumptions about population decline triggered much stronger colonial anxieties and interventions than in the 1870s. It argues that Portuguese perceptions and reactions resulted from, and are illustrative of, major shifts that were affecting the political and economic, ideological and medical foundations of Portuguese colonialism in Angola in the last quarter of the nineteenth century. These shifts, which were closely linked to broader developments in European colonialism, redefined Portuguese views on the African population and its role in colonisation, thus setting the stage for new policies towards the 'native' population in Angola in the twentieth century, aimed at increasing both its 'quantity and quality'.

Sleeping Sickness in Luanda's Hinterland

To understand Portuguese reactions, one must remember that the sleeping sickness epidemic of the mid-1890s particularly struck the historical and economic heartland of colonial Angola. Many of the affected *concelhos* situated to the east of Luanda between the Bengo and Cuanza rivers, such as Golungo Alto, Cazengo, Cambambe, Massangano, Muxima and Calumbo, had been under nominal Portuguese rule since the seventeenth century, when the Portuguese defeated the Mbundu kingdom of Ndongo and turned local rulers (*sobas*) into vassals.[24] Until the mid-nineteenth century, the region had been a major supplier of slaves for the transatlantic slave trade. With an estimated 2.8 million slaves embarked between 1582 and 1850, Luanda was by far the trade's foremost port of departure.[25] While most of these people probably came from regions beyond direct Portuguese influence, many were also enslaved in areas under nominal Portuguese control.[26] With the end of the transatlantic slave trade from Luanda, its hinterland – alongside coastal areas

---

[24] Heintze, *Studien*. See also Thornton, *History of West Central Africa*.
[25] Eltis and Richardson, 90; 143.
[26] Silva, 'Atlantic Slave Trade'; Silva, *Atlantic Slave Trade*, esp. 93–5 and Ferreira, *Cross-Cultural Exchange*, 52–87.

under Portuguese control further south such as Dombe Grande, Novo Redondo (now Sumbe), Benguela and Moçâmedes – became a hotspot of agricultural colonisation and 'legitimate' trade, as more and more European settlers set up commercial coffee and sugar cane plantations as well as trading houses in the region. The influx of many hundreds of European farmers and traders, mostly men, particularly in the 1880s and 1890s, went hand-in-hand with massive land expropriation, the dispossession of African smallholders and the mass employment of 'indentured' labourers (*serviçães/serviçais* or *contratados*), held almost as slaves on European estates.[27]

This ongoing economic transformation is crucial to understanding why the recrudescence of sleeping sickness in the region in the late 1890s provoked so much anxiety in comparison to the 1870s. Much worse than previously, the depopulating effects of the disease were perceived as a serious threat to the prosperity of European planters and trading companies. By the late nineteenth century, the area between the Bengo and Cuanza rivers had become more than ever the 'core of Portuguese colonial occupation'.[28] Conversely, the economic transformation of Luanda's hinterland was one of the main reasons that sleeping sickness reached epidemic proportions. Some Portuguese colonial doctors later identified such a causal nexus: with hindsight, they blamed the spread of the disease on the influx of thousands of migrant workers during the 1870s to 1890s for the construction of the Ambaca railway, which connected Luanda with Lucala and later Malange.[29] This specific increase in Angolan mobility might indeed have contributed to the proliferation of the disease, by forcing people through infested areas and by moving infected bodies and trypanosomes to regions with still uninfected tsetse flies. Besides the railway workers, this also concerned the many thousands of *serviçais* who were forcibly employed on the plantations during the same period, an even more critical side of colonial rule in Angola that these doctors did not mention. However, labour migration is unlikely to have been the only cause for epidemic outbreaks in a region that had been crisscrossed by slaves and trade caravans for centuries.[30] Other socio-economic, political and ecological consequences of the colonisation process were probably as important.

As Jill Dias has shown, the enforcement of Portuguese rule in the region during the last decades of the nineteenth century weighed heavily on the local Mbundu population, as it involved massive land appropriation for large-scale plantation agriculture, the collapse of political order with the gradual

---

[27] Birmingham, 'Coffee Barons'; Dias, 'Changing Patterns'; Freudenthal, *Arimos e Fazendas*; Ferreira, 'Agricultural Enterprise'.

[28] Dias, 'Changing Patterns', 285 (quote).

[29] Mora, *Luta*, 1 and Sarmento, 'História breve', 25. On the railway construction, see Freudenthal, 'Angola', 325–6.

[30] On mobility in Angola, see generally Heintze and Oppen (eds.), *Angola on the Move*.

destitution of the old Mbundu elites and the imposition of both hut tax and labour conscription.[31] Arguably, these developments reduced the physical separation between humans and tsetse flies that had long protected the local population against infection. This happened in various ways. As the Portuguese appropriated fertile farmland, African farmers had to open new fields for cultivation in new, potentially tsetse-infested, areas. Others, being forcibly recruited or trying to pay their taxes, might have been infected while clearing tsetse-infested bushes from expanding European plantations. Still others moved into heavily infested areas, such as the densely vegetated (and since 1872, notoriously rebellious) Dembos region, situated further north between the Bengo and Dande rivers, to escape Portuguese control.[32]

If one follows the epidemiological model defended by John Ford and James Giblin for East Africa, the same previously cited political and economic changes might also have triggered epidemics of sleeping sickness in a somewhat different way. Ford and Giblin argue that precolonial African societies actively controlled sleeping sickness, not by completely avoiding contact with infected tsetse flies or the wild animals serving as trypanosome reservoirs, but by modifying their environment and carefully shaping their contact with these animals to acquire some level of immunity. Colonial conquest largely disabled such ecological control, as it provoked political crisis, social disruption, famines and population decline.[33]

Applying this explanatory model to the Cuanza region in the late nineteenth century moves social, ecological and demographic changes to the fore. Arguably, massive land appropriation led to the impoverishment of the vast majority of the local Mbundu population. Occurring together with a series of natural disasters and European preference for cash crops over food crops, colonisation exacerbated malnutrition and famines, thus reducing Africans' general resistance to disease. Tellingly, both upsurges of sleeping sickness in the mid-1870s and the late 1890s to the early 1900s coincided with periods of severe drought and famine.[34] Consistent with this view is the fact that Africans themselves, and for instance also missionaries and medical officers further north in the Cabinda enclave, identified under-nutrition and malnutrition as important reasons for the spread of the disease.[35]

Furthermore, famines, in combination with the deadly smallpox epidemics that over and again ravaged Luanda's hinterland in the 1870s to early 1900s,

---

[31] Dias, 'Changing Patterns', 304–13.

[32] Ibid., 309. On revolts and military campaigns in the Dembos region (1872–1919), see Pélissier, *História das campanhas*, vol. I, 321–49.

[33] See Ford, *Role of the Trypanosomiases* and Giblin, 'Trypanosomiasis Control'.

[34] Dias, 'Famine and Disease', 367–9 and Dias, 'Changing Patterns', 304, 309.

[35] Azevedo, *Algumas palavras*, 33; *Bulletin de la Congrégation du Saint-Esprit* 21 (1901–2), 718; Silva, 'Doença do somno'.

the ongoing labour drain from the region to São Tomé and Príncipe (on both, see below) and sleeping sickness itself caused considerable population decline. According to Dias, the population between the Dande and Cuanza rivers had already declined almost 50 per cent between 1876 and 1898, prior to the peak of the sleeping sickness epidemic.[36] If one follows Ford and Giblin, this ongoing depopulation disrupted the 'intricate balances among people, flora, fauna, tsetse flies and trypanosomes' that Africans had preserved for decades or even centuries. The breakdown of ecological control would have allowed bush vegetation and tsetse flies to encroach upon formerly cultivated areas and tsetse-free settlements.[37] The disease therefore spread not only because humans entered tsetse-infested areas, but also because tsetse flies invaded areas inhabited by humans. These explanations – the increase of direct physical contact between people and tsetse flies and the breakdown of ecological control – overlap, each pointing to the social, political and ecological disruption caused by colonialism as the root causes for epidemic sleeping sickness. There is hence good reason to align with John Ford, Maryinez Lyons and Heather Bell, who argue that it was colonialism itself, which, before setting out to 'rescue' the 'victimised' Africans from a 'new' disease, had transformed it from endemic to epidemic.[38]

Epidemic sleeping sickness also facilitated the expansion of Portuguese political control in various ways. It not only caused local African polities to lose population, and hence wealth and power, but arguably also questioned the political legitimacy of their rulers *(sobas)*, which, in Mbundu societies as in many other places in Africa, was closely tied to their ability to protect their subjects against illness and other misfortunes such as war and drought.[39] Alongside Portuguese economic expansion, sleeping sickness and other disasters further eroded the power basis of these *sobas*, ultimately leading to a more direct form of colonial rule east of Luanda.[40] Sapping the forces of resistance, epidemic sleeping sickness also helped the Portuguese to subjugate the Dembos region north of the Bengo river between 1907 and 1919.[41] More generally, efforts to monitor and control the disease would, in the long term, enhance territorial knowledge and colonial control over African societies.[42]

---

[36] Dias, 'Famine and Disease', 370.   [37] Lyons, *Colonial Disease*, 55 (quote).

[38] Ford, *Role of the Trypanosomiases*, 9–10; Lyons, *Colonial Disease*, 3–4; 34–5; 54–6; Bell, *Frontiers of Medicine*, 130–5.

[39] See, for instance, Dias, 'Famine and Disease', 352; Dias, 'Black Chiefs', 264–5. Compare with Feierman, *Shambaa Kingdom*; Hokkanen, 'Contestation', 121–3; Webel, *Politics of Disease Control*, 14–5 and 118–38.

[40] Dias, 'Changing Patterns', 304–13.

[41] Dias, 'Famine and Disease', 375; Dias, 'Changing Patterns', 312–3; Pélissier, *História das campanhas*, vol. I, 326–49, esp. 330, 341 and 349.

[42] See Chapters 2 and 3.

However, much more than the disease's potential political gains, Portuguese administrators, doctors and businessmen around 1900 were concerned with the economic and demographic ravages of the disease. During his mission in 1900–1 through the *concelhos* of Golungo Alto, Cazengo, Cambambe, Massangano, Muxima and Calumbo, medical officer Alberto de Maia Leitão spoke to dozens of Portuguese administrators, plantation managers and residents as well as African *sobas* and village headmen. Not all of them had witnessed cases of sleeping sickness and some were ostensibly reluctant to admit its presence, but most of his interlocutors mentioned that several people on their plantation or in their village, sometimes entire families, had died over the past few years, or that nearby villages had almost entirely been wiped out. For Maia Leitão, this was consistent with the generalised decrease of the workforce observed on almost every plantation he visited, and which reduced agricultural production and trade in the region.[43]

In Muxima, for instance, he was told that many of the European trading houses had recently been abandoned due to lack of business and people.[44] The consequences were even worse in the *concelho* of Cazengo, a major coffee producing area, where the epidemic had first been noticed among African plantation workers in 1895, at a time when international coffee prices were high and almost 5,000 people (most of them *serviçais*) worked on the 28 plantations in the region.[45] While Maia Leitão himself used less dramatic terms, other observers pointed to the incredible loss of life and the 'damage caused to the plantation owners with the death, sometimes *en masse*, of their *serviçães*'. According to the British Consul, Nightingale, plantation owners had 'lost more than two-thirds of their people within the last two years' and had been forced 'to abandon a part of their crops for want of hands to pick the coffee'.[46]

Most agreed that the district most severely hit was the *concelho* of Cambambe and its capital Dondo. On the right bank of the Cuanza river, Dondo had in the last decades of the nineteenth century become the 'most important commercial centre of the interior'.[47] From here, coffee and other goods were shipped to Luanda. However, visitors and medical officers also considered Dondo one of the unhealthiest places in Angola. Due to the hot and humid climate, the many swamps and the town's lack of cleanliness, malaria and other diseases reigned supreme.[48] Dondo had already been hit by sleeping sickness in the 1870s, but the havoc wrought by the disease in the late 1890s and early 1900s was of a different magnitude. Sleeping sickness contributed to

[43] Leitão, *Relatório da visita sanitária.*   [44] Ibid., 90.
[45] Dias, 'Famine and Disease', 372; Birmingham, 'Coffee Barons', 529.
[46] Quotes from José Pereira do Nascimento, in Leitão, *Relatório da visita sanitária*, 116 and Nightingale, *Report*, 8. Compare with Leitão, *Relatório da visita sanitária*, 49–73; 127.
[47] Dias, 'Black Chiefs', 248. See also Collaço, 'Relatório Dondo (1877)'.
[48] See, for instance, Xavier, 'Relatório Dondo (1881)'.

staggering mortality rates that were said to depopulate the city. According to Correia Mendes, one of the commission members who revisited the city in 1904, 240 people had officially died from sleeping sickness between 1901 and 1903, and the total population of the city declined from 2,000 to 1,200.[49] The shortage and higher cost of African labour that sleeping sickness caused in the region had lasting economic effects. Reinforced by the collapse of international coffee prices, the plantation sector in the region entered a prolonged crisis in the 1900s, from which it did not recover until the 1940s.[50]

Sleeping Sickness and the Making of a Demographic Crisis

For contemporaries around 1900 as well as for historians today, it was – and is – impossible to measure the exact demographic impact of sleeping sickness on Angola. With much caution, one can assume that the disease killed tens of thousands of people in Angola between 1895 and 1910, during what was probably the worst phase of the epidemic. However, that is necessarily a very rough estimate, based on the extrapolation of all available and – for various reasons problematic – quantitative and qualitative information discussed below. It is also and deliberately a much more prudent and inexact figure than the 250,000–300,000 victims that historians usually and uncritically take for granted as the death toll for the Uganda sleeping sickness epidemic between 1901 and 1905 (sometimes also until 1903, 1910 or 1920), without reflecting much upon the epistemological (im)possibility of such a narrow estimate for early twentieth-century Africa.[51] The reasons for this prudence are twofold. On the one hand, mortality statistics for Angola around 1900 are extremely scarce and always gross underestimates. On the other, censuses at the time only covered a small part of the colony. Moreover, where they exist, the data do not allow scholars to quantify the share of sleeping sickness in the population loss they attest, as the disease occurred in tandem with other depopulating factors, such as famine, smallpox, war, forced migration and flight.

As this section shows, contemporary doctors, administrators and other observers struggled with the same epistemological doubts. While they knew that mortality statistics were partial, they also doubted the accuracy of census

---

[49] Mendes, 'Glossinas de Angola', 67. See also Leitão, *Relatório da visita sanitária*, 74–80, 127.
[50] Dias, 'Famine and Disease', 375; Clarence-Smith, *Third Portuguese Empire*, 97.
[51] The Uganda mortality figures have been advanced by Harvey Soff and Maryinez Lyons. While they are based on various estimates by contemporary doctors and administrative bodies, the epistemological basis for these estimates is unclear or shaky. See Soff, 'Sleeping Sickness', 257–9, 262 and Lyons, *Colonial Disease*, 70–1. For the further circulation of these numbers, see, for instance, Hoppe, *Lords of the Fly*, 27; Webel, *Politics of Disease Control*, 12 and Ehlers, *Europa und die Schlafkrankheit*, 9 and 50.

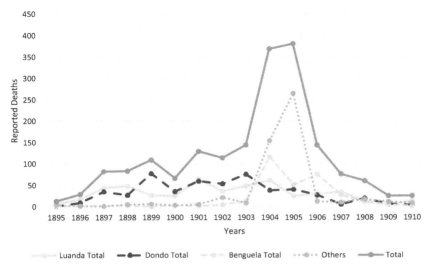

Figure 1.1 Registered sleeping sickness deaths in Angola, 1895–1910.
Source: *Boletim Oficial de Angola*, 1895–1910

data and sometimes privileged factors other than sleeping sickness to explain population decline. Rather than relying on exact figures, fears that sleeping sickness was depopulating some of the colony's most fertile areas originated from a continuous stream of appalling reports and estimates by travellers, settlers, administrators and doctors.

Around 1900, mortality statistics were published every month in the colony's official gazette, the *Boletim Oficial (do Governo Geral) de Angola*. These were part of the monthly health bulletins (*boletins sanitários*) that the director of the health services in Luanda collated on the basis of the monthly reports he received (or sometimes did not receive) from the district medical officers (*delegados de saúde*) in the colony. These mortality statistics, however, were very incomplete. Rather than quantifying the disease's death toll, they reflect the extent of medical control the Portuguese exerted in Angola. Thus the number of sleeping sickness casualties mentioned in these health bulletins rose to about 100 per year in the late 1890s, culminated at almost 400 in 1905 and then gradually fell again to 25 in 1910, totalling about 1,850 for the period 1895–1910 (see Figure 1.1). However, the vast majority of deaths went unregistered, for three main reasons.

First, most deaths probably occurred in regions not under effective Portuguese control. By 1900, Portugal had already laid claim to territory that, with minor border rectifications, would become colonial Angola, but most of that territory was not yet conquered, let alone under firm administrative control. This process of military 'pacification' and administrative occupation would last until the late 1910s and even then territorial control remained uneven.[52] In 1900, Portuguese-ruled Angola consisted of five districts (*districtos*): Luanda, Benguela, Moçâmedes, Congo and Lunda. In theory, they covered the whole territory, but apart from the eastern hinterland of the capital Luanda, administrative control was mostly limited to coastal areas and some 'islands of rule' in the interior.[53] There is hence almost no quantitative data for the interior of the Congo district (including Cabinda), the hinterland of Benguela or the Quiçama and Libolo regions south of the Cuanza river, all regions where the disease was known to be raging before 1910.[54] This also means that, if contemporary reports about sleeping sickness focused on Luanda's hinterland, this was not necessarily because it was the region most affected, but because administrative structures, economic interests and the geographical proximity to the capital allowed for, and required, a much more substantial flow of information. Conversely, this also explains why the existence of sleeping sickness in the Congo district drew far less official attention until the end of the First World War. Here, Portuguese investments were still modest, and the economy was dominated by African smallholders and traders as well as northern European export factories.[55]

Second, even in areas under effective colonial control, such as Luanda's hinterland, there were hardly any Portuguese doctors who could have reported the disease's death toll. On the eve of the epidemic, in 1894, the colonial health services in Angola only employed 17 doctors, of whom several were usually on furlough in the metropolis and most of the others were stationed in the colony's major urban centres, such as Luanda, Benguela and Moçâmedes, or in areas where the disease did not occur.[56] Moreover, the two or three medical officers who, during the late 1890s, were stationed in the *concelhos* east of Luanda – most continuously in Dondo, where there was also a military lazaret, and sometimes also in Golungo Alto and Cazengo – had little accurate knowledge about what happened outside the town centres where the Europeans lived. They did not seek African patients and Africans usually did not seek European medical assistance. Rather than exposing themselves to potentially painful and – until the introduction of atoxyl around 1906 – fully

---

[52] Pélissier, *História das campanhas*. See also Chapter 6.
[53] See, for instance, the census data in *Annuário Estatístico da Província de Angola* 4 (1900). On the idea of 'islands of rule', see Pesek, *Koloniale Herrschaft*.
[54] See, for instance, for Congo and Cabinda, Casement, *Report*, 10–1; Silva, 'Doença do somno', and for Quiçama, see Barradas, 'Relatório'.
[55] See, for instance, Vos, 'Of Stocks and Barter' and Vos, *Kongo*, 19–59.
[56] 'Relatório nominal dos facultativos e pharmaceuticos do Quadro de Saúde', 31 October 1894, AHU, SEMU, 2970–2.

ineffective biomedical treatments, most Africans stuck to their own healers and practices.[57] As sleeping sickness was an eminently rural disease, only a very small portion of those affected came to Portuguese attention. This explains why even the many hundreds of victims referred to in Maia Leitão's report on Luanda's hinterland were not captured in the mortality statistics, and why medical officers in their monthly reports stated countless times that sleeping sickness was wreaking havoc in the interior of their districts without giving death rates.[58] When, exceptionally, they did give figures for rural areas, as did the medical officer in Golungo Alto in 1904–5, they were staggeringly high: amounting to 144 (1904) and 252 (1905), mortality figures for the Golungo Alto district alone accounted for more than half of the total of registered sleeping sickness deaths in these years.

Finally, even for towns provided with medical officers, the sleeping sickness mortality numbers in the *Boletim Oficial* were still underestimates. The health bulletins primarily quantified the deaths (and causes of death) that had occurred in the colony's six state hospitals and lazarettos (Luanda, Benguela, Moçâmedes, Ambriz, Cabinda and Dondo). Sometimes, they also enumerated non-hospital deaths, but this was not consistent. Where they did, or where we have other reports detailing total sleeping sickness mortality, such as for Dondo, they show that the proportion of sleeping sickness patients who died outside hospital was huge (see Figure 1.2). Certainly, this was not specific to sleeping sickness: from the 508 persons officially buried at the public cemetery in Dondo in 1896, only 19 had died in the lazaret.[59] But this state of affairs complicated the statistical registration of sleeping sickness deaths: while some of the non-hospital deaths were attributed to sleeping sickness, many other cases were probably missed, as causes of death were often not registered. Even in Luanda, where medical surveillance was tighter, this was often impossible as the long-standing health director José de Brito Freire e Vasconcellos complained, because their relatives 'never give the doctor, who verifies the deaths, information that allows [him] to acknowledge, even in an approximate manner, the cause of death'.[60] In 1903, for instance, almost a third of all deceased people in Luanda, that is 260 (of which 25 were 'whites') out of 754, did not have their cause of death specified and Vasconcellos suspected that many of them had

---

[57] See, for instance, *Annuário Estatístico da Província de Angola* 4 (1900), xv and especially Chapter 2.

[58] See, for instance, the health bulletins in *Boletim Oficial de Angola* (hereafter *BOA*) (1897), 68 (Cazengo); (1903), 323–4 (Novo Redondo) and 600 (Golungo Alto); (1904), Suplemento ao n. 42, 2 (Ambriz).

[59] Collaço, 'Relatório Dondo (1896)'.

[60] 'Boletim Sanitário, Setembro 1905', *BOA* (1905), Appenso 39, 3.

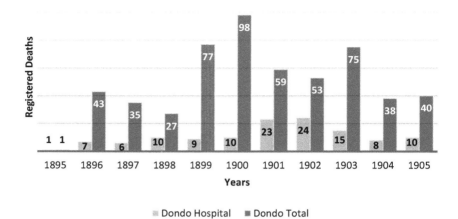

Figure 1.2 (Hospital vs. total) reported sleeping sickness deaths in Dondo, 1895–1905.
Sources: Boletim Oficial de Angola, 1895–1905; Collaço, 'Relatório Dondo (1896)' and Leitão, *Relatório da visita sanitária*, 76. Collaço mentions 43 sleeping sickness deaths for 1896 (against 9 in BOA) and Maia Leitão 98 for 1900 (against 35 in BOA)

died from sleeping sickness as well.[61] Overall, this state of affairs was not exceptional. In Angola as in the rest of sub-Saharan Africa, accurate population statistics, especially for rural areas, would remain a problem throughout most of the colonial period (see also Chapter 4).

The fixed idea that, prior to the epidemic, the hinterland of Luanda had been much more densely populated was also backed by demographic estimates and censuses. As one of the few regions in tropical Africa, colonial census-taking in Angola dated back to the 1770s, when the Marquês de Pombal, the 'enlightened' prime minister of Portugal, had ordered the first population surveys in the Portuguese Empire. From the late eighteenth to the mid-nineteenth century, censuses were carried out almost every year in coastal regions under Portuguese control, with Luanda's hinterland figuring prominently among them. After the end of Angola's official participation in the transatlantic slave trade in the 1840s, interest in demography waned, with only

[61] Monthly Bulletins for 1903 in *BOA*, February 1903–January 1904. For Vasconcellos' hunch, see 'Boletim Sanitário, Abril 1903', *BOA* (1903), 323.

a few censuses taken in the 1860s and 1870s.[62] Yet, towards the end of the century, the colonial state resumed the regular collection and publication of demographic data, due to the growing importance of the African population for the colonial endeavour and the emerging international imperative of scientific colonialism, which required that 'modern' colonial states govern on the basis of secure, scientific knowledge.[63] In 1897, the colonial administration in Angola began to collect and publish demographic data in statistical yearbooks and, in 1900, following the 1899 census law for the entire Portuguese Empire, it proceeded with a first, more comprehensive census operation, with a mixed system of counting and estimates.[64]

The total population numbers in nineteenth-century censuses varied widely, from almost 400,000 in 1846 to more than a million in 1898 and fewer than 800,000 two years later (see Table 1.1). Rather than reflecting demographic change, the huge variation in these numbers, especially between the 1870s and 1890s, was caused by two other factors: censuses had different levels of accuracy, as they relied on different counting and estimating methods; and they covered different geographical areas, that is, changing portions of what was to become colonial Angola in its consolidated twentieth-century borders. In all cases, only a small part of the later territory of ca. 1.25 million square kilometres was included, due to the lack of territorial control over the rest. To grasp what the total population might be, geographers in the late nineteenth century used another procedure: they determined the density of areas for which presumably good data existed and extrapolated these data in a reasoned manner for the whole territory. In 1896, army captain and geographer Ernesto de Vasconcelos thus assumed an average density of 3.3 inhabitants per square kilometre (much less than the 7.3 which Josef Chavanne had calculated a decade earlier) to arrive at an estimated 4,181,730 inhabitants.[65] Most other estimates were much higher, from 5 to 12 and even 19.4 million.[66]

Yet, while total population figures fluctuated wildly, nineteenth-century censuses conveyed a more stable and comparable set of demographic data for the sleeping sickness-ridden area between Luanda and Malanje north of the Cuanza river, the prime historical nucleus of colonial occupation (see Table 1.1). Certainly, these data were also far from perfect. The substantial

[62] See, for instance, Curto, 'Sources'; Santos, 'Administrative Knowledge' and, for the Portuguese Empire in general, Matos, 'Counting'. See also the database http://colonialpopulations.fcsh.unl.pt/.

[63] On scientific colonialism, see Kwaschik, 'Verwissenschaftlichung'.

[64] On the 1900 census, see Diniz, 'Contribuição', 36–8 and Lemos, 'Introdução ao primeiro censo', 20–7. The data are compiled in Annuário Estatístico da Província de Angola 4 (1900).

[65] Vasconcelos, Colonias portuguezas, 162.

[66] See retrospectively Athayde, 'Perigo do despovoamento', 229 and Annuário Estatístico da Província de Angola 1 (1897), x. See also Chapter 4.

Table 1.1. *Population numbers in Angolan censuses, 1844–1900*[67]

Years	Total population	Population Luanda District[68]
1844	387,463	246,356
1861	559,296	365,345
1869	433,397	274,562
1877	373,474	276,268
1897	828,963	191,168
1898	1,083,360	208,127
1899	946,301	230,697
1900	789,946	172,928

Sources: Lima, *De Angola e Benguella*, 4A; *BOA* (1863), 218–9; *BOA* (1870), 596–7; Secretário Geral de Angola, 'Mappa estatistico da população da Província de Angola', 20 February 1878, AHU, SEMU-DGU 648.1; *Annuário Estatístico da Província de Angola* 1 (1897), 15–44; 2 (1898), ix–x and 1–66; 3 (1899), vol. II, 3–76; 4 (1900), xvi–xvii and 3–180.

differences between the annual numbers in the late 1890s, for instance, can hardly have reflected real changes; rather, they must have resulted from changing methods and levels of accuracy in particular *concelhos*. Even in 1900, when the census for this area was said to be nominative (see Map 1.2), local census commissions faced great difficulties, ranging from logistical problems with personnel and census bulletins to the avoidance strategies of Africans who did not want to be counted.[69]

However, the 1900 census data seemed to confirm the progressive depopulation of the region, and were also used for that purpose by its compiler. Comparing the 1900 population figures for the 18 *concelhos* in the Luanda district with those from earlier censuses, Francisco Pereira Batalha, also director of the telegraph services, concluded that, between 1869 and 1900, the population in this area had fallen by 92,010–172,928.[70] Significantly, the

[67] I would like to thank Paulo Teodoro de Matos for sharing the 1861, 1869 and 1877 data.

[68] The Luanda district is defined as in the borders of 1900 (see Map 1.2). The numbers refer to the 18 *concelhos* Alto Dande, Ambaca, Ambriz, Barra do Bengo, Barra do Dande, Calumbo, Cambambe, Cazengo, Dembos, Encoge, Golungo Alto, Icolo e Bengo, Loanda, Massangano, Muxima, Novo Redondo, Pungo Andongo and Zenza do Golungo. They do not include Libolo, whose population was estimated only in 1900.

[69] See, for instance, Administrador de Icolo e Bengo to Secretaria Geral do Governo da Província d'Angola, 20 March and 31 July 1901, ANA, Cx. 5055. See also Lemos, 'Introdução ao primeiro censo', 26–7.

[70] *Annuário Estatístico da Província de Angola* 4 (1900), xiv–xvi. Batalha assumed that the population of the Luanda district (in its 1900 borders) was 264,938 in 1869 and not 274,562, as I have calculated (see Table 1.1).

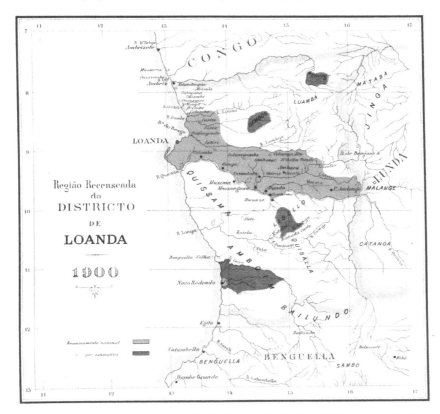

Map 1.2 Parts of the Luanda district included in the 1900 census, either by nominative census or estimate.
Source: http://purl.pt/1434/3/. See also *Annuário Estatístico da Província de Angola* 4 (1900), xxii
Image courtesy of the National Library of Portugal

concelhos with the greatest registered population decrease were also those designated by Maia Leitão and others to be those most affected by sleeping sickness: Cambambe, Cazengo, Golungo Alto, Icolo e Bengo, Massangano, Muxima and Zenza do Golungo.[71] This does not mean that the 'missing people' in 1900 had all died from sleeping sickness. Many Africans had probably abandoned their villages to escape the disease, thereby also contributing to its spread.[72] Many others, as already indicated, had left the region to

[71] Compare with Leitão, *Relatório da visita sanitária*, 127 and footnote 79.
[72] Dias, 'Famine and Disease', 372; Correia, 'Doença do sono', 164.

avoid growing colonial control or had died from famines and other diseases, most notably smallpox.

Batalha advanced yet another explanation for the apparent demographic decline in the Luanda district. He did not doubt that, along with smallpox, sleeping sickness was one of the main causes, even if it was, as he admitted, impossible to gauge the precise demographic impact of these diseases. Yet he also pointed at the steady flow of *serviçais* to the cocoa plantations on São Tomé and Príncipe. Assuming that, since 1869, 6,000 contract labourers had thus left Angola every year, half of them from the Luanda district, he calculated that this stream alone covered the registered population loss of the last three decades.[73] Batalha was right in addressing the considerable size of this forced migration movement. Beginning in the 1850s after the legal abolition of the transatlantic slave trade, it involved several tens of thousands of Angolans in the second half of the nineteenth century and triggered growing international critique.[74] However, his figures were probably exaggerated and are much higher than those published in official statistics or compiled by James Duffy in his seminal book on the subject: for roughly the same time period, they average around 2,200 forced emigrants per year.[75] Moreover, many of them did not come from the Luanda district, but were Ovimbundu from the central highlands shipped via Novo Redondo or Benguela further south.[76]

Batalha was not the only one who questioned the demographic impact of sleeping sickness and pointed at other causes of depopulation. Despite the hundreds of cases he had personally examined or heard about, Maia Leitão did not consider the disease to be the primary cause of population decline either. In his opinion, staggeringly high infant mortality rates of up to 90 per cent, the *serviçais* trade to São Tomé and Príncipe, and low fertility among local plantation *serviçais* contributed more to the ongoing depopulation of Luanda's hinterland than did sleeping sickness, which he listed as fourth amongst the depopulating factors.[77] For both Batalha and Maia Leitão, sleeping sickness was a major and obvious cause of depopulation but only one element in a much broader demographic crisis, a view that gained strength over the next decades. Particularly after 1918, the colonial government would also increasingly investigate and tackle the other depopulating factors they mentioned: further diseases (see Chapter 3), low fertility and high infant mortality rates (see Chapters 4 and 5) and the (forced) emigration of *serviçais* and other 'natives' (see Chapter 6).

---

[73] *Annuário Estatístico da Província de Angola* 4 (1900), xv.

[74] For more detail, see Chapters 2 and 6.

[75] Duffy, *Question of Slavery*, 98; *Annuário Estatístico da Província de Angola* 2 (1898), x.

[76] See, for instance, Duffy, *Question of Slavery*, 135–7, 172–4, 180–1; *Annuário Estatístico da Província de Angola* 2 (1898), 72–3; Vos, *Kongo*, 49.

[77] Leitão, *Relatório da visita sanitária*, 127–8.

In the 1900s, however, sleeping sickness was and remained the most important driver of depopulation anxieties in Angola, fed by a continuous stream of alarming reports about the disease's debilitating and depopulating effects, mentioning cachectic and dying people, deserted villages, empty regions and innumerable casualties.[78] Some of these reports contained horrendous estimates that undoubtedly captivated contemporary minds, although they were sometimes probably exaggerated as they greatly exceeded census figures. The *moradores* ('citizens') of Barra do Bengo thus wrote to the government in Luanda that 'the *concelho* of Zenza de Golungo [had] almost been entirely wiped out, as 15,000 people had died [there] over the last ten years' and that 'the *concelhos* of Dondo [*sic*], Massangano, Muxima, Calumbo, Golungo Alto and Icolo e Bengo [had] lost about half of their original population'. Like a 'formidable cataclysm', they concluded, sleeping sickness had depopulated and destroyed previously flourishing centres of trade and agriculture.[79]

Moreover, many reports in the early 1900s suggested that the epidemic was still gaining strength. According to Annibal Correia Mendes, for instance, who crossed the *concelhos* east of Luanda in August 1904, the situation had drastically worsened since his visit as a member of the Bettencourt research mission three years before. While hundreds had died in Dondo, probably as much as 20 per cent of the inhabitants in Golungo Alto were now infected, he claimed.[80] Many others indicated that the disease was increasingly wreaking havoc in other parts of Angola as well, such as the area around Novo Redondo, the hinterland of Benguela, the Portuguese Congo around São Salvador and Cabinda.[81]

As long as the aetiology of the disease and the role of the tsetse flies in its transmission were not well understood, contemporaries could not know how far this incurable and fatal disease would spread. This not only concerned Angola. 'The whole centre of Africa is already contaminated, from the Zambezi to the Sudan', the Portuguese consul in France Almada Negreiros stated in 1903, continuing that even Egypt and the Transvaal were threatened. 'If one does not succeed in circumventing this terrible disease, the negro race is in jeopardy of disappearing soon.'[82] Some British doctors feared that the

---

[78] See, for instance, footnotes 1, 2, 3, 58 and 81.
[79] Residents of Barra do Bengo to Governor-General, 3 March 1905, ANA, Cx. 3721. The censuses of 1897–1900 only mention a total population of 1,500 inhabitants for Zenza do Golungo. See the sources of Table 1.1.
[80] Mendes, 'Glossinas de Angola', 67–9.
[81] Aguiar, 'Maladie du sommeil'; Bastos, 'Monographia de Catumbella', here 30 (1912), 74 and 77; *Portugal em África* 10 (1903), 347. See also Dias, 'Famine and Disease', 373. On alarming missionary reports from Cabinda and São Salvador, see Chapter 2.
[82] J. S. A., 'Hygiene colonial', 690 (quotes).

disease might also spread to India.[83] Moreover, as Ayres Kopke, one of the members of the Portuguese commission in 1901–2, later recalled, there were fears at the time that the disease might even become endemic in non-tropical climates, such as Europe.[84]

Sleeping Sickness and the Emergence of Population Politics

Around 1900, epidemic sleeping sickness, as I have argued, threatened to ruin the economy of one of Angola's most important regions and jeopardised other regions. In and of itself, however, this cannot explain the sustained campaigns against this disease over the next decades. To understand why the disease and, with it, the presumed decrease of the 'native' population in Angola, triggered much stronger depopulation anxieties and colonial interventions than in the 1870s, one must consider various fundamental shifts in Portuguese colonialism in Angola. They relate to the domains of national and international politics, colonial ideology and medicine.

The Political and Economic Reconfiguration of the Portuguese Empire

In a very general way, the strong reaction to epidemic sleeping sickness was a consequence of the renewed importance the colonies had acquired, not only for planters and traders in Angola, but also for political, economic and intellectual elites in Portugal in the last quarter of the nineteenth century. In the first half of that century, the independence of Portugal's main colony Brazil in 1822 and the decline of Portuguese participation in the transatlantic slave trade after its legal abolition in 1842 had debased the economic and political importance of the empire for the metropole. These changes particularly affected Angola, which had been strongly tied to Brazil both economically and culturally as its prime supplier of slaves.[85] Certainly, there were plans to turn the remaining colonies into economically prosperous 'new Brazils', spearheaded by the Viscount (later Marquess) of Sá da Bandeira. However, despite some modest agricultural enterprises in areas like Luanda's hinterland, metropolitan governments and entrepreneurs were initially reluctant to invest, both politically and economically, in the empire. It was only the international 'scramble' for Africa from the 1870s to the 1890s that triggered a renewed and broad interest in colonial Africa in Portugal.[86]

---

[83] Lyons, *Colonial Disease*, 71.   [84] Kopke, *Estudo da doença do sono*, 2.

[85] See Introduction and footnotes 25 and 26 in this chapter.

[86] See especially, at the end of a long and controversial debate between both authors, Marques, *Sounds of Silence*, 193–248 and Alexandre, 'Portuguese Empire'.

The scramble generated strong feelings of colonial nationalism and victimisation in Portugal. Newly established colonial pressure groups such as the Geographical Society of Lisbon (founded in 1875) and an increasingly pro-colonial press condemned other European powers' attempts to acquire or expand colonial possessions in Central Africa as infringements of Portugal's 'historical rights' in the region. To secure these rights, Portuguese governments adopted a two-pronged approach. While they tried to secure the country's territorial claims on the diplomatic stage, they also commissioned explorers, mostly military men, to survey, map and formally occupy the territories in the interior of Angola and Mozambique to comply with the new imperative of 'effective occupation'. The journeys, and later book-length travel accounts, of Serpa Pinto, Capelo and Ivens received broad and usually very positive coverage at home. By contrast, the increasingly nationalist and pro-colonialist public opinion was often very critical of the diplomatic results, even though Portugal was able to secure vast new territories 'out of all proportion to its economic and political standing in Europe'.[87]

This particular pro-colonial mindset was both exhibited and reinforced by the so-called British ultimatum of 1890 when the British government forced its Portuguese counterpart, through a short memorandum, to give up its claims to the territory between Angola and Mozambique, indicated on the so-called pink map (*mapa cor-de-rosa*) of 1886. The ultimatum sparked fierce diplomatic and public indignation in Portugal.[88] It caused a further entanglement of nationalism and colonialism and contributed to what Valentim Alexandre has called the 'sacralization of the empire': for a large part of Portuguese public opinion, the colonies not only symbolised the country's glorious past, but also its future. For them, the survival of the Portuguese nation had come to depend on its empire.[89]

Economic interests were not completely alien to this imperial revival. In contrast to Richard Hammond, who in the 1960s argued that Portuguese imperialism had not been economically driven, but rather motivated by political and cultural factors such as national pride and widely shared colonial enthusiasm, various historians have underlined economic factors.[90] Valentim Alexandre has thus stressed that the idea of an economic 'Eldorado' underwrote discussions about the empire from the 1830s. He and other historians such as William Gervase Clarence-Smith and Pedro Lains have argued that Portuguese colonies indeed offered substantial economic opportunities for

---

[87] Axelson, *Portugal and the Scramble*; Alexandre, 'Nação e império'; Clarence-Smith, *Third Portuguese Empire*, 82 (quote). On the scramble in general, see Wesseling, *Divide and Rule*.

[88] See particularly Teixeira, *Ultimatum inglês*.

[89] Alexandre, 'Política colonial'. See also Castelo, *Passagens para África*, 43–5.

[90] Hammond, *Portugal and Africa*.

entrepreneurs and generated income for the Portuguese metropolitan state. In the 1880s and 1890s, investments in both settler agriculture and trade with African producers rose considerably and, aided by high international prices, the export of commodities such as cocoa, rubber and coffee from Angola and São Tomé and Príncipe boomed. In 1892, a protectionist reform of colonial tariffs also turned the colonies into important export markets for metropolitan products such as wine and cotton.[91] Hence, at the turn of the twentieth century, Portuguese colonies were not only reframed as an inalienable part of the Portuguese nation, a status further elaborated by the *Estado Novo* from the 1930s onwards,[92] but the empire was also considered crucial for Portugal's economic welfare.

Both nationalist-imperialist and economic expectations and projections centred on Angola. 'The province of Angola is certainly the possession from which justifiably we have to expect the most', the Minister of Maritime and Overseas Affairs Dias Costa stated in 1898, 'not only because of the exceptional conditions of fertility that allow for a broad and prosperous development, but [also] because of the intimacy of the relations that tie Angola to the metropole and that have turned it into the market of some of our most valuable industries'.[93] As the pro-colonial thinker and Portuguese consul in France, António Lobo de Almada Negreiros, worded it, Angola was not only the colony where 'the colonising activity of Portugal has asserted itself in the most evident way' but also the Portuguese possession, which 'because of its vastness, its material importance and its high population number [is] the most important of all Portuguese colonies'. 'One can say,' he added, 'that the province of Angola is today the Portuguese Brazil.'[94] Due to its long colonial history, its close ties with the metropole and its huge economic possibilities, Angola had taken centre stage in the Portuguese imperial imagination. Now, arguably, by depopulating and ruining the colony's most prosperous region, sleeping sickness was not only threatening the future of Angola, but also the empire and hence Portugal itself.

The Acclimatisation Problem and the New Importance of the African Population

The urge to resolve the sleeping sickness problem also reflected shifting views on the position of the 'native' African population in the colonisation process.

---

[91] See particularly Alexandre, *Origens*; Clarence-Smith, 'Myth'; Clarence-Smith, *Third Portuguese Empire*, 81–115; Lains, 'Causas'; Alexandre, 'Portuguese Empire', 129–30. See also Vos, 'Of Stocks and Barter'.
[92] Polanah, 'Imperial Mystique'. See Introduction.   [93] Costa, *Relatório (1898)*, 56.
[94] Negreiros, *Angola*, 5.

Across empires, colonialists were acknowledging the necessity of preserving the African population, and even promoting their health and well-being, if modern colonialism, particularly in the tropics, were to be viable and legitimate. By the late nineteenth century, most colonialists were convinced that the possibilities of white settlement in the tropics were very limited due to the so-called acclimatisation problem, and that hence, the economic future of tropical Africa depended on a healthy, growing African population. For Portuguese intellectuals, it was obvious that the policies that had, deliberately or not, led to the disappearance or extreme marginalisation of the 'native' populations in the United States, Australia or even at the Cape were not to be replicated in Portugal's African possessions. 'Our politics with regard to the Negro', António Francisco Nogueira, a member of the Geographical Society in Lisbon, concluded, 'is hence inevitably one of preservation'. Nogueira, who spent 25 years in south-west Angola, continued: 'If we thrust away or annihilate the Negro, we would only make a desert around us, we would only create ... sterility.'[95]

During the nineteenth century, scientific views on human acclimatisation in the tropics had completely shifted. In the eighteenth and early nineteenth century most European scientists still believed that human bodies, like plants and animals, could in principle be transferred to and thrive in other climes by means of physical adaptation and creolisation processes.[96] During the second half of the nineteenth century, however, the possibility of acclimatisation, and hence settlement, for white Europeans in the tropics had been increasingly questioned and repudiated by doctors and anthropologists. This rejection was not only based on a Hippocratic understanding of disease causation, which stressed the (im)balance between organisms and their environment and which had also underwritten positive acclimatisation theories, but also and mainly on new theories of 'biological-geographical' or 'racio-climatic determinism'.[97]

Tying in with new, more rigid concepts of race, these theories posited that Europeans could not adapt to tropical climate and its pernicious disease environment without degenerating. Individuals were still considered malleable, yet the physiological and mental hybridisations they would experience in the tropics were no longer seen as steps towards successful acclimatisation, but as pathological and degenerative. Some, like the influential German physician and anthropologist Rudolf Virchow, maintained that even if individual acclimatisation were possible in some cases, the 'race' would inevitably perish

---

[95] Nogueira, *Raça negra*, 7–12 (quotes 11). For similar views, see Guimarães, *Corrente do colonialismo*, 62–3. On the relationship between settler colonialism and genocide, see the contributions in Moses (ed.), *Empire, Colony, Genocide*.

[96] See Harrison, *Climates and Constitutions*; Osborne, 'Acclimatizing the World'.

[97] Livingstone, 'Tropical Climate'; Grosse, *Kolonialismus*, 54–96, quote 57; Jennings, *Curing the Colonizers*, 8–39 (quote 30).

either through the accumulation of degenerate traits from generation to generation or through practices of miscegenation or racial mixing.[98]

Focusing on Portugal and Angola, it appears that anti-acclimatisation discourse was not monolithic. Some observers believed that southern Europeans in general or the Portuguese more specifically had a greater potential to acclimatise in the tropics than northern Europeans, since they were less 'white' and 'Aryan', as Virchow's racialist explanation in 1885 went, or simply came from a different climate, as the Portuguese hygienist Augusto dos Santos Júnior put it two years earlier.[99] Such discourses of exceptionalism, however, did not prevent medical practitioners in Angola rallying with mainstream anti-acclimatisation positions: Joaquim Cardoso Botelho, the later Viscount of Giraúl, for instance, after examining the Portuguese settlers and their descendants around the city of Moçâmedes in the mid-1890s, concluded that they showed signs of degeneration. In order to survive, their descendants should not intermarry, but seek out 'uncorrupted whites coming from Europe'.[100]

Yet, according to Santos Júnior or his mentor, Manuel Ferreira Ribeiro, acclimatisation in the tropics was not impossible per se for another reason: they argued that there was not a 'single' tropical climate, but a great variety of tropical climates with different characteristics and hence conditions for white settlement. It was their task as colonial hygienists to identify adequate places and monitor the physiological and mental development of settlers. With regard to Angola, Santos Júnior, Ferreira Ribeiro or other doctors such as José Pereira do Nascimento were convinced, much in line with international discussions about the value of tropical plateaus and hill stations, that the temperate highlands of Huíla and Benguela offered good conditions for permanent settlement. Here, acclimatisation would not mean adaptation to a quintessentially hot and humid tropical climate, but to climatic conditions similar to those in southern Europe.[101]

These regions, however, to which studies in the first decades of the twentieth century would also add the highlands of Malanje and the coastal areas south of the 12° parallel, only covered a small area.[102] Most of the colony consisted of genuinely tropical and malaria-stricken lowlands that, against the backdrop of persisting beliefs in climatic determinism, were considered unsuitable for European settlement until well into the twentieth century.[103] In these areas,

---

[98] Virchow, 'Acclimatement'.   [99] Ibid., 742; Junior, *Acclimação*, xxii–iii.

[100] Bastos, 'Migrants, Settlers and Colonists', esp. 43–5 (quote 45).

[101] Junior, *Acclimação*; Ribeiro, *Colonisação luso-africana*; Nascimento, *Districto de Mossamedes*. On Ribeiro's work on acclimatisation and hygiene, see Roque, *Antropologia e Império*, 307–24; Bastos, 'Corpos, climas, ares e lugares', 35–42.

[102] See, for instance, Nascimento and Mattos, *Colonização de Angola*, 19–20, 37–42; Machado [de Faria e Maia], 'Zonas colonisáveis'.

[103] For the longevity of climatic determinism, see Jennings, *Curing the Colonizers*, 32–5; Crozier, 'What Was Tropical'.

which included northern Angola where sleeping sickness was raging, colonisation and economic exploitation was necessarily reliant on 'native' populations perceived as able to withstand the physical demands of manual labour under such climatic conditions.[104]

Persisting climatic fears were crucial in keeping the overall migration of Portuguese settlers to Angola low until after the Second World War and at least partially explain the lack of state funding for planned migration schemes most of the time and the continuous preference of Portuguese emigrants for destinations such as Brazil and the United States.[105] In 1900, there were, according to the census of that year, only 9,198 'whites' in the colony. Besides planters, many of these were temporarily stationed in the colony as soldiers or civil servants, or were (former) convicts (*degredados*), exiled from Portugal or its African colonies to Angola as punishment.[106]

Inter-Imperial Competition

In late nineteenth-century discourse not only the viability but also the legitimacy of colonialism in (tropical) Africa depended on the preservation and transformation of a large and healthy 'indigenous' population. Tapping into older abolitionist discourse, European powers had, at the Berlin conference in 1884–5, legitimised the political and economic occupation of the African continent with a humanitarian 'civilising mission'.[107] Even if their promise to 'watch over the conservation of the indigenous populations and the amelioration of their moral and material conditions of existence' was hollow if one considers the violent conquest and brutal subjugation of these very populations, the 'humanitarian argument' was crucial in debates about the legitimacy of empire. How empires lived up to this promise became the object of international scrutiny and inter-imperial rivalry.[108] Accordingly, the decision in 1901 to send a high-profile medical commission to Angola and Príncipe to investigate sleeping sickness was in part driven by the fear that it would cause an international scandal were Portugal to remain passive. In the late 1890s, intelligence about the sleeping sickness epidemic in Angola was already reaching other metropoles. Both the British and the German consuls in Luanda reported it to their governments in increasingly alarming terms and the reports of the German consul played a direct causal role in the creation of the Portuguese commission.[109]

---

[104] Giraúl, *Ideas geraes*, 13–4.   [105] Castelo, *Passagens para África*.
[106] *Annuário Estatístico da Província de Angola* 4 (1900); Coates, *Convict Labor*, 45–7.
[107] Compare with Osterhammel, 'Great Work'.
[108] Jerónimo, *Civilising Mission*, 11–6; 'General Act of the Conference of Berlin', art. 6 (quote).
[109] For the British consuls, see footnotes 3 and 46.

In July and August 1899, Otto Gleim visited the sleeping sickness-ridden eastern hinterland of Luanda. During his previous stay in the German colony of Cameroon, state doctor Hans Ziemann had informed him of the existence of sleeping sickness in Angola and encouraged him to further investigate.[110] In his letters to the Colonial Department of the Foreign Office in Berlin, Gleim painted a gloomy picture of decimated populations and deserted villages, accusing Portugal of not undertaking any action to check the disease and urging a German medical expedition to Angola.[111] That mission was eventually cancelled,[112] but on the demand of the Imperial Health Council (*Kaiserliches Gesundheitsamt*), Gleim's reports were published in the *Archiv für Schiffs- und Tropenhygiene*, Germany's leading journal of tropical medicine, together with a more general article on sleeping sickness in Angola and the Congo Free State by the journal's editor Carl Mense, who had practised medicine in the Congo in the mid-1880s.[113] These articles were deemed so important that dozens of offprints were subsequently sent to Germany's colonies and many of its consulates in Africa.[114]

These articles caused quite a stir in Portugal. They were reviewed by Miguel Bombarda, an official collaborator of the *Archiv*, in Portugal's leading medical journal, *A Medicina Contemporânea*.[115] At the turn of the century, Bombarda was one of the most influential doctors in Portugal. He was the medical superintendent of Lisbon's psychiatric hospital Rilhafolles, co-founder and long-time director of *A Medicina Contemporânea* and a leading member of the *Sociedade das Sciências Médicas de Lisboa*, the presidency of which he held from 1900 to 1903.[116] With Gleim's observations in hand, Bombarda tried to convince the *Sociedade* and the Overseas Ministry to send a study mission to Angola. On-the-spot research, he argued, would be more fruitful than further discussion and laboratory research in Portugal. He noted that other colonial powers had increased their medical expeditions to Africa and Asia (and even some parts of Europe) and thus unravelled the aetiology of other 'tropical' diseases such as malaria. Portugal had no choice but to follow,

---

[110] Gleim, 'Berichte über die Schlafkrankheit', 358; Ziemann, 'Schlafkrankheit der Neger', 414.

[111] Gleim to Reichskanzler Hohenlohe-Schillingsfürst, 10 August 1899 and 26 April 1900, BArch, R1001/5886, 3r–5r and 12r–16r.

[112] F. W. (Kolonialabteilung des Auswärtigen Amtes) to Präsident des Kaiserlichen Gesundheitsamtes, 25 June 1900, BArch R1001/5886, 27; Ziemann, 'Schlafkrankheit der Neger', 414, 423.

[113] Gleim, 'Berichte über die Schlafkrankheit'; Mense, 'Bemerkungen'.

[114] Präsident des Kaiserlichen Gesundheitsamtes to Direktor der Kolonialabteilung des Auswärtigen Amtes, 13 July 1900, BArch R1001/5886, 28. For the list of separata, dated 4 January 1901, see BArch R1001/5886, 37.

[115] Bombarda, 'Doença do Sono'.

[116] See Araújo, *Miguel Bombarda* and the contributions in Pereira and Pita (eds.), *Miguel Bombarda*.

Bombarda concluded. There were also compelling humanitarian and economic reasons for this intervention: 'As it is increasingly spreading in our prime colony, [the disease] is wiping out thousands of lives', Bombarda stated, so that 'the race that is the main lever of our colonisation and of our colonial possessions is being destroyed in a cruel manner'. Moreover, national dignity was at stake. Apparently assuming that sleeping sickness was ravaging mainly Portuguese possessions, Bombarda warned that it would be embarrassing for Portugal as a 'free country' were others to accomplish what was Portugal's responsibility.[117] Bombarda wrote this before the writings of consuls, journalists and philanthropists on the atrocities in the Congo Free State and slave-like labour conditions in Angola and São Tomé and Príncipe generated major colonial scandals in European and North American public opinion.[118] He rightly sensed that, through these very same actors, colonial administrations and public opinions were already observing how other colonial powers dealt with the 'native' populations under their rule and were increasingly sensitive to colonial conditions that contradicted Europe's self-declared civilising mission.

At the turn of the century, Portugal could not afford to attract more international criticism. Although it was not an exposed imperial 'newcomer' like Germany, Belgium or Italy, its position as a colonial power had been considerably weakened by the persistent economic and financial crisis of the metropole, the country's failure to enforce its coast-to-coast territorial claims in Central Africa against Great Britain and repeated accusations of colonial underdevelopment and mismanagement.[119] Such accusations included references to the continuation of slave-like labour, mostly exported from Angola, on the cocoa plantations of São Tomé and Príncipe.[120] Moreover, observers increasingly questioned the racial and cultural fitness of the Portuguese as modern colonisers. Many traveller accounts portrayed the Portuguese in Africa not only as uncivilised and backward, a view that was also present in the writings of many Portuguese intellectuals at the time, but often as Africanised and/or miscegenised. Racial scientists even cast doubt on the whiteness and hence Europeanness of the Portuguese in general.[121] Against this backdrop, some of Portugal's competitors called into question the legitimacy of Portuguese rule in Africa. In 1898, Germany and England even negotiated a 'secret' treaty in which they partitioned the Portuguese colonies in anticipation of an eventual declaration of bankruptcy by Portugal.[122]

---

[117] Sociedade das Sciências Medicas, 'Representação' (quotes). Similarly Bombarda, 'Doença de somno'.

[118] See Hochschild, *King Leopold's Ghost*; Burroughs, *Travel Writing*; Higgs, *Chocolate Islands*.

[119] Freeland, 'Sick Man of the West'; Teixeira, *Ultimatum inglês*. For accusations of underdevelopment, see also Kingsley, *West African Studies*, 283–4.

[120] See also Chapter 6.

[121] Newitt, 'British Travellers' Accounts'; Williams, 'Migration and Miscegenation', 161–2.

[122] See the extensive account in Tschapek, *Bausteine*.

Aware of the country's vulnerability, Portuguese elites were very sensitive to how Portugal and its colonial project were discussed abroad. When Bombarda wrote that it was Portugal's duty as a 'free country' to organise a sleeping sickness commission, he reflected widespread anxieties among Portuguese elites regarding Portugal's position in the world and the possible loss of its colonies. At the same time, the research mission was a chance to show that Portugal was keeping up with, or even outpacing, its competitors and hence deserved its place among the colonising nations. The commissioners (as shown in Chapter 2) tried hard to live up to these expectations.

Colonial Medicine and African Health

The 'scientific scramble for sleeping sickness' also illustrates a doctrinal shift in the role of medicine in European colonialism around 1900. Governments, doctors and pro-colonial publicists no longer thought of Western biomedicine as a mere 'tool of empire' enabling European domination by protecting white soldiers, administrators and settlers, as had been the main objective in the nineteenth century.[123] Medicine was increasingly viewed as an appropriate instrument with which to implement the practical and ideological imperatives of African population improvement, as a crucial means to foster 'the numerical increase and the improvement of the native race, the indispensable auxiliary of tropical colonization', as Eduardo da Costa, an influential colonial official and future Governor-General of Angola, worded it at the First National Colonial Congress in Lisbon in 1901.[124] This new 'mission' of colonial medicine gained broad currency at Portuguese and international colonial congresses at the turn of the century. 'Medical assistance' to the African population responded to the double rationale of modern colonialism: serving the colonising nations' own vested economic interest and fulfilling the moral duties of the civilising mission.[125]

The underlying idea that Africans needed European medical assistance was itself the result of three fundamental and intertwined shifts. First, anxieties about the possibility of European acclimatisation in the tropics did not prevent European colonialists and racial theorists from believing in the fundamental racial superiority of white Europeans and the social and biological inferiority of the African race. Against the backdrop of late nineteenth-century theories of racial difference and Social Darwinist ideas about the survival of the fittest,

---

[123] On medicine as 'tool of empire', see Introduction.

[124] Costa, *Estudo sobre a administração*, 187–9 (quote 187).

[125] See, for instance, Telles, 'Assistência aos indígenas' and Treille, 'Mesures', esp. 108–15 and 121–2. See also the discussion on Treille's paper in the same volume 'Condition matérielle des indigènes' and the recommendations in Exposition Universelle Internationale de 1900, *Congrès International de Sociologie Coloniale*, 34–6.

(tropical) Africans were increasingly, though often in a confused and totalising manner, conceptualised as an endangered race that would not survive without the help of European biomedicine and other forms of civilising action.[126] This was exactly what medical doctor and Secretary-General of the Geographical Society of Lisbon, Francisco Xavier da Silva Telles, called for at the Colonial Congress in Lisbon in 1901. Without assistance, he stated, colonialism would result in the progressive disappearance of the indigenous population.[127]

Second, such racialist views dovetailed with the growing pathologisation of the 'native' and colonised body.[128] In nineteenth-century European discourse, as Warwick Anderson has argued, disease susceptibility in tropical environments was strongly linked to the idea of 'racial immunities'. This idea, which also underpinned acclimatisation theories, posited that 'races' – and not individuals – had, through strong exposure, acquired biological immunity to certain diseases over the course of generations.[129] Consequently, Africans were thought to be more immune than Europeans to tropical diseases such as malaria, but particularly vulnerable to imported diseases like tuberculosis and smallpox.[130] However, as the occupation of the continent advanced and produced more information about the actual disease incidence among Africans, belief in racial immunities became more and more blurred. Colonial regimes grew convinced that Africans also suffered terribly from a wide range of tropical diseases and had very high general morbidity and mortality levels.[131] At the same time, the explanation partly shifted from biology to culture: many Europeans believed that it was the primitiveness of African customs, including a general lack of hygiene, that predisposed Africans to certain diseases.[132] Moreover, the same lack of precautions also made them carriers of communicable diseases against which Europeans had to defend themselves, either by treating their diseases or physically separating them from Europeans. Segregationist policies to prevent the spread of diseases like bubonic plague and malaria beset, to some extent, all colonial powers in the late nineteenth and early twentieth centuries. They were mostly conceived and implemented in colonial cities, but, as the example of sleeping sickness in the next chapter shows, were also applied to the African countryside.[133]

---

[126] On this discourse of extinction, see Brantlinger, *Dark Vanishings*.
[127] Telles, 'Assistência aos indígenas', 26.   [128] See Vaughan, *Curing Their Ills*.
[129] Anderson, 'Immunities of Empire'.
[130] For such ideas in Angola, see Giraúl, 'Prophylaxia do paludismo', 201; Roque, 'Prophylaxie du paludisme', 155.
[131] Treille, 'Mesures', 108–15; Telles, 'Assistência aos indígenas', 26.
[132] Vaughan, *Curing Their Ills*, 12–4, 200–2. Similarly, for 'native' Filipinos, Anderson, *Colonial Pathologies*.
[133] See Swanson, 'Sanitation Syndrome'; Eckart, 'Malariaprävention und Rassentrennung'; Goerg, 'From Hill Station'.

Arguably, the way in which sleeping sickness was framed in the late nineteenth century both reflected and further entrenched this view. As I have already mentioned, many observers characterised sleeping sickness as a 'racial' disease that only affected Africans, due to their backward customs or biological differences. They thereby willingly ignored or dismissed evidence of European casualties. Both in Angola and on Príncipe, various Portuguese observers including medical doctors had reported cases of sleeping sickness in white Europeans in the late 1890s and early 1900s.[134] Others, however, questioned the validity of their diagnosis, for lack of 'conclusive' scientific proof that the victims had died of sleeping sickness, or, like the German consul Gleim, stated that the victims must have been 'half-bloods' (*mestiços*), thus reiterating doubts about Portuguese whiteness.[135] Despite repeated Portuguese doubts, it would take the formulation of the trypanosoma theory and Patrick Manson's description of a white patient in London in 1903 for the broader European scholarly community to accept the idea of white casualties.[136]

Finally, the rise of biomedical interventionism also rested on the growing belief in the superiority of European medicine over African healing systems. Until well into the nineteenth century, colonial doctors often did not assume that their methods were better suited to cure diseases in the tropics.[137] As various case studies have shown, doctors in the Portuguese colonies in Africa, India or Brazil were not averse to adopting 'indigenous' practices and medications, leading to multiple medical hybridisms.[138] Towards the end of the nineteenth century, however, belief in the supremacy of 'European medicine' grew much stronger, first and foremost among colonial decision-makers and doctors in the European metropoles and more gradually also among colonial practitioners. This was mainly due to the emergence of germ theory in what has often been called the bacteriological revolution and its influence on the emerging discipline of tropical medicine.[139]

In practice, the doctrinal shift towards African healthcare was slow to be implemented 'on the ground', especially in the countryside, due to the lack of doctors and medical infrastructure and competing African healing practices.[140] Yet, in many colonies in tropical Africa, including Angola and Príncipe, the fight against sleeping sickness would be the main testing ground before the

---

[134] Maldonado, 'Doença do somno'; Leitão, *Relatório da visita sanitária*, 100, 110; *BOA* (1898), 13 and 225, (1901), 244, (1902), 219 and (1903), 250.

[135] Bettencourt, Kopke, Rezende and Mendes, *Maladie du sommeil*, 11–2; Gleim, 'Berichte über die Schlafkrankheit', 360–1. See also Coghe, *Population Politics (2014)*, 74–6.

[136] See Ehlers, *Europa und die Schlafkrankheit*, 92–6.

[137] Comaroff, 'Diseased Heart', 315; Fischer-Tiné, *Pidgin-Knowledge*.

[138] See, for instance, Bastos, 'Medical Hybridisms'; Walker, 'Acquisition and Circulation'; Havik, 'Hybridising Medicine' and Kananoja, *Healing Knowledge*.

[139] See later in this chapter.   [140] See Chapter 3.

1920s. As Maryinez Lyons has stated, study missions and health campaigns against this disease constituted 'the first real effort made by the Europeans to deal with the health of the Africans'.[141]

The focus on sleeping sickness, however, is not self-evident. In late nineteenth-century Angola, other serious diseases afflicting the African population figured prominently in medical reports and statistics as well, notably respiratory diseases such as pneumonia and tuberculosis.[142] Most importantly, sleeping sickness was matched and perhaps even outweighed in frequency, extension and mortality by smallpox. Smallpox had been known in Angola since the seventeenth century, when it was most likely introduced by Portuguese soldiers, but it gained prominence from the 1850s onwards, when expanding commercial networks, mounting labour migration flows and military campaigns facilitated the spread of infectious disease. After the devastating epidemic of 1864, smallpox epidemics were reported every five to 10 years in various parts of the colony. They often included Luanda and its hinterland and claimed many thousands of lives.[143] Smallpox was considered an eminently African disease in Angola, but for different reasons and in a less absolute manner than sleeping sickness. Europeans were believed to be less vulnerable because they were vaccinated or had acquired immunity through contact with milder forms of the disease.[144] At the time, the demographic impact of smallpox was believed to be considerable. Around 1900, observers often attributed deserted villages in northern Angola to both sleeping sickness and smallpox.[145]

Since the 1860s, Portuguese health services had set up vaccination campaigns in Luanda and a few larger towns in its hinterland.[146] However, these campaigns, which became increasingly regular by the end of the century, were mostly of limited success, since many Africans did not believe in the protective power of vaccination and only agreed to be vaccinated in greater numbers during epidemics. Moreover, the vaccine lymph that the few medical officers in the interior received was often insufficient in both quantity and quality, as the heat diminished or destroyed its potency. This further frustrated doctors' attempts to convince Africans of the benefits of vaccination and they often fell

---

[141] Lyons, *Colonial Disease*, 102 (quote).
[142] See the monthly health bulletins in the *Boletim Oficial de Angola* during the 1890s and medical reports such as Collaço, 'Relatório Dondo (1896)', 2 and Joaquim Bernardo Cardoso Botelho, 'Relatório Médico do Districto Sanitário de Mossamedes (1896)', 23 December 1896, 19–20, both AHU, SEMU, DGU 942.
[143] See particularly Dias, 'Famine and Disease', 359, 362–9, 374 and the detailed historical accounts in Correia, 'Varíola' and Correia, 'Clima', 405–7, 453–9.
[144] Dias, 'Famine and Disease', 362; Correia, 'Varíola', 445.
[145] Monteiro, *Angola and the River Congo*, vol. 1, 143–4; Leitão, *Relatório da visita sanitária*, 16, 30; Brandão, 'Diario da marcha', 224, 409.
[146] Dias, 'Famine and Disease', 369.

back on arm-to-arm inoculation.[147] Between 1902 and 1904, some vaccine was produced directly in Luanda, but production difficulties eventually stopped this service.[148] Only in the 1920s was the disease brought under control by mass vaccination campaigns that made use of new freeze-dried vaccines and that, in northern Angola, were increasingly conducted during sleeping sickness screening campaigns.[149]

If, in comparison, the medical establishment in Lisbon and Luanda prioritised the fight against sleeping sickness, this had much to do with another shift in colonial medicine: unlike smallpox, which was a well-understood disease that could be prevented through vaccination, sleeping sickness constituted a real scientific challenge for the emerging discipline of tropical medicine. Its powerful representatives would put it at the top of their agenda.

The Rise of Tropical Medicine

Sleeping sickness research and campaigns in the early twentieth century thrived on, and greatly contributed to, the increasing institutionalisation of tropical medicine in Europe. Responding to growing European interest in understanding and fighting tropical pathologies that impeded the development of empire in the tropics, this new medical specialty was closely linked to the ascendancy of germ theory, which was gradually revolutionising 'Western' views on disease causation, prevention and treatment.[150] For its proponents, tropical diseases were no longer the product of a hostile climate, as older theories about diseases in the tropics had posited, but were caused by bacteria, parasites or other micro-organisms invading the human body, just as diseases in temperate climates did. Tropical medicine thus relied on microbiological knowledge and on the laboratorial and microscopic examination of bodily fluids and tissues.[151]

Accordingly, by the time the Portuguese sleeping sickness mission was organised in 1901, a considerable segment of the international medical community believed that causation theories blaming 'racial' habits were obsolete and had started looking for micro-organisms. Patrick Manson, often considered the 'father of tropical medicine', assumed that the *filaria perstans*

---

[147] See, for instance, Curto, 'Relatório do Chefe do Serviço de Saúde de Angola', 323–5; Filippe Nery Collaço, 'Relatorio sobre o serviço de saúde em Noqui (1896)', 31 December 1896, 6–7, AHU SEMU, DGU 942 and the health bulletins in *BOA* (1895), 586 and 737.

[148] See the correspondence in ANA, Cx. 361, Pasta 2 and Cx. 391, Processo 361/42.

[149] Correia, 'Varíola', 446–50; Mora, 'Serviços de Saúde em Angola (1928)', 90–1. See also Chapter 3.

[150] Worboys, 'Bacteriological Revolution'; Latour, *Pasteurization*, 140–5.

[151] On the long rise of tropical medicine, see Arnold (ed.), *Warm Climates*; Worboys, 'Germs' and Neill, *Networks*.

worm that he had found in the blood of a sleeping sickness patient in London was the pathogenic agent of the disease.[152] In Portugal, various scientists (António Carvalho de Figueiredo in Lisbon in 1889–90 and António Olympio Cagigal and Charles Lepierre in Coimbra in 1897) had identified bacteria in patients' blood as the cause of the disease.[153] These unconfirmed aetiological assumptions underwrote the decision to send out some of Portugal's finest microbiologists in 1901. The fact that they would identify another bacterium and not find the parasite that was later accepted as the cause of the disease (see Chapter 2) reveals that tropical medicine was still in its formative stage. The importance of parasites as pathogens had not yet been fully recognised and the parasite-vector-model, which was first confirmed for malaria in 1897, would only become the core explanation for tropical diseases in the first decades of the twentieth century.[154]

As Deborah Neill has shown, the institutionalisation of tropical medicine as a new medical specialty in Europe in the late nineteenth and early twentieth centuries was closely entangled with sleeping sickness research. Institutionalisation involved the establishment of schools, journals and medical societies specialising in tropical medicine in Europe's imperial metropoles, alongside the organisation of special sections at international medical conferences. In this process, the new schools of tropical medicine founded in Liverpool (1898), London (1899), Hamburg (1901) and other imperial cities replaced and expanded the courses in tropical medicine taught in some universities and naval schools. While sleeping sickness research benefited from this ongoing institutionalisation process, it also accelerated the process as scholars rallying around this disease consolidated the epistemic foundations of the new discipline and used public attention to acquire funding for research and schools.[155]

The interdependence between sleeping sickness research and the institutionalisation of tropical medicine can also be observed in the Portuguese case. On the one hand, the medical and political challenge posed by epidemic sleeping sickness led to a more tangible institutionalisation of tropical medicine in Portugal. There had been a course in 'exotic pathology' at Lisbon's Naval School since 1887, but as it was not mandatory, most doctors did not enrol in

---

[152] Haynes, 'Framing Tropical Disease'. On Manson's role in developing the discipline of tropical medicine, see Haynes, *Imperial Medicine*. For more critical views, see Arnold, 'Introduction', 1–4 and Worboys, 'Germs'.

[153] Amaral, 'Bacteria or Parasite', 1283–4.

[154] On the slow separation of parasitology and tropical medicine from bacteriology, see Worboys, 'Germs'.

[155] Neill, *Networks*, esp. 5–72. See also Ehlers, *Europa und die Schlafkrankheit*, 29–65. For the institutionalisation of tropical medicine in Germany and Belgium, see also Eckart, 'From Questionnaires to Microscopes'; Mertens and Lachenal, 'History'.

it before leaving for the colonies. Overall, research in tropical diseases remained marginal in nineteenth-century Portugal.[156] In 1901–2, influential doctors like Miguel Bombarda and António Ramada Curto, the former health director and Governor-General of Angola who now directed the Overseas Ministry's Health Department, capitalised on the much-reported labours of the Portuguese sleeping sickness mission to advocate the establishment of a fully-fledged school of tropical medicine for research and training. The advantages of such a school would largely outweigh the considerable costs, they argued, as it would reduce death rates among colonisers and colonised alike. Moreover, Portugal was, in their view, bound to follow more advanced colonial powers like Great Britain, France and Germany, which had already recognised the value of tropical medicine for colonisation and established such schools.[157] The Overseas Ministry endorsed their demand and in 1902 the *Escola de Medicina Tropical (EMT)* was founded in Lisbon, together with the *Hospital Colonial*, where patients with tropical diseases from the colonies would be accommodated, treated and studied. From 1905 onwards, the EMT also published Portugal's first journal of tropical medicine, the *Archivos de Hygiene e Pathologia Exoticas.*[158]

The creation of the EMT and the Colonial Hospital, which both played an eminent role in Portuguese sleeping sickness research in the following decades, reflected the importance that the Portuguese government and medical establishment attached to tropical medicine as a 'tool of empire'.[159] Inter-imperial competition and learning were key to this development, as the practical organisation of the EMT shows. In 1902, Ayres Kopke was sent to Bordeaux, Marseille and London to observe local courses and schools of tropical medicine. Upon his advice, which was critical of French efforts, the EMT was modelled on the London School of Tropical Medicine of Patrick Manson.[160] It was much smaller, however, with initially only three professors and a dozen graduates per year until the end of the First World War.[161] At an organisational level, the school was deeply entangled with empire: it was an integral part of the colonial administration, partly funded by the colonies and its first director was António Ramada Curto, the director of the Health Department in the Overseas Ministry.[162]

---

[156] Lencastre, 'Ensino', i–iii. See also Azevedo, *Cinquenta anos*, 10.

[157] Bombarda, 'Criação'; Ramada Curto in 'Acta da Sessão, 09.11.1901', 408–9. On Ramada Curto's career, see Lapa, *Conselheiro Ramada Curto.*

[158] On the institutionalisation of tropical medicine in Portugal, see Amaral, 'Emergence'; Castro, *Escola de Medicina Tropical*; Azevedo, *Cinquenta anos*, 9–17.

[159] For such an interpretation, see also Shapiro, *Medicine.*

[160] Kopke, 'Escola portugueza'. See also Castro, *Escola de Medicina Tropical*, 37–9.

[161] See the list of graduates in Azevedo, *Cinquenta anos*, 97–124.

[162] Ibid., 12–3; Amaral, 'Emergence', 307–10.

On the other hand, the institutionalisation of tropical medicine was also instrumental in turning sleeping sickness into 'a top priority and a focal point for scientific research and colonial intervention'.[163] In the early twentieth century, it gave birth to a transnational epistemic community of medical scientists, who shared common values and beliefs and who influenced colonial policy-making via a small group of distinguished gatekeepers. Eminent medical scientists like Patrick Manson, Alphonse Laveran and Robert Koch – alongside Miguel Bombarda and later Ayres Kopke for Portugal – used their medical prestige and political connections to convince colonial administrations to fund sleeping sickness research. They were seconded by young scientists, whom they had often trained themselves, keen to do the necessary fieldwork. Because of the complex aetiology of the disease and considerable academic and public interest, sleeping sickness research was a rewarding career choice for young scientists, allowing them to further increase the prestige of their mentors. At the same time, the 'scramble' for a cure for sleeping sickness was also the result of scientists' ability to mobilise nationalism, by invoking rivalry between the emerging national communities of tropical medicine and staging it as part of a larger inter-imperial competition.[164]

This competition partly explains why the dominance of sleeping sickness research in the field of tropical medicine was particularly strong in the Portuguese case. Before the First World War, all schools of tropical medicine in Europe devoted great attention to sleeping sickness, through expeditions and control programmes. However, while the research programmes of these schools generally included study missions on other tropical diseases as well, such as malaria, yellow fever and beriberi, the School of Tropical Medicine in Lisbon focused almost entirely on sleeping sickness. The four medical missions that it organised and supervised between 1902 and 1914 were all dedicated to this disease, even if Ayres Kopke's mission in 1904 also included a small study of beriberi on São Tomé.[165] From the outset, Miguel Bombarda and later especially Ayres Kopke legitimised this 'specialisation' with the inter-imperial competition between Portuguese and other national medical communities. Since the fight against sleeping sickness quickly became the most important medical intervention of European colonialism in Africa as well as the standard by which to measure medical progress (and good governance), it made sense for Portugal, whose main colonies were in Africa, to concentrate its scarce resources on this single tropical disease.

---

[163] Hoppe, *Lords of the Fly*, 27.

[164] Neill, *Networks*; Haynes, 'Framing Tropical Disease', 483–91; Hoppe, *Lords of the Fly*, 29.

[165] See Amaral, 'Emergence', 313 and, for more details, Chapter 2. By way of comparison, from the 32 missions organised by the Liverpool School of Tropical Medicine before 1914, only six concentrated on sleeping sickness. See Liverpool School of Tropical Medicine, *Historical Record*, 73–5.

Conclusion

Known among Portuguese colonial doctors in Angola since the 1870s, a new epidemic of sleeping sickness starting in the mid-1890s triggered unprecedented fears of depopulation among Portuguese colonialists. The disease was reported to be carrying off the 'native' population in the hinterland of Luanda, the heartland of Portuguese colonisation in Angola, and increasingly in other parts of the colony. This fed depopulation anxieties with gloomy reports about deserted villages and horrendous estimates, founded on common assumptions that the regions where sleeping sickness was raging had been much more populous in the past. Such assumptions were partly backed by census data, but colonial officials were wary of attributing population loss to sleeping sickness only. They pointed at additional causes such as smallpox, low birth and high infant mortality rates and the continuous flow of Angolan labourers to the cocoa plantations on São Tomé and Príncipe. While these factors contributed to the sense of a demographic crisis, it was sleeping sickness that, until well into the interwar years, would receive most attention from Portuguese colonial doctors and policy-makers.

That a sleeping sickness epidemic and the presumed decrease of the 'native' population triggered strong colonial interventions in the early twentieth century was, in turn, a result of various ongoing and mutually reinforcing shifts in Portuguese and European colonialism in the last quarter of the nineteenth century: the political subjugation and economic transformation of Luanda's hinterland, which probably contributed to the epidemic outbreak in the region; the key role political, intellectual and economic actors in the metropole attributed to the colonies for safeguarding the political and economic future of the Portuguese nation; the growing consensus about the necessity to actively promote the preservation, increase and improvement of Angola's indigenous population; the rise of tropical medicine as a new discipline with powerful gatekeepers committed to understanding and controlling sleeping sickness; and the inter-imperial competition and collaboration between Portugal and other European powers regarding many of these issues. Taken together, all these factors explain why sleeping sickness became the object of a panoply of medical, pharmaceutical and administrative interventions, analysed in the next chapter.

2   Tropical Medicine and Sleeping Sickness Control Before 1918

In the early twentieth century, the fight against sleeping sickness became the most important medical intervention and a crucial aspect of Portuguese population politics in Angola. Despite the vast and still growing historiography on this disease, however, the long history of sleeping sickness in Angola, and the Portuguese colonies in general, has received very little scholarly attention. While there are a few articles by scholars based in Portugal,[1] international studies, even those with comparative and transimperial approaches, have virtually ignored it, thus implying that nothing noteworthy happened.[2] This neglect is all the more surprising given that Portuguese colonial entanglements with the disease already started in the 1870s, varied in some important respects from the story commonly told and left a considerable paper trail in Portuguese, French and English. Together with Chapter 1, which focused on the disease's early history, demographic impact and broader context, and Chapter 3, which deals with the 1920s and 1930s, this chapter fills this historiographical lacuna. It analyses the multi-faceted medical and administrative efforts to check sleeping sickness in Angola until the end of the First World War. It sheds light on the varied practices, multiple conflicts and intra- and transimperial flows of knowledge that were part and parcel of anti-sleeping sickness policies in early twentieth-century Angola and shows why this 'Portuguese story' matters for international historiography.

---

[1] See Varanda, 'Cavalo de Tróia'; Amaral, 'Bacteria or Parasite' and Castro, *Escola de Medicina Tropical*. For Príncipe, see Silva, *Land of Flies*, for Guinea, Havik, 'Public Health and Tropical Modernity'.

[2] From the vast literature, see particularly Ford, *Role of the Trypanosomiases*; Giblin, 'Trypanosomiasis Control'; Lyons, *Colonial Disease*; Worboys, 'Comparative History'; Bado, *Médecine coloniale*; Bell, *Frontiers of Medicine*, 127–62; Eckart, 'Colony as Laboratory'; Hoppe, *Lords of the Fly*; Isobe, *Medizin und Kolonialgesellschaft*; Bado, *Eugène Jamot*; Neill, *Networks*; Tousignant, 'Trypanosomes'; Mertens and Lachenal, 'History'; Lachenal, *Médicament*; Mertens, *Chemical Compounds*; Webel, *Politics of Disease Control* and Ehlers, *Europa und die Schlafkrankheit*. A notable, yet brief and incomplete exception is Headrick, 'Sleeping Sickness Epidemics'. See also, for Príncipe, McKelvey, *Man against Tsetse*, 107–24 and for Angola, Coghe, 'Sleeping Sickness Control'.

The chapter argues that Portuguese doctors played an important role in the European 'scramble for sleeping sickness'. Driven by fears of depopulation and economic ruin, and by inter-imperial competition, they actively contributed to the transimperial efforts to understand, cure and eradicate this deadly disease, through research missions, drug research and medical campaigns. Nevertheless, practical disease control policies in Angola remained fragmentary prior to the 1920s, particularly compared to Príncipe and some other colonies. This was due partly to factors also faced by other colonial powers: many Africans continued to distrust Western biomedicine and colonial health services lacked the resources, manpower and sometimes also skill to implement disease control policies on a vast scale. However, it was also due to the Portuguese imperial preference for eradication measures undertaken on the island of Príncipe. The chapter also reveals other important particularities of Portuguese dealings with the disease, such as the pivotal role of the Colonial Hospital in Lisbon for the treatment of African patients and related drug experiments, and the great reliance on vector control to check the disease in (West African) Príncipe. Taken together, these show that including the 'Portuguese case' not only adds new empirical detail, but also nuances some of the over-generalising findings on 'European' dealings with the disease in recent historiography.[3] This chapter also rejects the idea of 'national' styles in the fight against sleeping sickness, by showing that disease control measures varied greatly between Portuguese colonies.

Unravelling the Aetiology: Of Bacteria, Parasites and Scientists

In August 1901, after only three months of investigation in Príncipe and Angola, the Portuguese commissioners announced that they had probably found the causative agent of the disease. In the cerebrospinal fluid of many patients, both *intra-vitam* and *post-mortem*, they had detected a bacterium described as 'diplo-streptococcus'.[4] This discovery, though based on tenuous evidence, sparked great enthusiasm in Portugal's medical press. Most commentators, including the Overseas Minister and Miguel Bombarda, stated that a long-standing enigma was now being deciphered and proudly proceeded to celebrate a 'colossal triumph for Portuguese medicine', 'one of [its] most precious glories'.[5] A year later, the commissioners bolstered their claims with

---

[3] Compare with Neill, *Networks*; Ehlers, *Europa und die Schlafkrankheit*.

[4] Ministério da Marinha e Ultramar (ed.), *Doença do somno*, 13–40, esp. 32–3. On Portuguese contributions to the aetiology of the disease, see also Amaral, 'Bacteria or Parasite' and Castro, *Escola de Medicina Tropical*, 33–4, 40–2.

[5] Teixeira de Sousa to Bombarda, 1 October 1901, and Bombarda to Teixeira de Sousa, 7 October 1901, *Jornal da Sociedade das Sciências Médicas de Lisboa* 65 (1901), 417–9 (first quote 417); Lopes, 'Chronica' (second quote). Similarly, Ferreira, 'Doença do somno', 301.

a new and more extensive report stating that additional research, conducted in Angola and at the Royal Bacteriological Institute in Lisbon, had confirmed their initial findings. In all examined patients, they had found the same bacterial microorganism, which they now fancily baptised 'hypnococcus', a contraction of hypnosis, a term often used for sleeping sickness (from the Greek word *hypnos* for sleep), and streptococcus.[6]

The reports of the Portuguese sleeping sickness commission also received much international attention: they were reviewed and some of them published in translation in Europe's leading medical journals.[7] In October 1902, Carl Mense even presented preparations and cultures of the hypnococcus, which he had received from Portuguese commission member Ayres Kopke, to a medical section of the German Colonial Congress in Berlin.[8] To assure an international audience, the commission published its final report in French.[9] Although this procedure delayed the dissemination of research results, it ensured that language did not hinder international circulation. In the following decades, important Portuguese sleeping sickness reports were generally made available in French or English.

However, the international community of tropical medicine experts was not convinced by the Portuguese results. Other leading researchers were not able to confirm the presence of the 'hypnococcus' in their cases. They either did not find any bacterium at all, like Warrington in Liverpool, or found a different one, like Broden in the Belgian Congo in 1901 and Castellani in Uganda in 1902. Still others stuck to competing theories that did not involve bacteria. Hans Ziemann, for instance, continued to believe in his manioc food-poisoning theory, while Patrick Manson was not yet disposed to abandon his *filaria perstans* theory.[10] He believed that the Portuguese commissioners' failure to find this parasitic worm in their sleeping sickness patients was due to 'unsuitable technique'.[11] That Manson himself could not find the 'hypnococcus' in the brain of a deceased sleeping sickness patient in London did not increase his respect for the work of his Portuguese colleagues.[12] In the third edition of his

---

[6] Bettencourt, 'Doença do somno (1902)'.

[7] See, for instance, *Journal of Tropical Medicine* 5, 10–12 (1902), 149–51, 171–2, 185–6; *The Lancet* 4126 (27 September 1902), 885–8; 4160 (23 May 1903), 1438–40 and 4213 (28 May 1904), 1507–8; *British Medical Journal* 2207 (18 April 1903), 908–10 and 2265 (28 May 1904), 1258; *La Presse Médicale* (24 June 1903), 468; *Centralblatt für Bakteriologie, Parasitenkunde und Infektionskrankheiten* 35 (1903), 45–61, 212–21, 316–23 and *Archiv für Schiffs- und Tropenhygiene* 6 (1902), 43–4 and 7 (1903), 382, 398–9.

[8] Mense, 'Deutscher Kolonialkongress', 56.

[9] Bettencourt, Kopke, Rezende and Mendes, *Maladie du sommeil*.

[10] Warrington, 'Note'. Broden's bacillus is commented upon in Bettencourt, 'Doença do somno (1902)', 227–9. For Castellani and Ziemann, see later in this chapter.

[11] Manson's introduction to Cook, 'Sleeping Sickness'.

[12] Upon receiving part of this patient's brain from Manson, the Portuguese commissioners also proved unable to find the hypnococcus. See Bettencourt, 'Doença do somno (1902)', 290.

authoritative manual on tropical diseases, published in March 1903, Manson
stated that 'until further evidence has been collected, it is impossible to say if
either of these bacteria is the germ of sleeping sickness'.[13]

The most serious blow to the hypnococcus, and the bacterial hypothesis in
general, occurred shortly thereafter, when Aldo Castellani, a member of the
Sleeping Sickness Commission sent to Uganda by the British Royal Society in
1902, published his research. First, in March 1903, Castellani announced the
discovery of another streptococcus as the cause of the disease. The Portuguese
commissioners hastened to claim, in the Portuguese and British medical press,
that this streptococcus was identical with their hypnococcus, but this discussion was quickly outpaced by new developments.[14] In May, Castellani stated
that neither 'his' nor other streptococci, but trypanosomes, probably of the
same *gambiense* kind that had previously been discovered in a different
context by Forde and Dutton in Gambia, caused sleeping sickness. He had
found these parasitic protozoa in 20 out of 34 patients.[15]

Although this trypanosoma theory quickly received support from other
researchers such as Bruce, Nabarro, Sambon and Brumpt, it was also met with
scepticism, particularly from Manson, who now (ironically) supported the
bacterial hypothesis.[16] The Portuguese commissioners, too, were reluctant to
abandon the hypnococcus. When they re-examined some of their blood slides,
they found trypanosomes in 4 out of 12 cases.[17] In response to this rather
inconclusive result, Annibal Correia Mendes, commission member and since
1902 director of the Bacteriological Laboratory in Luanda's Hospital Maria
Pia, began to bring in sleeping sickness patients from infested regions and to
search for trypanosomes in their blood and cerebrospinal fluid.[18] In addition,
the School of Tropical Medicine in Lisbon (EMT) sent Ayres Kopke, who had
been appointed Professor of Bacteriology and Parasitology, on a new research
mission to Angola and Príncipe.

By the time Kopke arrived in Angola in July 1904, the most essential parts
of the trypanosoma theory had already been formulated and partly proved.
This included the role of the *Glossina palpalis*, a particular type of tsetse fly
that, through its bite, transmitted *Trypanosoma brucei gambiense*, and the
existence of two disease stages: a first stage, in which trypanosomes could

---

[13] Manson, *Tropical Diseases (1903)*, 342.
[14] Castellani, 'Etiology'; Bettencourt, 'Doença do somno (1903)'; Bettencourt, Kopke, Rezende
and Mendes, 'On the Etiology'.
[15] Castellani, 'Trypanosoma'.
[16] Manson et al., 'Discussion on Trypanosomiasis'; Bruce et al., 'Discussion on
Trypanosomiasis', 379. See also Sambon, 'Elucidation', 72–3.
[17] Bettencourt, Kopke, Rezende and Mendes, *Maladie du sommeil*, 273–6.
[18] See the epidemiological bulletins of June, July and August 1903 in *BOA* (1903), 447, 516
and 599.

be found in the blood and lymph, with no or few symptoms such as fever and the swelling of the cervical lymph glands; and a second stage with strong and disease-typical neurological symptoms after the trypanosomes had invaded the brain. Kopke could merely confirm the trypanosoma theory. In collaboration with Correia Mendes in Luanda and António Damas Mora, the medical officer on Príncipe, Kopke examined more than 40 new cases of sleeping sickness, finding trypanosomes in the blood or cerebrospinal fluid of almost all of them. Moreover, with the help of Correia Mendes, who inspected Luanda's hinterland, and local medical officers who provided fly specimens, Kopke verified that the *Glossina palpalis* existed in the regions where patients had probably been infected. Finally, in addition to these microbiological and epidemiological confirmations of the trypanosoma theory, he showed that the diplo-streptococci only invaded the brain long after the trypanosomes had done so, and only in about half of his new cases. With this finding, Kopke implicitly adhered to the emerging consensus that the bacteria identified by Portuguese and other researchers were not the cause of sleeping sickness, but a secondary infection in the final stage of the disease.[19]

Although their hypnococcus theory died a silent death, the work of the Portuguese commissioners had not been completely in vain. Years later, Carl Mense still praised their elaborate descriptions of the symptomatology and anatomical pathology of the disease, which were based on the observation of a far greater number of cases than earlier studies.[20] Yet, their failure to find the true cause of sleeping sickness provoked scathing critique in Portugal, much of it directed at the composition of the commission. Had the endeavour been organised by 'suitable persons from all three study centres of the country', the Coimbra-based bacteriologist Charles Lepierre opined, 'one can suppose that in a joint effort they would have thought about the role that protozoa (so high on the agenda) could possibly have been playing in the aetiology of the disease.'[21] Lepierre made clear reference to the rivalry between the medical schools of Lisbon, Coimbra and Porto and the exclusion of the latter two from the mission. His criticism of Lisbon's dominance was also motivated by his personal disappointment that, despite his own path-breaking bacteriological study on sleeping sickness and long-standing experience in the field, he had not been selected for the study mission.[22] Lepierre had been one of the most vociferous critics of the work of the sleeping sickness commission in Portugal, along with António de Padua, professor in medicine at the same University of

---

[19] Kopke, 'Investigações'; Mendes, 'Glossinas de Angola'. See also, with hindsight, Kopke, *Estudo da doença do sono*, 3–34.
[20] Mense, 'Menschliche Trypanosomenkrankheit'.
[21] Padua and Lepierre, *Doença do somno*, 88.
[22] See also Amaral, 'Bacteria or Parasite', 1281–2.

Coimbra. They had consistently claimed that the hypnococcus was identical to (or at best a small variation of) the meningococcus discovered by Weichselbaum, the causative agent of cerebrospinal meningitis, and as such unlikely to be the cause of sleeping sickness.[23] The tone of this rivalry is reminiscent of the fierce competition between the London and Liverpool Schools of Tropical Medicine, or between Berlin and Hamburg-based experts around the same time. According to Deborah Neill, competition within national scientific communities was one of the principal reasons for experts in tropical medicine seeking to establish transnational networks.[24]

Whether the inclusion of scholars from Coimbra and Porto would have changed the results of the commission is uncertain, but Lepierre arguably had a point in attributing the commission's failure to epistemological neglect of parasitology. Although the doctors had also looked for Manson's *filaria perstans*, they were convinced *a priori* that the disease was bacterial. It was this presumption and, as Kopke later admitted, their bacteria-centred laboratorial education that prevented them from finding the trypanosomes in the blood and cerebrospinal fluid of almost 70 cases of sleeping sickness during their two years of research.[25] Manson, who had also systematically overlooked the trypanosomes, pointed to the technical difficulties of microscopical work, which required the scientist seeking 'parasites, filaria embryos, trypanosomes, malaria parasites, spirilla, bacteria' to be already 'intent on finding the particular form of organism he is in quest of'.[26] Indeed, research questions and techniques went hand-in-hand. It was only by combining a new aetiological presumption, inspired by Bruce's work on nagana or livestock trypanosomiasis, with a novel technique of centrifuging the cerebrospinal fluid that Castellani had developed that he was able to detect and eventually cared to further investigate the trypanosomes under his microscope in Uganda.[27]

By the end of 1904, the basic assumptions of the trypanosoma theory had been accepted by the medical community in Europe. Some questions regarding the transmission process, however, continued to be discussed for years to come. These included whether the *Glossina palpalis* was the only vector of the disease or whether sleeping sickness could be transmitted by other blood-sucking insects, or even through sexual intercourse. In the early 1910s, a distinct strain of sleeping sickness was discovered in Southeast Africa, caused by another trypanosome, labelled *Trypanosoma brucei rhodesiense*, and transmitted mainly by another tsetse fly, the *Glossina morsitans*. While this

---

[23] Their articles (1901–2) in the Coimbra-based journal *Movimento Médico* were later reprinted in Padua and Lepierre, *Doença do somno*. See also Amaral, 'Bacteria or Parasite', 1288–90.
[24] Neill, *Networks*, 29–31.   [25] Kopke, 'Estudos Moçambique', 234.
[26] Manson et al., 'Discussion on Trypanosomiasis', 646.
[27] See, for instance, Boyd, 'Sleeping Sickness', 102–3.

trypanosome could (and can) not be distinguished from *gambiense* on a morphological basis, experts pointed to its different geographical distribution and clinical manifestations. The East and South African *rhodesiense* form of the disease has a much shorter incubation period and much more rapid development, often causing death in a few months rather than years, as was the case with the more chronic *gambiense* form predominant in West and Central Africa. It also depended more strongly on animal reservoirs for transmission than its *gambiense* counterpart, which was mainly transmitted between humans. Moreover, the *Glossina morsitans* mainly responsible for the spread of *rhodesiense* was known to live in savannah fly-belts, while the *Glossina palpalis* preferred shady riverbanks and shores of lakes. These differentiations, which are not absolute but commonly accepted today also because biochemical methods later allowed the trypanosomes to be distinguished, contributed to the development of diverging disease control measures between *gambiense* and *rhodesiense* regions, with a stronger focus on the control or eradication of domestic animals and game in *rhodesiense* areas and the employment of different drugs and drug-use strategies.[28]

Contesting Trypanosomes: The (Non-)Circulation and (Non-) Acceptance of a Scientific Theory in an African Colony

Despite the consensus among medical experts in Europe, many people in Angola, including some European doctors, continued to adhere to incompatible aetiological views, thus hindering effective action against the disease. The necessarily slow circulation of medical knowledge in a colonial setting like early twentieth-century Angola might explain some of the early cases of ignorance or contestation. Yet the persistence of 'deviant' beliefs points to more fundamental conflicts between knowledge systems: between biomedical views and popular medical beliefs held by Europeans and Africans, and between different factions within the medical community. As Bruno Latour and other sociologists of knowledge have argued, scientific 'facts' are objects of controversy and negotiation; their acceptance by (scientific) communities does not follow the internal logic of evidence or reason, but is governed by power relations and social struggles for legitimacy.[29]

First, medical practitioners in the colonies did not accept the trypanosoma theory at the same pace and to the same degree as metropolitan experts in

---

[28] See Lyons, *Colonial Disease*, 51–3, 61–3 and White, 'Tsetse Visions', 222–4. On biochemical distinctions and different drugs used, see also Gibson, Stevens and Truc, 'Identification of Trypanosomes'; De Koning, 'Drugs of Sleeping Sickness' and www.who.int/mediacentre/factsheets/fs259/en/ (last accessed 13 March 2021).

[29] See, for instance, Latour, *Pasteurization*; Pestre, 'Histoire sociale et culturelle'.

tropical medicine. When, in early 1905, the Colonial Ministry asked medical officers in Angola to describe the major diseases in their district and the best ways to cope with them, the responses of some doctors in sleeping sickness-ridden areas still expressed ignorance, doubt or even overt rejection of the trypanosoma theory. Thus, the medical officer in Cazengo did not know which one of the 'causal agents' under discussion was the 'true' one and asked for more information. He was also convinced that vaccination campaigns against smallpox contributed to the spread of sleeping sickness. His colleague in Golungo Alto knew about the role of tsetse flies and trypanosomes, but was convinced that sleeping sickness was also contagious, having observed how entire families fell ill after contact with infected people. Similarly, because of the disappearance of entire villages, the government doctor in Ambriz also believed in the 'infectious-contagiousness' of the disease.[30]

Certainly, it may be argued that many doctors in the interior of Angola did not have regular access to scientific journals and that it was only a matter of time until they would acknowledge the 'true' aetiology of the disease. Yet, there is ample evidence to suggest that the persistence of alternative aetiologies was also symptomatic of a more fundamental antagonism between colonial practitioners and the growing group of experts in tropical medicine. Many colonial practitioners had difficulties in accepting that their authority with regard to tropical diseases was being challenged by scientists based in Europe and their new methods, and clung to theories based on their own field observations. As Eric Jennings's work on the persistence of *climatisme* (i.e. climatic explanations for tropical diseases such as malaria) in twentieth-century French colonial medicine has illustrated, new microbiological evidence did not lead colonial doctors and hygienists to immediately and completely abandon entrenched beliefs about the influence of climate, environment, lifestyle and nutrition.[31] Rather, both views, the microbiological and the hygienic, often coexisted, reflecting the competition between two paradigms of disease causation and, in consequence, prevention and treatment: the older and broader view that linked disease to environmental conditions and general well-being and for which sanitation and social improvement were key solutions; and a new, more narrow model for understanding disease, which focused on eliminating micro-organisms and their vectors and which 'largely excluded from vision the broader social and economic contexts within which malaria occurred'.[32]

---

[30] Reports by Américo Herculano Campos (Cazengo), [1905]; C. C. Rodolpho Nogueira (Golungo Alto), 9 March 1905 and José Maria da Silveira Montenegro, 5 March 1905, AHU, SEMU, DGU 3025.

[31] Jennings, *Curing the Colonizers*, esp. 32–5.

[32] See the summary in Packard, *Making of a Tropical Disease*, 115–7 (quote 115).

In this vein, Manuel Ferreira Ribeiro, who had brought sleeping sickness to the attention of the Society of Medical Sciences in Lisbon in 1871 and since became one of Portugal's leading colonial hygienists, maintained that sleeping sickness could not be attributed to the tsetse fly 'as some bacteriologists asserted', since he had never encountered it during his long stays and travels in the sleeping sickness-ridden hinterland of Luanda.[33] From 1904 onwards, Francisco da Silva Garcia, who had served in various regions of Angola and São Tomé and Príncipe since 1891, became the most notable opponent of the trypanosoma theory in Portuguese Africa. Describing his theories in internal reports and Portuguese medical journals, Garcia did not deny the presence of trypanosomes in many sleeping sickness cases, but refused to accept that they entered the body via tsetse flies, which he had thus far not observed in Angola, or that they were the only causative agent of sleeping sickness. He even suggested that trypanosomes might be the 'protecting and supporting agent of the resistance that natives have against malaria'. Garcia firmly believed that sleeping sickness was caused by toxic substances in badly processed dried fish.[34]

This idea was reminiscent of earlier food intoxication theories. In 1876, the French naval doctor Armand Corre suggested that sleeping sickness might be caused by poisonous cereals, and although he rejected this 'armchair hypothesis' soon after as incongruent with the disease's long incubation period, it was still cited decades later.[35] In the late 1890s, his Portuguese colleague Pereira do Nascimento blamed the consumption of raw manioc, a thesis also defended by Hans Ziemann in 1902–3.[36] In the late nineteenth century, food intoxication was a popular explanation for diseases. At the time, pellagra and beriberi – nowadays defined as vitamin deficiency diseases – were also linked to the consumption of food staples, maize and rice respectively.[37] Garcia's theory was the product of this context and of his own long-standing interest in nutritional issues.[38]

---

[33] Ribeiro, *Lições práticas*, 265–70 (quote 266).

[34] Francisco da Silva Garcia, 'Resposta ao questionnario', 24 March 1905, AHU, SEMU, DGU 3025; Garcia, 'Contribuição' and Garcia, 'Apontamentos', 289 (quote). On his career, see 'Livro Mestre do Quadro de Saúde de Angola (1858–1913)', 50, AHU, SEMU, DGAPC 895.

[35] Compare Corre, 'Contribution', 563 with Corre, 'Recherches', 353. For later references to his first hypothesis, see, for instance, Azevedo, *Algumas palavras*, 34 and Sambon, 'Elucidation', 62–3.

[36] For a discussion and refutation of Nascimento's raw manioc thesis, see Leitão, *Relatório da visita sanitária*, 116–9 and Bettencourt, Kopke, Rezende and Mendes, *Maladie du sommeil*, 21–6. See also Ziemann, 'Schlafkrankheit der Neger'; Ziemann, 'Bericht über das Vorkommen'.

[37] Mense, 'Bemerkungen', 365.   [38] See Garcia, *Vinho do Porto*.

Similar to Ribeiro, Garcia grounded his fish intoxication theory in observations he had made in Angola and São Tomé and Príncipe over the years, particularly in Benguela, where he had been stationed since 1902. Two observations in particular had raised his suspicions: endogenous sleeping sickness cases in the Benguela district, which he wrongly believed to be free from tsetse flies, and the striking coincidence between the geographical distribution of sleeping sickness in Angola and the areas where local diets contained much dried fish. The case of Benguela was particularly illuminating, he argued, since endogenous cases of sleeping sickness only appeared after the devastating rinderpest epidemic of 1898, which provoked a shift in local diets from fresh meat to dried fish.[39] Like many earlier theories, including Manson's *filaria* hypothesis, Garcia's aetiological theory relied on geographical distribution patterns: the concurrent presence of sleeping sickness and a specific pathogen. However, he was also able to offer a plausible explanation for how the disease and its symptoms were caused. Similar to nicotine and alcohol, he claimed, the toxins in badly prepared dried fish accumulated and slowly poisoned the human body, thus causing the nervous lesions commonly described in sleeping sickness. He did not blame African cooking methods, as Pereira do Nascimento and Ziemann had, but the unhygienic processes of the Portuguese fishing industry in the coastal cities of southern Angola (Moçâmedes, Porto Alexandre and Baía dos Tigres). He urged the Portuguese government to halt the distribution and consumption of dried fish until the shortcomings in the fish-drying factories were resolved. As proof of his theory, Garcia also stated that he had cured 12 out of 32 sleeping sickness patients in the Benguela hospital with a 'toxin neutralising' iodine-iodide syrup, cold showers and a rich diet.[40]

Garcia's theory stirred controversy within Portuguese medical circles. While Ribeiro and others emphasised its merits, others contested it.[41] His colleague António Bernardino Roque, for instance, also used geographical distribution patterns to contest dried fish (and raw manioc) as possible causes, arguing that there were no endogenous cases of sleeping sickness in the coastal cities of southern Angola, although both foodstuffs were integral to local diets.[42] Moreover, Garcia later complained that he had been silenced by his superiors, who feared that his allegations might damage the international reputation of Angola's fishing industries. He did not abandon his theory, however. In 1911, as deputy head of the health services in São Tomé and Príncipe, he still defended his ideas before other government doctors and the local governor, causing great consternation among both his local colleagues and the

---

[39] Garcia, 'Apontamentos'.   [40] Ibid., 290.   [41] Ribeiro, *Lições práticas*, 266.
[42] Roque, 'Doença do somno'.

professors of the School of Tropical Medicine in Lisbon.[43] Interestingly, this scientific conflict did not compromise his colonial career. Promotions were generally awarded on the basis of seniority and, in 1913, Garcia became director of Angola's health services.[44]

Second, the trypanosoma theory was also slow to affect popular beliefs about sleeping sickness among Europeans in Angola. Thus, 18 *moradores* (European or Europeanised residents) of Barra do Bengo, a *concelho* in the sleeping sickness-ridden hinterland of Luanda, petitioned the Governor-General in March 1905 to prohibit mourning customs among the local African population. Ignoring the role of tsetse flies and trypanosomes, they still believed that sleeping sickness was contagious and that customs such as protracted bodily contact between the deceased and their closest family members greatly contributed to the spread of the disease.[45] Even more illustrative of the slow dissemination of medical knowledge are the cases of several Portuguese soldiers who were infected during the military campaigns in the Dembos region between 1907 and 1909.[46] When later interrogated by Ayres Kopke in Lisbon, they declared themselves unaware of the danger of tsetse-fly bites, until they had seen the educational leaflet composed by the Sleeping Sickness Bureau in London, translated into Portuguese by the EMT in 1910.[47]

Medical authorities in Angola knew about the importance of popular education in combating the disease, but had not been up to the task. In 1907, Annibal Correia Mendes urged the *Junta de Saúde* (Health Council), the directing body of the health services in Angola, to 'draw up a leaflet where it explains in a simple and clear language how sleeping sickness spreads through the tsetse fly', as proposed by the International Conference on Sleeping Sickness in London.[48] To promote public awareness, the same Health Council proposed to award a small sum of money (1 real) for every captured glossina presented to the medical officer or other colonial officials in infected regions and therefore wanted to teach doctors, administrators and missionaries how to recognise the flies.[49] While it took until 1910 to distribute the leaflet, there is no evidence that the other measures were implemented.

---

[43] Junta de Saúde Pública de São Tomé, 'Sessão extraordinaria', 9 February 1911; Garcia to Governor of São Tomé and Príncipe, 6 March 1911; Silva Telles (Director of EMT) to Director Geral das Colónias, 21 April 1911, AHU, MU, DGAPC 3473.

[44] Direcção Geral das Colónias, 'Processo 93/1913: Francisco da Silva Garcia', AHU, MU, DGAPC 3456.

[45] Residents of Barra do Bengo to Governor-General, 3 March 1905, ANA, Cx. 3721.

[46] On these campaigns, see Chapter 1.

[47] Kopke, 'Escola de Medicina Tropical de Hamburgo', 143–4; Kopke, *Estudo da doença do sono*, 99 and 101. For the leaflet, see *Doença do somno – como evitar a infecção*.

[48] Mendes, 'Subsídio', 400–1. On this conference, see later in this chapter.

[49] Junta de Saúde, 'Acta da sessão extraordinaria', 12 February 1907, ANA, Cód. 1867, 135r.

Third and finally, the trypanosoma theory clashed with ingrained beliefs in disease causation among the Angolan population. There is no evidence to suggest that, prior to 1904, people in Angola suspected a correlation between tsetse flies and human disease. Even on Príncipe, where tsetse flies were well-known as Gabon flies (they had probably been introduced with cattle from Gabon in the early nineteenth century), locals made no connection with sleeping sickness.[50] European observations indicate that Angolans, like many other people in West and West Central Africa, believed that the disease was either contagious, with transmission occurring through saliva and clothes and leading to diseased people being isolated outside their villages; hereditary, as it often killed entire families; or caused by spirits.[51]

That disease could be caused by spirits matches a by now common historiographical observation: in many parts of sub-Saharan Africa, including northern Angola, societies conceived of disease in ways that differed fundamentally from European biomedicine (but much less from early modern medical beliefs), insofar as they linked them not only to the individual, but also to the social body. Many societies divided illnesses into two groups: 'natural diseases' or 'diseases of God', which had a natural cause and were treated with herbs and other natural substances; and 'diseases of man', which were caused by other human beings through sorcery or by offended ancestral spirits, and which required community healing. Usually, the former would be addressed by so-called herbalists and the latter by so-called diviners, who communicated with the spirits to diagnose the causes of disease and misfortune and remedy them. In practice, however, many healers combined these functions, just as diseases could have multiple and shifting causes addressed by different therapeutic practices. Particularly serious illnesses that affected healthy adults often shifted to the spiritual domain.[52]

This explains why doctors, administrators and missionaries alike complained well into the twentieth century that their attempts to convince Angolans of the role of tsetse flies often met with overt and persistent scepticism. Francisco dos Santos Serra Frazão, who worked as local administrator in northern Angola between 1914 and 1919, later recorded how 'one of the most intelligent and civilised chiefs (sobas) of the region' reacted to his teachings by stating: 'Listen, sleeping sickness does not come from the flies... It comes

---

[50] Costa, *Sleeping Sickness (1913)*, 1–2. See also Harry Johnston's declarations in Sleeping Sickness Committee, *Minutes of Evidence*, 117.

[51] See Curto, 'Relatório do Chefe do Serviço de Saúde de Angola', 333; Bettencourt, 'Doença do somno (1902)', 217–8 and Silva, 'Doença do somno'. For West Africa, see similarly Corre, 'Recherches', 355 and Sambon, 'Sleeping Sickness', 207–8.

[52] See Janzen, *Quest for Therapy*, 1–11; Ranger, 'Godly Medicine'; Vaughan, 'Healing and Curing', 290–2. See also Coghe, 'Disease Control and Public Health' and Kananoja, *Healing Knowledge*, esp. 7–13.

from something else against which we cannot fight. ... The flies, well, the flies do not cause any harm, may the doctor say what he wants. ... The others, however, the others, yes.' By 'the others', Serra Frazão explained, the chief meant the spirits of the dead.[53]

Curing an Incurable Disease: Of Testicular Liquids, Cervical Gland Excisions and Magic Bullets

Before the causative agent was discovered, European doctors employed a wide variety of therapeutic measures to treat sleeping sickness patients. Their therapeutic choices were usually tied to how they conceived the disease, but many ended up trying all kinds of medications.[54] A profound sense of helplessness pervades medical reports on the issue. In 1887, Angola's health director António Ramada Curto lamented that he had used 'antiseptics, alterants, tonics, stimulants, etc.', but that none had saved his patients.[55] Similarly, the manager of the Sundy plantation (roça) on Príncipe, Angelo de Bulhões Maldonado, desperately enumerated, almost 15 years later, all the medications that had been tried on his serviçais: 'Following the instructions of our doctor, we have applied tonics in all their forms, cauterisation, stimulants like coffee, hydrotherapy, electricity, caustics in the back of the neck and the spine, changes of air, baths in the sea, baths of sand, stays at low and high altitude, modifications of diet, gold and silver salts, subcutaneous injections of stimulants, quinine, etc.'[56]

The Portuguese sleeping sickness commissioners were equally powerless. One after the other, their patients in the hospital of Luanda died, mostly within a few weeks or months. Of the 27 (African) patients they embarked with on their return to Portugal in December 1901, six died during the voyage, while all the others, who were accommodated in a small clinic annexed to the Bacteriological Institute, passed away within a year of arriving in Lisbon. Most of the drugs used by the commissioners targeted the symptoms and complications of the disease only, but they also tried experimental medications, such as repeated injections of dead 'hypnococcus' cultures and of the anti-streptococcic serum of Marmorek, without notable success, however.[57] Due to such failures, European doctors in the early 1900s continued to view

---

[53] Serra Frazão, 'Reabilitação dos Negros. Estudo crítico sobre diversos aspectos de Angola', 1942, 133, AHU, T 215. Similarly, Mercier Gamble in Sleeping Sickness Committee, *Minutes of Evidence*, 188.

[54] See, for instance, Corre, 'Recherches', 356; Azevedo, *Algumas palavras*, 64–77.

[55] Curto, 'Relatório do Chefe do Serviço de Saúde de Angola', 334.

[56] Maldonado, 'Doença do somno', 97.

[57] See the detailed patient histories in Bettencourt, Kopke, Rezende and Mendes, *Maladie du sommeil*, 116–270.

sleeping sickness as incurable. As Louis Sambon, an experienced lecturer at the London School of Tropical Medicine and close collaborator of Manson, stated, 'the physician that cures is death'.[58]

Certainly, accounts of cures sometimes appeared in the medical press, but these were eventually proven false or dismissed for epistemological reasons. A good example of the first category is the case of João Novaes, the Portuguese medical officer in Landana, a coastal town in the Cabinda enclave. In 1893, he reported to have cured an African employee of the local Catholic mission with repeated hypodermic injections of testicular liquid extracted from a ram.[59] After its rejuvenating effects had been described and praised by the renowned physiologist Charles-Édouard Brown-Séquard in 1889, the injection of testicular extracts had become a fancy, though highly contested, treatment in Europe and the United States for nervous diseases and ageing. Brown-Séquard's sensational findings provoked many scathing reactions in the medical community, but also prompted others, like Novaes, to conduct further experiments with this 'elixir of life', as some had dubbed it.[60] In Luanda, health director Ramada Curto received Novaes's report with a mixture of enthusiasm and caution. He praised the application of Brown-Séquard's method to sleeping sickness as a rational decision, given the nervous nature of the disease and the lack of contraindications for this kind of medication. Yet he also warned that a single apparent cure did not yet prove the scientific validity of the treatment and encouraged all doctors in the colony to repeat the experiment.[61] In consequence, 300 grams of testicular liquid was sent from Europe to Angola, but there are no published accounts of further testing. The limited empirical evidence notwithstanding, Novaes's 'cure' was referenced in the medical press in Portugal and also began to circulate among European experts: it received support from Carl Mense in Germany and even found its way into the first edition of Patrick Manson's manual on tropical diseases in 1898.[62] Doubts remained, however, and the method was definitively discredited when, in 1901, Novaes himself, who had retired to Europe for health reasons shortly after his experiments, publicly admitted that his 'cured' patient had eventually died, following a period of apparent recovery.[63]

---

[58] Sambon, 'Sleeping Sickness', 208.

[59] Novães to Ramada Curto, 1 December 1893, *BOA* (1894), 150–1.

[60] Brown-Séquard, 'Des effets'. For the context and impact of Brown-Séquard's study and its role in founding modern endocrinology and hormone replacement therapy, see Olmsted, *Brown-Séquard*, 205–33; Aminoff, *Brown-Séquard*, 235–60 (quote 239).

[61] Ramada Curto to Novaes, 26 December 1893 and Ramada Curto, 'Circular', 22 December 1893, both *BOA* (1894), 151.

[62] *Jornal da Sociedade das Sciências Médicas de Lisboa* 57 (1893), 204; Mense, 'Bemerkungen', 367–8; Manson, *Tropical Diseases (1898)*, 255–6.

[63] Novaes, 'Doença do somno em Angola'. See also Silva, 'Doença do somno', 422.

Epistemological boundaries, then, hindered local African treatments from being incorporated into Western biomedicine. Despite the constant failure of their own methods, European doctors around 1900 invested little in studying African healing practices and rarely adopted them. In Angola, some doctors knew that local healers put pepper or the juice of certain leaves in the eyes of the sick to keep them awake, or prepared concoctions with similar ingredients. They also were aware that healers and patients used necromantic rituals against spirit possession.[64] As in many other parts of sub-Saharan Africa, the combined use of spiritual possession ceremonies and medicinal herbs to combat disease was not considered contradictory by northern Angolans, but reflected the coexistence of the two basic disease explanations and groups of healers mentioned earlier: the *adivinhos* (diviners/witchdoctors) and *curandeiros* or *quimbandas* (healers).[65]

These therapeutic practices, however, were unlikely to be adopted by the Portuguese (and European) medical community in the early 1900s. Whereas, from the sixteenth to the late nineteenth century, medical doctors, colonial officers, naturalists and missionaries in the Portuguese colonies had shown considerable interest in local medicines and therapies, the rise of Western biomedicine and tropical medicine had induced European doctors to believe in the superiority of their own knowledge system and to increasingly disregard indigenous knowledge.[66] The development of modern pharmacology, with its growing focus on chemically-synthesised, industrially-produced and -standardised pharmaceuticals, further diminished interest in local medicinal plants and 'empirical' healing methods.[67] In the early twentieth century, such local knowledge was still included in botanical and ethnographic writings, and sometimes even in medical publications.[68] However, this knowledge lacked detail and practical relevance, as it was usually excluded from academic discussions about how European colonial doctors should combat tropical diseases.[69] Interest in medical 'ethnobotany' in Angola only rose in earnest after decolonisation, with the first detailed study on the use of 'traditional'

---

[64] Joaquim Antonio d'Oliveira, 'Relatório do delegado de saúde de Ambrizette', 1898–9, 31 December 1899, 9, AHU, SEMU, DGU 944; Mercier Gamble in Sleeping Sickness Committee, *Minutes of Evidence*, 189; Weeks, *Among the Primitive Bakongo*, 228.

[65] See footnote 52 and, for twentieth-century Angola, Correia, 'Processos práticos', 191–3; Diniz, *Missão civilisadora*, 12; Santos, *Medicina e magia*, 13–5, 153–7.

[66] See Chapter 1.

[67] See Gradmann and Simon (eds.), *Evaluating and Standardizing*; Quirke and Slinn, 'Introduction', 7–9.

[68] See, for instance, Junior, *Subsídios* and Noronha, 'Algumas plantas medicinais'.

[69] See, for instance, Manson, *Tropical Diseases (1898)* and Mense (ed.), *Handbuch der Tropenkrankheiten*.

herbal remedies for sleeping sickness in northern Angola published in 2020.[70] Using Londa Schiebinger and Robert Proctor's concept of agnotology, that is the study of the non-circulation of knowledge and the production of culturally-induced ignorance, one can say that colonial arrogance and prejudice served as 'agnotological roadblocks' to the circulation of African healing knowledge.[71]

Moreover, even when such knowledge circulated, European doctors hesitated to 'go native', as the following example shows. As early as the 1870s and well into the twentieth century, European observers reported that African healers in the Gulf of Guinea removed the enlarged lymph glands in the neck of the sleeping sick, since these were considered to be both the cause and a premonitory sign of the disease.[72] Although these operations were almost invariably said to be successful, European doctors were reluctant to emulate them. The main hindrance was probably that academic medicine did not believe in such treatments. Manson, for instance, firmly dismissed the possibility of achieving a cure in this manner.[73] The Portuguese commissioners displayed great scepticism as well. In the few instances in which they did extract swollen cervical lymph glands, this seems to have been in order to study the glands and not to cure their patients.[74] Significantly, it was only after Manson's younger colleague Louis Sambon recommended closer investigation of this 'bold surgical interference' that various Portuguese doctors described their own experiments with this indigenous method.[75] In Angola, health director Vasconcellos mentioned that the Portuguese medical officer in Ambaca had performed such an operation in January 1904.[76] Around the same time, his colleagues on Príncipe, António Damas Mora and Vicente Bernardino Collaço, reported the removal of the cervical glands of more than a dozen patients, a fact that was also mentioned straightforwardly by Ayres Kopke. Appearing to have beneficial effects, the operations initially stirred enthusiasm among doctors and patients on the island. However, the operations did not prevent patients from dying and did not enter the canon of Western therapeutic practice.[77]

The scientific marginalisation of indigenous healers did not diminish their popularity in African communities. However, since European doctors,

---

[70] Vahekeni et al., 'Use of Herbal Remedies'. For broader overviews, see van-Dúnem, *Plantas medicinais* and Bossard, *Médecine traditionelle*.

[71] Proctor and Schiebinger (eds.), *Agnotology*; Schiebinger, *Secret Cures*, 158.

[72] See, for instance, Corre, 'Recherches', 356 and Sambon, 'Sleeping Sickness', 208–9. For Príncipe, see Maldonado, 'Doença do somno', 97. In Portuguese Guinea, this practice was still mentioned by European doctors in the 1920s and 1930s, see Havik, 'Public Health and Tropical Modernity', 645, 647.

[73] Manson, 'Clinical Lecture', 128.

[74] Bettencourt, Kopke, Rezende and Mendes, *Maladie du sommeil*, 61–2, 128, 136 and 141.

[75] Sambon, 'Sleeping Sickness', 208 (quote).   [76] *BOA* (1904), 155.

[77] J. S. A., 'Hygiene colonial', 689–90; Kopke, 'Investigações', 26–8.

missionaries and administrators believed that healers, whom they often decried as 'witchdoctors', were the main obstacle to the diffusion of Western biomedicine, Christianity and socio-cultural progress at large, circumscribing their influence became an integral part of the colonial project. In the early twentieth century, some colonial states regulated or prohibited their activities, particularly divining and witchcraft practices. Other, mainly herbal, forms of healing, however, were less affected. Even in South Africa, which banned all other African healers in the 1920s, *inyanga*-herbalists were excepted.[78] Like some other British colonies in the region, however, the colonial government in Angola did not impose legal restrictions on African healers. In 1931, in a general bill on medical practices, it even planned to officially condone their practices, provided they only treated 'natives'. This clause was one of the reasons that the Health Department in the Colonial Ministry eventually stopped the law from being promulgated. Its director argued that, while it was acceptable for colonial administrations to turn a blind eye to African healing practices, it was wrong to officially legalise them.[79] Overall, Portuguese decision-makers did not believe in legal bans, as these would be difficult to implement. The best way to diminish the influence of African healers was, in their opinion, promoting and expanding the competing system of 'rational' Western biomedicine. The superiority of its methods and drugs would, they hoped, eventually eclipse 'traditional' healing methods.[80]

In the case of sleeping sickness, this entailed the large-scale and often forced use of new synthetic drugs developed in European laboratories. For Western biomedicine, sleeping sickness therapy changed dramatically when trypanosomes were identified as the causative agent. Doctors and pharmaceutical researchers in Europe, aided by colleagues in Africa upon whom they relied for clinical tests, could now develop 'trypanocidal' drugs that would destroy these particular parasites in the human body. Due to the biological complexity of the disease, however, the quest for a safe and effective drug was challenging (and remains so).[81] Even the drugs that were eventually commercialised and used by the European colonial health services were all contested due to their damaging side effects.[82]

Portugal's pharmaceutical science and industry did not play any significant role in the creation of these drugs, either before or after the First World War.

---

[78] Hokkanen, 'Contestation', 124–9; Flint, 'Competition'.
[79] Gôverno Geral de Angola, 'Regulamento do exercício da arte de curar em Angola', 7 May 1931, *BOA Série II* (1931), 2.° Suplemento ao n. 18, 1–22, art. 6; 'Processo 247' (1931), AHU, DGCO 373.
[80] See also Correia, 'Processos práticos', 191–4; Diniz, *Missão civilisadora*, 12–3. For this dilemma, see also Flint, 'Competition', 204–5.
[81] De Koning, 'Drugs of Sleeping Sickness'.
[82] See particularly Mertens, *Chemical Compounds* and Lachenal, *Médicament*.

The most important pharmaceutical laboratories and scientists were located at the School of Tropical Medicine in Liverpool, the Institut Pasteur in Paris and especially in Frankfurt, at the Institute for Experimental Therapy and the Georg-Speyer-Haus for Chemotherapy, where later Nobel Prize-winner Paul Ehrlich integrated the search for trypanocidal drugs into his broader research on chemotherapy.[83] Ehrlich's aim was nothing less than to create a 'magic bullet', a substance that would kill pathogenic micro-organisms like trypanosomes or bacterial spirochetes (the cause of syphilis, yaws and relapsing fever) without damaging the host and preferably in a single 'shot' or dose to avoid the emergence of resistant strains. Ehrlich's systematic search for such a miracle therapy received worldwide attention at the time and he has come to be considered the 'founder of modern chemotherapy'.[84]

Locating Portuguese Drug Research: Ayres Kopke's Transimperial Networks and the Scientific Marginalisation of the Colonies

The lack of potent pharmaceutical laboratories and industries on national soil did not bar Portuguese researchers from participating in sleeping sickness drug therapy research. As various authors have shown, this research was, in the early twentieth century, an eminently transimperial endeavour, in which networks developed between research institutes, doctors and colonial health services from different nations. To test their drugs on sleeping sickness patients, researchers crossed national boundaries. Ehrlich, for instance, supplied doctors in the German colonies, British Uganda, French Equatorial Africa and the Belgian Congo.[85] Although much less noted by historiography, Ayres Kopke also participated in these transimperial networks. Using his position as Professor of Bacteriology and Parasitology at the EMT in Lisbon, Kopke tested a whole series of new trypanocidal drugs on his patients in the Colonial Hospital attached to this school.

Kopke played a particularly prominent role in the testing of atoxyl, an arsenical compound that constituted the first major pharmaceutical breakthrough and, despite its severe side effects, became the most widely-used drug for sleeping sickness until well into the 1920s. Arsenical compounds had long been believed to ease the symptoms and slow the progression of sleeping

---

[83] Mertens, *Chemical Compounds*, 46–51.

[84] Bäumler, *Paul Ehrlich*, 174–206; Riethmiller, 'From Atoxyl to Salvarsan', 234 (quote). On Ehrlich, see also Hüntelmann, *Paul Ehrlich*.

[85] Neill, 'Paul Ehrlich'; Isobe, *Medizin und Kolonialgesellschaft*, 98–118; Mertens and Lachenal, 'History'.

sickness, but they were also known to be very toxic.[86] First described in the 1860s, atoxyl seemed to solve this problem, as it contained a high level of arsenic but with much reduced toxicity. In July 1905, right after Wolferstan Thomas and Anton Breinl at Liverpool School of Tropical Medicine obtained very promising results with atoxyl against trypanosomes in animals, Kopke started to use this drug on 10 of his patients at the Colonial Hospital. In his presentation at the 15th International Congress of Medicine in Lisbon in April 1906, he described how repeated atoxyl injections made the trypanosomes disappear temporarily from the peripheral blood circulation of his patients. Kopke was far from euphoric, however, because the drug did not eradicate trypanosomes in the cerebrospinal fluid. This meant that once trypanosomes had entered this fluid – and most patients were only diagnosed in this second stage – they invariably caused brain damage and death.[87] Moreover, at the First International Conference on Sleeping Sickness in London in 1907, Kopke also warned that atoxyl probably caused severe ocular lesions. Of the 29 patients he had treated, six had developed serious eye damage and four had gone blind.[88] Similar concerns were also raised by doctors who tested atoxyl in the Belgian Congo.[89]

Nevertheless, the international experts gathered in London proclaimed atoxyl the standard drug against sleeping sickness. This was to a great extent due to the enthusiasm of Robert Koch and other medical authorities like Patrick Manson and Alphonse Laveran, who felt the advantages outweighed the risks. Koch, one of the most eminent medical scientists of his time, had by then conducted extensive experiments with atoxyl in East Africa in 1906–7.[90] Even if he did not consider atoxyl a miracle drug, Koch firmly recommended its use for two reasons: there were simply no better drugs available; and in addition to its curative effects, atoxyl also had epidemiological advantages. By destroying the trypanosomes in the blood of infected patients, atoxyl turned them non-infectious. It was, hence, also a powerful preventive drug. As Guillaume Lachenal has shown, Koch developed this 'treatment as prevention' approach when studying malaria in German New Guinea and East Africa around 1900. Koch believed that with regard to infectious diseases, the generalised treatment of individual disease carriers would have a strong prophylactic effect at population level – and ultimately lead to disease

---

[86] Manson, *Tropical Diseases (1898)*, 255; Bettencourt, Kopke, Rezende and Mendes, *Maladie du sommeil*, 63.

[87] Kopke, 'Trypanosomiasis humaine (Congrès)'.

[88] 'Proceedings First International Conference', 28. On this episode, see also Neill, 'Paul Ehrlich', 70–1.

[89] Mertens, *Chemical Compounds*, 55–8.

[90] Koch, 'Schlussbericht'. On Koch's mission, see Webel, *Politics of Disease Control*, 73–107.

eradication.[91] While practical implementation failed for malaria, this model of 'therapeutic prophylaxis' guided anti-sleeping sickness campaigns in large parts of West and Central Africa from the 1910s onwards and especially during the interwar period (see Chapter 3).

Hence, Kopke's early trials may not have been decisive for atoxyl's 'success story', but Kopke repeatedly emphasised in publications and public lectures that he had been the first to test the drug on humans.[92] This claim was widely accepted by the international community at the time.[93] For decades, Portuguese colonial officials also mentioned this 'first' to underscore Portugal's important contribution to the fight against sleeping sickness and African healthcare in general.[94] Moreover, Kopke's work on atoxyl raised his prestige within the emerging transimperial networks of tropical medicine, giving him access to other experimental drugs. At the international conference in London in 1907, Kopke met Ehrlich, with whom he was already corresponding.[95] In 1913, he also visited Ehrlich's Institute for Experimental Therapy in Frankfurt on behalf of the EMT.[96] Capitalising on these personal and institutional connections, Kopke was able to test Ehrlich's most promising new compounds on his patients in Lisbon until Ehrlich's death in 1915. Beyond the synthetic dyes Trypan Red and Parafuchsine, these included the arsenobenzols Arsacetine (306),[97] Arsenophenylglycin (418), Salvarsan (606) and Neosalvarsan (914).[98] Kopke also contacted other researchers to obtain their newest creations, trying out several medications proposed by Alphonse Laveran, the French discoverer of the malaria parasite who had started working on trypanosomes, and Félix Mesnil from the Institut Pasteur in Paris. He also tested injections with emetic proposed by Plimmer and Thompson, aryl-stibinic acids developed by Anton Breinl in Liverpool and Galyl from the

---

[91] Lachenal, 'Genealogy', 76–80.

[92] See, for instance, 'Proceedings First International Conference', 27; Kopke, 'Conferência Internacional', 503.

[93] See, for instance, Mense, 'Menschliche Trypanosomenkrankheit', 653; Laveran and Mesnil, *Trypanosomes et trypanosomiases*, 189; van Hoof, 'Thérapeutique', 87, 100.

[94] Azevedo, 'Anglo-Portuguese Contribution', 706; Azevedo and Faria, *Quatre siècles*, 84.

[95] See, for instance, Ayres Kopke to Paul Ehrlich, 17 April 1907, STABI, Slg. Darmstadt 3d 1906: Kopke, Ayres.

[96] See Kopke, 'Escola de Medicina Tropical de Hamburgo', 144–5.

[97] The numbers in parentheses are serial numbers. Ehrlich made hundreds of slightly different chemical drugs, each of them having a serial number. The serial numbers of his most famous drugs were very well known in the medical community – and they were often even used instead of the names of the drugs.

[98] Kopke, 'Trypanosomiasis humaine (Congrès)', 240–1; Kopke, 'Traitement (1909)', 223, 226; Kopke, 'Sobre a doença do somno', 228; Kopke, 'Traitement de quelques cas'; Kopke, *Estudo da doença do sono*, 104–8.

French doctor Mouneyrat.[99] By testing these new compounds and different administration methods, and publishing the results in Portuguese and French, Kopke sought to contribute to international efforts to find a drug with fewer side effects than atoxyl that could also eliminate the trypanosomes in the cerebrospinal fluid.

Partly due to Kopke's personal ambition, Portuguese experiments with trypanocidal drugs reveal some important particularities. Whereas, in other colonial empires, researchers *in the colonies* (for instance at the Institut Pasteur in Brazzaville or the Bacteriological Laboratories in Léopoldville and Entebbe) did most of the testing,[100] Portuguese drug therapy research was mainly conducted by Ayres Kopke himself in Portugal. Between 1904 and 1922, Kopke observed some 130 individuals in the Colonial Hospital in Lisbon, of which about 115 were treated, from August 1905 onwards, with atoxyl and other trypanocidal drugs. On the majority, he published lengthy and detailed patient records in medical journals and international conference proceedings, containing personal data (name, age, sex, 'race', place of birth and place of residence) as well as details about the treatment, the course of the disease and, if applicable, autopsy results.[101] Kopke's patients far exceeded the number of those treated in other European metropoles and while the colonial hospitals in London, Paris and Hamburg seem to have admitted only European sleeping sickness patients, Kopke's patients in the Colonial Hospital in Lisbon were predominantly African: from his approximately 130 patients until 1922, only 14 were reported as 'white' and at least 67, probably many more, explicitly as 'black'.[102] The volume and detail of this work was also far superior to drug research in the Portuguese colonies. Although Kopke shared some of the newer drugs with his colleagues in Príncipe and Angola, they do not seem to have conducted extensive experiments before 1918 – or at least did not publish on them. The only notable exception were the drug trials during the sleeping sickness mission on Príncipe in 1907–8 that was supervised by Kopke (analysed below).[103]

Doing drug therapy research in Lisbon had various practical and ethical implications. First, it was difficult to secure a steady flow of sleeping sickness

[99] See Kopke, 'Investigações', 30; Kopke, 'Trypanosomiasis humaine (Congrès)', 241; Kopke, 'Tratamento (1907)', 9–10; Kopke, 'Traitement (1909)', 226–7; Kopke, 'Trypanosomiase gambiense'; Kopke, *Estudo da doença do sono*, 108–12 and Kopke, 'Ensaios com o galil'.
[100] See Mertens and Lachenal, 'History'; Neill, 'Paul Ehrlich'.
[101] See Kopke, 'Investigações'; Kopke, 'Trypanosomiasis humaine (Archivos)'; Kopke, 'Traitement (1907)'; Kopke, 'Traitement (1909)'; Kopke, 'Traitement de quelques cas' and Kopke, *Estudo da doença do sono*.
[102] See previous footnote. Compare with Martin and Darré, 'Résultats éloignés'; Daniels, 'Cases of Trypanosomiasis' and Mannweiler, *Geschichte*, esp. 145; 151–2.
[103] Short references to further drug experiments can be found in Castro, 'Cura?' and McCowen, 'Note on Sleeping Sickness', 193.

patients from the colonies. Research missions constituted good opportunities for this. As the research commission had done in 1901, Kopke brought a dozen patients with him upon his return from Angola and Príncipe in 1904.[104] During the EMT research mission to Príncipe in 1907–8, more than 20 African patients were sent to Lisbon.[105] Kopke and the EMT direction also used connections with doctors in the colonies and administrative channels. Generally, the Overseas (from 1910: Colonial) Ministry was receptive to their argument that the school's scientific reputation was at stake and repeatedly urged the governors of Angola and São Tomé and Príncipe to send more (preferably first-stage) sleeping sickness patients to Lisbon. Colonial administrations, however, were not always willing or able to comply.[106] Patients in Angola often did not want to leave for Lisbon and whether colonial administrations were allowed to send them off against their will was a contested issue. While in 1903, the Governor-General of Angola prohibited the use of force in some cases, it was condoned on another occasion in 1906.[107] The vast majority of patients who eventually arrived in Lisbon were second-stage, hence with very limited chances of being cured, and all suffering from the *gambiense* form, the only one in Angola and Príncipe.[108]

Second, hospital conditions allowed Kopke to monitor his patients quite closely, yet his published patient records suggest that he could not keep them for longer periods against their will. In 1923, he complained that of the 115 cases he had treated with trypanocidal drugs in Lisbon, he had only been able to follow seven of them long enough to consider them cured. While 67 had died, he had lost track of the remaining 41. Most of these patients had not wished to continue treatment or observation in Lisbon and Kopke had been obliged to discharge them. Though non-documented forms of coercion cannot be excluded, it seems that Europeans and Africans alike were entitled to leave the hospital at will and return to their country of origin, where they

---

[104] Kopke, 'Relação dos doentes que seguem para Lisboa abordo do paquete Benguela', 9 September 1904, ANA, Cx. 1546. See also Kopke, 'Investigações', 6–35.

[105] See their detailed case descriptions in Kopke, 'Traitement (1909)', 240–69.

[106] See, for instance, Secretaria Geral do Governo, 'Processo 225/6' (1906), ANA, Cx. 4784; Silva Telles to Director Geral do Ministério das Colónias, 27 March 1911 and 16 May 1911 and José Serrão (Head of Health Department in Colonial Ministry), 'Parecer', 24 May 1911, AHU, MU, DGAPC 3473.

[107] Compare Director Geral do Ultramar to Interim Governor-General of Angola, 14 September 1903 and Delegado de Saúde Sergio Moreira da Fonseca to Chefe do Concelho do Alto Dande, 3 November 1903, ANA, Cx. 98 with Chefe do Concelho de Golungo Alto to Secretaria-Geral do Governo Geral d'Angola, 10 October 1906, ANA, Cx. 4784. On this, see also Castro, *Escola de Medicina Tropical*, 44–5.

[108] Kopke, *Estudo da doença do sono*, 103 and 112.

eluded long-term medical control.[109] Such was not always the case for African patients on colonial territory, where, before the 1920s, they were mostly treated in so-called segregation or concentration camps in tsetse-free areas. As recent historiography has emphasised, these camps not only served preventive and curative purposes, but were also the sites of most drug therapy research. Camp regimes varied greatly and also changed over time, as I will show later, with some allowing patients to come and go, but others forcibly incarcerating them.[110]

Third and finally, with about 115 patients between 1905 and 1922, Kopke's drug trials were far less comprehensive and systematic than those in foreign colonies. Moreover, given that almost all his patients were second-stage, with trypanosomes in the cerebrospinal fluid, his experimental research was increasingly geared towards finding a way to eliminate these. To get the drugs behind the blood-brain-barrier, he injected them not only subcutaneously and intravenously, but sometimes also, following a lumbar puncture, directly into the subarachnoid space of the spinal cord. While this experimental method did not trigger satisfactory results with most drugs, it caused severe 'accidents' with some of the newest compounds: subarachnoidal injection of Neosalvarsan and Galyl between December 1912 and February 1914 was probably the direct cause of death of four of his patients, who died days after the injection. Kopke, who had felt encouraged to continue 'his' method after the famous German doctor Wechselmann had successfully adopted it in syphilis therapy, seems to have abandoned it thereupon, but others continued using it to test other drugs.[111]

These 'accidents' are part and parcel of a long and sad tradition of sleeping sickness drug therapy research, in Africa and (as Kopke's research shows) in Europe.[112] They resulted from the risks that, in his quest for a cure, Kopke was willing to take with his experimental treatments. Nevertheless, his research was not merely human experimentation, but treatment as well. As Gradmann has pointed out in his insightful article on the experimental treatment of a German patient, presumably infected with sleeping sickness, in Berlin between 1906 and 1908, 'contemporaries employed no distinction between therapeutic and human experiment' and accusations of human experiments usually

---

[109] Kopke, 'Tratamento (1923)', 60. See also Kopke, 'Trypanosomiase gambiense', 224, 237, 245 and 262; Kopke, *Estudo da doença do sono*, 102 and the cases of 13 Africans repatriated in 1914 detailed in AHU, DGU 446.

[110] See particularly Isobe, *Medizin und Kolonialgesellschaft*, 71–117, 178–201 and 238–65; Neill, 'Paul Ehrlich'; Mertens and Lachenal, 'History' and Webel, *Politics of Disease Control*.

[111] See Castro, 'Cura?'; Kopke, 'Traitement de quelques cas', 291 and Kopke, *Estudo da doença do sono*, 103–12. Compare with Sicé, *Trypanosomiase humaine*, 211–2.

[112] See, for instance, Eckart, 'Colony as Laboratory', 76–7; Neill, 'Paul Ehrlich', 69–75.

emerged only when therapy failed.[113] Therapeutic rationales also explain why Kopke continued to use atoxyl in second-stage patients after his own research and that of others had shown that it could not heal them: he did so because it was widely acknowledged to improve the patients' clinical condition and, hence, to prolong life.[114] Further, in line with Gradmann's argument, there is no conclusive evidence in Kopke's publications that 'white' Portuguese patients were treated differently: new medications and administration methods were used on them as well. However, even if African patients in Lisbon could refuse further treatment and, under certain conditions, return home, it is more than probable that Kopke's therapeutic choices did not always depend on their informed consent, as this issue was only beginning to be discussed in Europe.[115] Overall, they were certainly more vulnerable than Portuguese patients, who more often left the hospital against Kopke's advice or were taken home by their families.[116]

Because of the practical problems of getting and keeping enough patients, Lisbon was not meant to remain the centre of Portuguese drug research. Although they had been supportive of Kopke's demands and ambitions, both Ramada Curto and, after 1910, the new director of the EMT Silva Telles, wanted to shift the focus to the colonies.[117] However, bacteriological laboratories in Portuguese Africa were poorly equipped and lacked qualified staff. Correia Mendes complained in 1913 that a continuous series of other assignments had kept him from scientific research for over a year and he had lost two of three laboratory assistants without replacement.[118] Another obstacle was that, compared to their French, German, British and Belgian competitors, Portuguese colonial health services were slow in creating sleeping sickness segregation camps, where experimental treatments could be tested on a large scale, as I will show below. As only a dozen sleeping sickness patients were admitted to the Colonial Hospital between 1914 and 1922, Portuguese sleeping sickness drug research virtually halted.[119]

Overall, whether in Lisbon or the European colonies in Africa, drug trials before 1918 did not have the desired outcome. While patients had to endure often painful and debilitating side effects and sometimes even died from the drug treatments themselves, none of the new compounds proved more effective or much less dangerous than atoxyl, including Salvarsan and Neosalvarsan,

---

[113] Gradmann, 'It Seemed about Time', 84 (quote). See also Neill, 'Paul Ehrlich', 74.
[114] Kopke, *Estudo da doença do sono*, 104–5. See also Neill, 'Paul Ehrlich', 70.
[115] Gradmann, 'It Seemed about Time', 84 and 95–6.
[116] See, for instance, Kopke, 'Traitement (1909)', 256, 264 and 266.
[117] See Silva Telles to Director-General of Colonial Ministry, 27 March 1911, AHU, DGAPC 3473.
[118] Correia Mendes to Colonial Minister, 26 June 1913, AHU, DGAPC 3456.
[119] Kopke, 'Troubles oculaires'; Kopke, 'Tratamento (1923)'.

Ehrlich's compounds that revolutionised syphilis treatment.[120] Based on their patient records, Kopke and other doctors believed that atoxyl could heal first-stage patients, but until the introduction of new drugs in the 1920s, the disease remained incurable when diagnosed in the second stage, as was usually the case.[121]

No Portuguese doctors played any significant role in the further quest for better drugs. The absence of stable research facilities in the colonies compromised Portugal's position in international sleeping sickness research. After World War I, Portuguese colonies were not invited to participate in inter-colonial drug testing schemes with promising new drugs such as Bayer 205, tryparsamide or, in the 1940s, pentamidine, for which the Belgian Congo became the most important testing-ground due to its prestigious medical laboratories and well-connected researchers.[122] This scientific marginalisation meant that the introduction of new trypanocidal drugs in the Portuguese colonies hinged on their creation by foreign pharmaceutical researchers and industries and clinical tests conducted in other colonies.

Studying and Practising Eradication: The Case of Príncipe

Once the trypanosoma theory and the existence of tsetse flies in Angola were confirmed, the colonial health authorities began to develop a comprehensive plan to tackle sleeping sickness. In 1907, the *Junta de Saúde* and the colony's foremost sleeping sickness experts, Annibal Correia Mendes and Alberto de Souza Maia Leitão, proposed a host of similar measures. While they wanted ongoing efforts to map the distribution of tsetse flies in Angola to continue, they recommended a three-pronged attack to check the disease: the reduction of human-fly contact, by forcibly relocating African villages from infested river banks to higher places free of flies, isolating the sick and using mechanical barriers (protective clothing and metallic grids in front of windows); the eradication of tsetse flies by destroying the bushes in which they lived; and the curative and preventive treatment of the diseased with atoxyl.[123] These measures were aligned with international recommendations and were very similar to those advocated in other European colonies.[124] Compared to British and German East Africa or the Belgian Congo, however, implementation was slow

---

[120] Bäumler, *Paul Ehrlich*, 207–93; Parascandola, 'Mercury', 16–7.

[121] See, for instance, Kopke, *Estudo da doença do sono*, 66; 102–4; 113; Broden and Rodhain, 'Atoxyl'.

[122] Mertens and Lachenal, 'History', 1263–5; Lachenal, *Médicament*, 29–56.

[123] Junta de Saúde, 'Sessões extraordinárias', 12 February 1907 and 5 March 1907, ANA, Cód. 1867, 133v–5v and 136v–8r; Mendes, 'Subsídio'; Leitão, 'Prophylaxia'.

[124] Compare with Worboys, 'Comparative History'; Neill, *Networks* and Ehlers, *Europa und die Schlafkrankheit*, 147–220.

and fragmentary until the 1920s. One of the main reasons was the division of labour within the Portuguese Empire. In 1907, the EMT sent a study mission to Príncipe to clarify remaining doubts about the transmission of the disease and test modes of prophylaxis and treatment, before they were to be applied on a larger scale in Angola. Moreover, Ayres Kopke nominated Correia Mendes to lead it. The health services in Angola would have to wait for the findings of this mission (published in 1909) and the return of their main sleeping sickness expert.

The choice of Príncipe was not devoid of scientific logic. For Kopke, who elaborated the instructions for the mission, Príncipe offered nearly ideal conditions for a 'large-scale experiment': sleeping sickness ran rampant; the island was small (126 km²); and it had a limited number of inhabitants who could easily be monitored over a long period of time, given that most of them served long-term labour contracts as *serviçais* on the island's cocoa plantations. Furthermore, the prevalence of sleeping sickness on Príncipe stood in sharp contrast to the absence of endogenous cases on the nearby island of São Tomé. About 10 times as big and populous as Príncipe, São Tomé had very similar climatic, environmental and socio-economic features, including a large influx of indentured labourers, mainly from Angola. Identifying the reasons for the different disease patterns would mean confirming or dismissing current aetiological theories, as well as determining whether and how São Tomé could be protected.[125]

Beyond these unique experimental conditions, there were also economic and political motives for prioritising Príncipe and São Tomé. By the early 1900s, these islands had become one of the world's leading exporters of cocoa and the most prosperous colony in the Portuguese Empire.[126] This prosperity was not only threatened by epidemic sleeping sickness on Príncipe, but also by a long-standing and intensifying British campaign against labour conditions on the 'cocoa islands'. Since the 1850s, British diplomats had repeatedly accused the Portuguese government of continuing the (legally abolished) slave trade by sending Angolan *serviçais* to the islands, against their will and keeping them there in slave-like conditions.[127] The British Foreign Office did not want to put too much strain on its oldest European ally, but in the early 1900s, journalists, humanitarians and chocolate manufacturers like William Cadbury began to mount their own investigations.[128] In 1906, the publication of Henri Nevinson's travelogue *A Modern Slavery* brought the issue into the public

---

[125] 'Portaria nomeando uma missão médica para ir estudar o tratamento da doença do somno na Ilha do Príncipe', *COLP* (1907), 422–4 (quote 422).
[126] Clarence-Smith, 'Cocoa Plantations', 151–2; Higgs, *Chocolate Islands*, 9.
[127] The most complete account remains Duffy, *Question of Slavery*.
[128] Compare Stone, 'Foreign Office' with Higgs, *Chocolate Islands*, 9–25.

eye and ignited a broader campaign in Great Britain against Portuguese labour policies in West Africa.[129] Other British eyewitness accounts and investigative reports followed. These actions eventually resulted in the boycott of São Tomé and Príncipe cocoa by Cadbury and its allied enterprises in 1909, and it was not until 1916 (and Portugal's entry into the First World War on the side of the Allies) that British humanitarians somewhat relaxed their pressure on the British Foreign Office and the Portuguese government.[130] Virtually all of these reports drew attention to appalling mortality rates among the *serviçais*, attributed to poor hygienic and labour conditions, the stressful recruitment process and, in the case of Príncipe, where mortality was still much higher than on São Tomé, to sleeping sickness.[131] Undoubtedly, Portugal's study mission and later dealings with sleeping sickness on Príncipe were, along with other rationales, meant to show that international criticism was unjustified and that Portugal did care about the health and lives of its 'contract labourers'.

From a scientific perspective, the study mission to Príncipe (October 1907– November 1908) was a clear success. Composed by the directors of the bacteriological laboratories in Luanda (Annibal Correia Mendes), São Tomé (Bernardo Bruto da Costa) and Praia on the Cape Verde Islands (Arnaldo José Villela, later replaced by Alfredo Silva Monteiro) and local medical officer António Damas Mora, the mission gathered valuable information on the incidence and distribution of the disease, pending aetiological issues and the efficiency of specific drugs and administration methods. After examining 1,836 individuals, about half of the island's population, they found that 23.5 per cent were infected with trypanosomes and that morbidity rates were highest in the north of the island, which was also the area most heavily infested with *Glossina palpalis*.[132] Conversely, they were able to correlate the lack of endogenous cases of sleeping sickness in the most southern part of Príncipe and the whole of São Tomé to the absence of tsetse flies there. The fact that they had encountered all other blood-sucking insects living on Príncipe on São Tomé as well strongly supported the idea that the *Glossina palpalis* was the *only* vector of the trypanosomes.[133] The mission's data, hence, rebutted new and controversial theories postulating that sleeping sickness could also be transmitted through sexual intercourse (Koch) and the bite of stegomyia

---

[129] Nevinson, *Modern Slavery*. On Nevinson's report, see Duffy, *Question of Slavery*, 186–90 and Burroughs, *Travel Writing*, 98–121.

[130] For an overview, see Duffy, *Question of Slavery*, 186–229; Higgs, *Chocolate Islands*; Ball, 'Alma Negra' and Jerónimo, *Civilising Mission*, 38–76.

[131] See Nevinson, *Modern Slavery*, 190–2; Cadbury, *Labour*, 1–4, 55–6, 93 and the 1907 report by Burtt, reprinted in ibid., 103–31, esp. 109–12.

[132] Mendes, Mora, Monteiro and Costa, 'Maladie du sommeil', 276–80.

[133] Ibid., 340–1, 347–8.

mosquitoes (Martin).[134] These theories had ignited fears that the disease could become endemic in Europe. Kopke, for instance, had cautioned the Lisbon Society of Medical Sciences against these alternative ways of infection in 1908, given the presence of stegomyia around the Colonial Hospital where many sleeping sickness patients were treated. Only in the wake of the Príncipe mission would he downplay these dangers.[135]

The commissioners also conducted many experiments with atoxyl, varying dosage, intervals and administration methods and testing it in combination with other compounds, such as afridol blue and mercury. They also evaluated the effects of parafuchsine, one of Ehrlich's most promising dyes. The best treatment, they concluded, was double subcutaneous injections of 0.5 or 0.6 g. of atoxyl alone, with an interval of 48 hours, every 10 days, for about six months.[136] A slight variation on what Robert Koch had proposed, this became the standard treatment in Príncipe and Angola for many years.[137]

Finally, the commissioners drew up a set of prophylactic measures intended to rapidly reduce the incidence of the disease and eventually lead to its eradication on the island.[138] While some of these measures were aimed at curbing the circulation of the parasite by isolating the infected and preventing human and animal carriers of the parasite to enter the island, the commissioners particularly hoped to exterminate the disease vector. Correia Mendes and his colleagues were convinced that, on an island as small as Príncipe, it was possible to eradicate the *Glossina palpalis* and hence the disease. In addition to destroying the flies' habitat (bushes near water) and food (all kinds of mammals), they also recommended the direct capture of flies through a procedure that had been developed on one of the island's cocoa plantations (*roças*). In 1906, the manager of the Sundy plantation, Angelo de Bulhões Maldonado, had ordered some of his *serviçais* to cover their backs with black cloths coated with a layer of bird-lime, an idea based upon the frequently observed predilection of the fly for dark colours. By the end of 1907, the *serviçais* had thus captured more than 130,000 tsetse flies. Several other *roças* had already copied the procedure, but the commissioners now wanted to make it mandatory for all plantations on the island.[139]

---

[134] Koch, 'Schlussbericht'; Martin, Leboeuf and Roubaud, *Rapport*, 257–8. See also 'Review of A. Correia Mendes et al.'
[135] Compare *Jornal da Sociedade das Sciências Médicas de Lisboa* 72 (1908), 197–200 with Kopke, 'Sobre a doença do somno', 229–30.
[136] Mendes, Monteiro, Mora and Costa, 'Relatório preliminar', 16–33; Mendes, Mora, Monteiro and Costa, 'Maladie du sommeil', 282–318.
[137] Costa, Sant'Anna, Santos and Alvares, *Sleeping sickness (1916)*, 8; Rebêlo, *Atoxil*, 43–56. For Koch, compare with Isobe, *Medizin und Kolonialgesellschaft*, 92.
[138] Mendes, Mora, Monteiro and Costa, 'Maladie du sommeil', 341–6.
[139] 'Maneira prática de destruir as glossinas palpalis'; Mendes, Mora, Monteiro and Costa, 'Maladie du sommeil', 342.

Yet, despite the urgency of the situation, the eradication plan was not immediately implemented due to the opposition of the planters. Many of them did not believe in the efficiency of the proposed vector control measures and were unwilling to bear the important – though as Correia Mendes emphasised, one-off – costs they would entail. Some also argued that it was up to the government to provide the manpower needed for their execution.[140] Moreover, many feared the complete ruin of their plantations, as Correia Mendes, who had grown increasingly pessimistic about the chances of eradicating sleeping sickness, proposed even more radical vector control measures such as the necessity to kill all mammals and remove all human beings from the island for at least one year – measures that were probably inspired by the ongoing depopulation measures and vector research on the Lake Victoria islands.[141] Planters used their power to resist compulsory measures: while plantation managers exercised a great deal of influence over local politics, many of the owners lived in Lisbon, where they were well connected to Portugal's economic and political elites.[142] Assuming that control of the human reservoir would be easier, cheaper and less disruptive than vector control, many plantation managers only resorted to the massive, though mostly irregular, use of atoxyl injections.[143]

This delay took a heavy toll. Between 1908 and 1911, officially another 555 people died from sleeping sickness alone, a huge proportion of Príncipe's population of roughly 3,500.[144] The economic costs were tremendous as well. The planters not only had to bear the costs of medical treatment and falling productivity; they also had to secure the expensive (£30–£35 in the mid-1900s) and increasingly difficult recruitment of new *serviçais* (the Colonial Ministry suspended recruitment in Angola in 1909 and Mozambique, which replaced Angola as main supplier of contract labourers for the cocoa islands, only allowed labourers to work on São Tomé).[145] Finally, Portuguese inaction was a public relations disaster. While Cadbury had praised the work of the sleeping sickness commission on Príncipe,[146] Portuguese reluctance to implement the mission's recommendations was now criticised by more radical humanitarians, including John Harris, the new secretary of the Anti-Slavery and Aborigines' Protection Society. Having visited Príncipe in 1911, he

[140] See the letter by Pedro Augusto da Rocha, 24 February 1911, enclosed in Francisco Mantero to Dr. Serrão, 11 April 1911, AHU, MU, DGAPC 3473.
[141] See British Consul Robert Smallbones to Governor-General of Angola, 16 August 1912, ANA, Cx. 2946; McCowen, 'Note on Sleeping Sickness', 194. For the Lake Victoria islands, see Hoppe, *Lords of the Fly*, 55–79.
[142] Clarence-Smith, 'Hidden Costs', 166–7; Higgs, *Chocolate Islands*, 15–9.
[143] Silva, *Land of Flies*, 199–200.   [144] Costa, 'Estudos estatísticos', 74.
[145] Clarence-Smith, 'Hidden Costs', 155–7 and 163–4; Nascimento, 'Recrutamento', 183–4 and 192; Duffy, *Question of Slavery*, 206–7, 211 and 228–9. On the recruitment question, see Chapter 6.
[146] Cadbury, *Labour*, 12–3.

characterised it as 'doomed'. While the 'whites [were] leaving the island' to escape the ubiquitous 'horror of sleeping sickness', he wrote, many of the 'slaves' on the *roças* were 'stricken by disease, with emaciated bodies and gaunt features' and were well-aware that they were 'confined in a death-trap'.[147]

The regime change in October 1910 proved crucial in changing the status quo. The new political elites of the First Republic, among them many doctors, were even more sensitive to mounting international critique than their predecessors and saw resolute action against sleeping sickness on Príncipe as a way to gain international legitimacy.[148] In early 1911, the new republican governor of São Tomé and Príncipe decreed most of Correia Mendes's recommendations and appointed a new commission, led by former commission member and director of the bacteriological laboratory on the islands Bernardo Francisco Bruto da Costa, to oversee their implementation.[149] Some planters continued to resist, however, refusing to comply with the regulations and launching a slander campaign against the commission members through anonymous pamphlets and newspaper articles. Bruto da Costa even received death threats.[150]

However, against all odds, this second commission succeeded in eradicating both flies and disease from Príncipe until 1914. This was something even the Director of the Sleeping Sickness Bureau in London, Arthur Bagshawe, had not deemed possible.[151] The commission followed the original recommendations of Correia Mendes, without the later evacuation idea. Plantation owners were obliged to undertake sanitation measures in their domains. Their *serviçais* were aided by a state-sponsored sanitation brigade *(brigada sanitária)* of 100 (1911) to 300 (1914) men, mainly prisoners of war from Angola and Goa and convicted *serviçais* from São Tomé. They cleared bushes and drained swamps across the island, thus destroying the preferred habitat of the glossina. In addition, almost all pigs and dogs on the island were killed, as the glossina were proven, by blood examinations and other observations, to feed upon them. Moreover, on each plantation, groups of *serviçais* wore the black bird-lime-coated cloths mentioned earlier, trapping nearly 500,000 flies between 1911 and 1914. By then, the Maldonado method had received much

---

[147] Harris, *Dawn in Darkest Africa*, quotes 82, 133, 181 and 191. On Harris and the ASAPS, see Duffy, *Question of Slavery*, 212–24 and Miers, *Slavery in the Twentieth Century*, 62–5.
[148] See, in extenso, Silva, *Land of Flies*, 147–212.
[149] Costa, *Sleeping Sickness (1913)*, 3; Silva, *Land of Flies*, 215–6.
[150] Costa, Sant'Anna, Santos and Alvares, *Sleeping sickness (1916)*, 60–2; Bernardo Francisco Bruto da Costa, 'Breves considerações', 4 July 1915, AHU, FM 4442.
[151] See the letter from Bagshawe to the British Foreign Office, quoted extensively in British Consul Smallbones to Governor-General of Angola, 16 August 1912, ANA, Cx. 2946.

international attention and was copied by other colonial powers.[152] Compared to the other measures, however, Bruto da Costa and his colleagues did not credit fly-trapping with much impact on the extinction of the tsetse fly. In their opinion, the number of trapped flies was above all an indicator of the sanitation level. In 1913, this number declined rapidly, and the last fly was caught in April 1914.[153] Simultaneously, other measures had reduced infection risk. Ill inhabitants were isolated in the local hospital and treated with atoxyl. Atoxyl was also given prophylactically to people bitten by tsetse flies and to the members of the sanitation brigade, who were continually exposed to them. Moreover, when the first *serviçais* from Angola arrived after the end of the recruitment suspension in 1913, their blood was tested and those tested positive were sent back.[154]

In sum, the events on Príncipe had proven that, under certain favourable conditions, ecological control and vector eradication were possible. Although he was still sceptical as to whether the flies were completely extinct, Bagshawe praised the Portuguese accomplishment as a valuable experiment that British health officers should study. However, Bagshawe (and later other British officers) emphasised that the experience would not be easy to replicate, given the special circumstances of Príncipe as a small and isolated island, where the inhabitants were under firmer control than in most places on the African continent.[155] Nevertheless, the dealings with sleeping sickness on Príncipe would have an important impact on the fight against the disease in Angola.

Implementing Sleeping Sickness Control in Angola: A Fragmentary Response

Anti-sleeping sickness campaigns in Angola experienced similar delays and discussions about the right strategy to follow as in Príncipe. After his return to Angola in 1909, Correia Mendes drew upon his experiences on Príncipe to present updated plans for action to the *Junta de Saúde*.[156] Yet, partly due to the political instability following the Republican revolution in October 1910, it was not until 1912 that his recommendations received the political support of the Colonial Ministry and the central government in Luanda and were sanctioned in laws and decrees.[157] Even then, a protracted debate on which strategy

---

[152] See Hegh, *Notice sur les glossines*, 111–5 and Silva, *Land of Flies*, 223–30.
[153] Costa, Sant'Anna, Santos and Alvares, *Sleeping sickness (1916)*, 56–138.
[154] Ibid., 57, 68–9, 112, 116 and 120.
[155] Bagshawe, 'Review Bruto da Costa'; Tilley, *Africa*, 191–2.
[156] Junta de Saúde, 'Acta da Sessão Extraordinária', 30 May 1910 and 'Acta da Sessão Ordinária', 30 January 1911, ANA, Cód. 1867, 161v–6r and 189v–96r.
[157] For the bulk of this legislation, see Alto Comissariado da República em Angola, *Diplomas Doença do Sono*.

to choose, paired with the shortage of medical personnel, further delayed effective action.

In 1910, Correia Mendes had urged Angola to follow the example of other colonial powers, notably Belgium, Great Britain and Germany, establishing as quickly as possible a special medical service to combat sleeping sickness. Yet, he also emphasised that, before starting any comprehensive health campaign, it was still necessary to gather more precise information on the distribution of both the tsetse flies and the disease. Detailed maps of infected areas were indispensable to decide which measures were to be implemented where and to inform neighbouring colonies as to which border areas were infected. Cattle farmers in Angola were also seeking exact information on fly distribution to better protect their herds against infection. Acknowledging that the regular medical officers, who had been repeatedly asked to provide such maps, were neither numerous nor prepared, Correia Mendes advocated a study mission of four doctors to travel across the colony and gather this data.[158]

However, not all doctors accepted the priority given to further reconnaissance. In 1912, the Colonial Ministry finally approved a two-year study mission along the lines of Correia Mendes's proposal, but when it got delayed, the very idea of comprehensive reconnaissance came under increasing pressure from those who urged immediate combat, arguing that too much time had been lost already. Senator António Bernardino Roque, who had been a government doctor in Angola for many years (1890–1903), tried to convince both the Senate and Colonial Ministry in Lisbon that research commissions were useless if their sole task was to delimit the infested areas. Not only were the borders of these areas unstable, but Portugal could not afford to lose another two years to studies and preparation, he warned. The colony was rapidly losing its 'native' workforce and therefore the doctors of the mission should proceed with simultaneous delimitation and 'sanitary occupation'.[159]

Bernardino Roque eventually won his battle in Parliament. In July 1913, a new law created a medical mission of six doctors, divided into two teams and directed by Correia Mendes, to study and combat the disease contemporaneously.[160] Yet, the law was only partially implemented. Due to funding problems and a lack of volunteers, only one team was formed, consisting of three, and later two doctors.[161] From November 1914 to January 1915 and again from early 1916 to August 1918 (after the interruption caused by the military campaigns in southern Angola, for which two doctors had been

[158] Junta de Saúde, 'Acta da Sessão Extraordinária', 30 May 1910, ANA, Cód. 1867, 161v–6r.
[159] For the debate, see *Diário do Senado da República Portuguesa*, Sessions of 7 and 10 March; 10, 15, 22, 29 and 30 April; and 28 June 1913.
[160] Ministério das Colónias, 'Lei 84', 25 July 1913, reprinted in Alto Comissariado da República em Angola, *Diplomas Doença do Sono*, 57–9.
[161] Velho, 'Tripanossomose humana', 49–52.

requisitioned), João Gomes Salgado Júnior, Manoel do Nascimento de Almeida and Luís Baptista de Assunção Velho travelled across the central and southern districts of the colony. During this journey, they noted and mapped the presence of the *Glossina palpalis* in several restricted areas and discovered *Glossina morsitans* in Alto Zambeze near the southeastern border with Northern Rhodesia.[162] The doctors also confirmed what many already doubted: there were no tsetse flies south of the 13th parallel and most of the central and southern districts were not infected.[163] There was no money nor manpower left to examine northern Angola, nor did Correia Mendes consider this necessary, given that the presence of vector and disease was obvious in most parts of the Cuanza and Congo districts.[164] Here, knowledge of exact distribution remained fragmentary and unordered until the anti-sleeping sickness campaigns of the late 1920s, when the first comprehensive map was produced.[165] In the early 1920s, the lack of published and citeable geomedical maps would contribute to the growing marginalisation of Portugal in international sleeping sickness circles.[166]

Tying in with these geographical choices, the most systematic attack on the disease prior to the 1920s did not take place in northern Angola, but in the central district of Benguela. In 1914, the mission had confirmed suspicions that sleeping sickness, which had already raged in this area in the early 1900s, was on the rise again and that tsetse flies abounded in forests and on river banks near the important economic centres of Benguela, Lobito and Catumbela.[167] To prevent the disease from entering these towns and the rest of the Benguela district, first measures, mainly bush clearings, were initiated in 1915 and, in 1916, Correia Mendes used the recommendations of the mission doctors to conceive a detailed plan of how to tackle the disease. For him, these areas deserved absolute priority not only because of their economic importance and their large European and African population, but also because of the feasibility of the task. Given that the presence of the tsetse fly in the Benguela district was still limited to a few spots in forests and along rivers, Correia Mendes believed that it would be feasible to eradicate vector and disease by replicating the combined approach used on Príncipe.[168]

[162] Ibid., 53–178.
[163] Vicente Ferreira, 'Diploma Legislativo 463', 9 December 1926, *BOA* (1926), 647–52, preamble.
[164] Correia Mendes, 'Plano de Combate da Doença do Sono', 8 September 1916, 5, ANA, Cx. 391.
[165] See the critique in Neves, 'Relatório Congo (1919)', 172; Ornelas, 'Nós e a última conferência' and Almeida, 'Relatório Congo'. For the map, see Chapter 3.
[166] See Chapter 3.   [167] Salgado Júnior, 'Relatório', November 1914, ANA, Cx. 391.
[168] Correia Mendes to Governor-General of Angola, 24 August 1916 and Correia Mendes to Secretário Geral do Governo, 12 October 1916, ANA, Cx. 391.

Just like in Príncipe, Bernardo Bruto da Costa was, on his own demand, entrusted with carrying out Correia Mendes' plan.[169] Between 1916 and 1919, sanitation brigades sponsored by the state and local companies cleared brushwood and cut trees on several thousands of hectares, and a small group of workers trapped flies with the Maldonado method. Infected game and domestic animals were killed. In addition to this 'ecological' attack against the vector and its habitat, Bruto da Costa also sought to reduce human-fly contact. He ordered that people be removed from infected areas, particularly from the Cavaco forest, where many returned *serviçais* from São Tomé had settled after 1910,[170] and that the diseased be isolated in a 'concentration camp' and treated with atoxyl. These violent intrusions into local people's lives met with considerable resistance. Many refused to leave villages in the infected zones until they were destroyed by order of Bruto da Costa. Some also opposed a drug treatment they did not believe in and fled the concentration camp in which they had been forcibly incarcerated. The extent of African resistance is reflected in the fact that the sleeping sickness service needed to hire 30 *cipaios* ('African policemen') to enforce these measures and guard the camp.[171] Just as in Príncipe, there was also resistance on the part of some Europeans, who mainly opposed the killing of their livestock. A few launched a slander campaign and made death threats against the doctors.[172] Nevertheless, the eradication campaign, which continued after Bruto da Costa's departure in 1919, was largely successful. In the late 1920s, bush clearings would be extended to further areas in the Benguela district.[173]

In the far more heavily infested Cuanza and Congo districts (including Cabinda) further north, by contrast, campaigns were less systematic and successful. Existing legislation promoted an integrated strategy here as well, aimed at destroying the vector and its habitat, reducing human-fly contact and killing the trypanosomes in the human body.[174] Yet, in practice, vector control played a much less important role. Due to differences in environment and scale, no one believed that it would be possible to sanitise the entire Congo and Cuanza districts. Correia Mendes, who had already in 1907 emphasised the impracticability of exterminating all the flies in the Cuanza region, was very clear about it 10 years later. 'Obviously, it is not possible to use the plan of

---

[169] Correia Mendes to Secretário Geral do Governo, 1 September 1916, ANA, Cx. 391. For the following, see Velho, 'Tripanossomose humana', 49–52, 184–7; Costa, *Vinte e três anos*, 132–56.

[170] Salgado Júnior, 'Relatório', November 1914, 6–7, ANA, Cx. 391. On their 'repatriation', see also Chapter 6 and Coghe, 'Reordering Colonial Society', 40.

[171] Costa, *Vinte e três anos*, 149–50.

[172] Ibid., 136, 153–4 and Associação Comercial de Benguela to Governor-General, 20 September 1917, ANA, Cx. 391.

[173] Mora, *Luta*, 67–70.

[174] See Alto Comissariado da República em Angola, *Diplomas Doença do Sono*.

action that is being executed in Benguela for the Cuanza district', he wrote. 'Nobody will seriously consider destroying the forests that cover the valleys of the Cuanza and Bengo and their numerous tributaries, just as it would be utopian to believe that one could exterminate all the animals living in that region.'[175] Emphasising the difference in scale between Príncipe and Angola, and hence echoing British reservations about the replicability of the Príncipe experience, health director Alberto de Queiroz was equally adamant in dismissing the possibility of eradicating the tsetse flies in Angola.[176] Moreover, by the late 1910s, studies on the bionomics of the tsetse fly (its behaviour and relationship to the environment) were generating scepticism on both the possibility and desirability of vector control and 'species sanitation'. Not only had the behaviour of tsetse flies (and their many subspecies) proved too irregular for large-scale extermination campaigns, but the species was also increasingly conceptualised as a single element in a larger and complex 'web of life'. Eradicating the tsetse fly was both difficult and likely to lead to uncertain consequences.[177]

Accordingly, the focus of anti-sleeping sickness campaigns in northern Angola lay with the two remaining approaches: preventing human-fly contact and treating the diseased. Stopping human-fly contact implied bush clearing around villages and plantations as well as the relocation of villages, usually from fly-infested riverbanks to higher ground. Decreed in 1912 and confirmed in Correia Mendes's anti-sleeping sickness plan of 1916, these measures were to be carried out by the local health officers and the administrative authorities, in collaboration with plantation managers and the African population.[178] Such collaborations, however, were not always a given and the vastness of the areas and the lack of a special team like in Benguela, due to lack of money and staff, further worsened conditions.

Medical officers were still few and overburdened with other tasks: by early 1913, their official number had risen to 42, but, just as 20 years before, some were always on furlough and only few were stationed in sleeping sickness

---

[175] Correia Mendes to Secretário Geral do Governo, 1 October 1917, ANA, Cx. 391. Compare with Mendes, 'Subsídio', 397.

[176] Alberto de Queiroz, 'Serviço de Saúde de Angola', 28 May 1917, 26, AHU, MU, DGAPC 3449.

[177] See, for instance, Hegh, *Notice sur les glossines*; Schwetz, *Recherches sur les glossines* and, for the reception of these studies in Angola, Velho, 'Tripanossomose humana', 193–5. On the 'ecological' reframing of the tsetse problem by British scientists, see Tilley, 'Ecologies of Complexity', 29–30, 35–7. On 'species sanitation', see Packard, *Making of a Tropical Disease*, 119.

[178] See Alto Comissariado da República em Angola, *Diplomas Doença do Sono*, 35–40 and Correia Mendes, 'Plano de Combate da Doença do Sono', 8 September 1916, ANA, Cx. 391.

areas.[179] Entrusting them – and not a special service – with the anti-sleeping sickness campaign, Alberto de Queiroz complained in 1917, was doomed to failure, since their medical districts were too vast to simultaneously direct anti-sleeping sickness work and provide general healthcare to the populations.[180] Moreover, relations between doctors and administrators were often strained: doctors frequently complained that administrators refused to support them and did not recruit the workers for the sanitation brigades that were to clear bush around roads and villages.[181] Beyond a few 'islands of intervention', like Dondo in 1910, Golungo Alto in 1914 and Cazengo in 1919–21, hardly any sustained attack on the disease was carried out by colonial officers before the 1920s, despite frequent reminders and threats from the Governor-General.[182]

Many plantation owners and managers were also reluctant to implement prophylactic measures, invoking a lack of money or personnel. Thus, in 1913, the medical officers who inspected the plantations in the Cazengo and Ambaca districts, first in March/April and again in October/November, noted that these had implemented hardly any of the preventive measures decreed a year before.[183] The recommendations made during the first inspection were often ignored as well. Workers' camps, for instance, were usually still surrounded by abundant vegetation, although some had been relocated to higher grounds. Workers usually did not have protective clothes nor professional healthcare.[184] The situation was particularly dramatic on the plantations of the Companhia Agrícola de Cazengo, one of the biggest coffee companies in the region, which were often badly entertained and abounding with tsetse flies. The inspecting doctor described the Canhoca plantation as a 'living cemetery' and the Hôco plantation, where several workers had recently died from sleeping sickness, as 'an uninhabitable place' that should be closed or sanitised, as it would be a 'crime against humanity if it were to continue under current conditions'.[185] Companies' compliance with the anti-sleeping sickness regulations certainly varied from plantation to plantation and district to district. The medical officer

---

[179] 'Relação oficial dos oficiães médicos', 31 January 1913, AHU, MU, DGAPC 3487. See also Chefe dos Serviços de Saúde to Chefe do Gabinete do Governador Geral, 20 June 1913, ANA, Cx. 404. Compare with Chapter 1.

[180] Alberto de Queiroz, 'Serviço de Saúde de Angola', 28 May 1917, 27, AHU, MU, DGAPC 3449.

[181] See, for instance, Augusto de Vasconcelos to Chefe do Serviço de Saúde, 20 March 1913, ANA, Cx. 109 and the preamble of Vicente Ferreira, 'Diploma Legislativo 463', 9 December 1926, *BOA* (1926), 647–52.

[182] See Velho, 'Tripanossomose humana', 187–92 and Correia, 'Doença do sono', 172–4.

[183] Compare with Portaria 627, 14 May 1912, in Alto Comissariado da República em Angola, *Diplomas Doença do Sono*, 35–40, esp. art. 12 and 13.

[184] 'Processo 140 – Inspecções sanitárias' (1913), ANA, Cx. 1546.

[185] João Gomes Salgado Júnior, 'Relatório da inspecção às fazendas agricolas e industriaes da circunscrição civil de Cazengo', 5 November 1913, ANA, Cx. 1546, Processo 140.

in the *concelho* of Cacongo (in the Cabinda enclave), for instance, praised the anti-sleeping sickness efforts and the excellent hygienic conditions on the plantations of Hatton & Cookson, a Liverpool-based exporting company, conceding that for most companies the financial burden of the measures was too heavy.[186]

African villagers had their own rationales. In Cacongo, for instance, most of them had, by 1913, abandoned the tsetse-infested riverbanks and relocated their villages to higher grounds, leading to a strong decline in disease incidence.[187] But, just like in Benguela, such decisions were not always voluntary. As administrator Serra Frazão later recounted, villagers often opposed resettlement, even over short distances. Apart from the practical disadvantages of being far from water, dislocation meant abandoning ancestral grounds and risking losing contact with the dead for the sake of an aetiological theory they did often not believe in.[188] The success of resettlement measures hence depended on the power and influence of local administrators and doctors. For similar reasons, the practical impact of segregation camps was limited as well. In the fight against sleeping sickness, all colonial powers in Africa made use of such camps, believed to fulfil two pressing needs: to break the human-fly infection cycle by separating the sick and infectious from the healthy and by isolating the former in glossina-free places; and to heal the diseased with drug therapy. Concentration camps met with massive resistance from the African population almost everywhere. Many refused entry, interrupted treatment or, if forcibly 'detained', escaped.[189]

African resistance against the camps was fed mainly from two sources. First, both drug therapy and the isolation of the diseased did, in most cases, not conform with local aetiologies and therapeutic practices. As elaborated earlier, therapeutic practices for 'diseases of man' focused on community healing, treating the social body instead of the individual. Extracting the individual body from the social body by incarcerating sleeping sickness victims in concentration camps meant that community healing was not possible. In the camps, they were also out of reach for what Janzen has called the 'therapy managing group': kinsmen, friends and neighbours, who guide the patients through periods of illness and support them by cooking food, washing clothes,

---

[186] Alfredo da Silva Borges, 'Circunscrição de Cacongo – Relatório sobre assistência aos indígenas e profiláxia da varíola, paludismo e doença do sono', 1913, 24–27, ANA, Cx. 3374.

[187] Ibid.

[188] Serra Frazão, 'Reabilitação dos Negros. Estudo crítico sobre diversos aspectos de Angola', 1942, 132–3, AHU, T 215.

[189] See, for Belgian Congo, Lyons, 'Death Camps'; for Uganda Hoppe, *Lords of the Fly*, 73–6 and for the German colonies Eckart, 'Colony as Laboratory' and Isobe, *Medizin und Kolonialgesellschaft*, 71–91, 178–86, 238–64.

talking, etc.[190] Certainly, this disconnection did not apply to all the sleeping sickness camps before 1914, since some of them allowed family members to accompany the diseased. The level of coercion varied and, in some cases, Africans were inclined to try the new therapeutic possibilities and sometimes economic benefits (in the form of arable land, food and other goods) the camps offered as incentives, especially when they had previous positive experience of European medicine.[191]

Second, segregation camps usually failed to gain legitimacy (or quickly lost it), as few patients were effectively healed in them before the 1920s. Drug therapy, as already indicated, was painful but mostly ineffective if not started early. Mortality rates were very high and many camps became known as death camps.[192] Even the camp of Bugalla in British Uganda, which in 1906–7 initially attracted many hundreds of patients hoping to find a cure, saw most of them leave again after a few months because their 'expectations of therapy and healing were not met' and because they noticed that Robert Koch and other German doctors were experimenting.[193] Distrust of camps also rose when diagnosed patients did not feel ill yet. Due to the long incubation period of the *gambiense* form of HAT, some only showed symptoms when they were already staying in the camps. Such stories fed the rumour that it was the Europeans who, through the diagnostic punctures or drug injections, gave the disease to Africans.[194]

Medical authorities in Angola knew the bad reputation of the closed concentration camps in other colonies and when the first Angolan camps were created in Camoma (Cuanza district) and Noqui (Congo district) in 1912, Correia Mendes advised that they should adopt a more open village-like camp concept. It was hoped that allowing family members to settle with their diseased relatives would overcome African resistance to the camps.[195] The few concentration camps established in Angola had huge structural problems, however. In 1914, Camoma was closed because the site was not free of tsetse flies, and the three camps that were functioning in the Congo district in the second half of the 1910s (the 'Central Treatment Camp' in São Salvador and the two auxiliary camps in Noqui and Maquela do Zombo) were severely understaffed,

[190] Janzen, *Quest for Therapy*, 1–11; Lyons, *Colonial Disease*, 114, 190.
[191] See especially Webel, *Politics of Disease Control*.
[192] Lyons, *Colonial Disease*, 120; Hoppe, *Lords of the Fly*, 74.
[193] Webel, *Politics of Disease Control*, 100 (quote).
[194] Lyons, *Colonial Disease*, 188–9, 191.
[195] Junta de Saúde, 'Sessão ordinária', 30 January 1911, ANA, Cód. 1867, 192r–v; Governor-General Norton de Matos, Portaria 1.272', 23 October 1912 and 'Portaria 1.481', 27 December 1912, reprinted in Alto Comissariado da República em Angola, *Diplomas Doença do Sono*, 51–5. For the Belgian Congo, see Lyons, *Colonial Disease*, 125–6; Neill, *Networks*, 130.

underfunded and underused.[196] In 1916, Correia Mendes complained that Noqui only had 18 patients, although it was built for hundreds, partly because the camp doctor was not allowed to go looking for patients in the area.[197] They also enjoyed very little acceptance among the Bakongo population. Many did not believe in their usefulness and, given that the camps were somewhat eccentrically positioned, distances were probably too great for family members and others to accompany the diseased. Thus the Congo district's chief medical officer, José da Silva Neves, reported in 1919 that,

the native, who lacks any notion of the danger as well as the belief in the methods of scientific treatment, does not go looking for the doctor to be examined, since he knows very well that, in the case of being tested positive, he would be forced to go to the Central Treatment Camp in São Salvador, at a distance of five days, and that it would be impossible to return soon, if ever, to his family.[198]

It was only in the 1920s that segregation camps would be effectively remodelled into, and substituted by a larger network of, more open village-like *sanzalas-enfermarias* ('village-infirmaries'). These gained greater acceptance in the population as they paid more attention to the social needs of patients. Simultaneously, colonial health services in Angola (and many other colonies) increasingly preferred ambulant treatment: all but the most advanced cases would be treated with atoxyl or other trypanocidal drugs in or near their villages by itinerant medical teams.[199]

From a comparative perspective, missionaries contributed little to anti-sleeping sickness campaigns in Angola, unlike for instance in the Belgian Congo, where the Colonial Ministry obliged nearly two dozen Catholic and Protestant mission societies to participate in state efforts against the disease in 1910.[200] One of the main reasons was that, until after the Second World War, Catholic missions in Angola generally did not engage trained physicians.[201] Sleeping sickness was a complex disorder, and diagnosis and treatment required advanced technical skills, while missionaries had (at best) only received rudimentary training in nursing. The Congregation of the Holy Spirit, the only male Catholic order in Angola until the 1930s, thus ran two mission stations in the interior of the Cabinda enclave, in Lucula and Luali, where sleeping sickness raged in the 1900s. The missionaries bemoaned the ongoing depopulation of the region, but there was little they could do except

---

[196] On Camoma, see 'Processo 2/1914', ANA, Cx. 391. On the other camps, see Neves, 'Relatório Congo (1919)', 167–72 and Velho, 'Tripanossomose humana', 187–90.
[197] Correia Mendes, 'Plano de Combate da Doença do Sono', 8 September 1916, 2, ANA, Cx. 391.
[198] Neves, 'Relatório Congo (1919)', 172 (quote).
[199] See Almeida, 'Relatório Congo', 36–7 and Chapter 3.
[200] Lyons, *Colonial Disease*, 129. On such medical 'co-operations', see also Au, 'Medical Orders', 67.
[201] See Chapter 5.

administering palliative care to the dying. They also tried to baptise them to 'save their souls', a practice that sometimes met with great suspicion and resistance by villagers.[202] Protestant mission societies in Angola (and in colonial Africa and Asia at large), by contrast, had already begun to professionalise medical work at the turn of the century by engaging Protestant lay doctors, so-called medical missionaries. Most of their mission posts, however, were based in sleeping sickness free zones in Central, Southern and Eastern Angola.[203]

The one exception was the Baptist Missionary Society (BMS). In São Salvador, the ancient capital of the Kingdom of Kongo, where its oldest station in the Lower Congo region (since 1879) was located, the BMS started systematic treatment of sleeping sickness patients in December 1908, a year after the arrival of its first 'medical missionary'.[204] Under Mercier Gamble, a graduate of the University of Manchester and the London School of Tropical Medicine, this mission post became the most important medical centre in a region where state health services were virtually non-existent before the First World War.[205] Sleeping sickness constituted the core of the station's medical work. Attracted by the growing fame of Gamble's work, patients came from São Salvador and surrounding areas. By administering astonishingly huge doses of atoxyl, often 4 g. on an almost daily basis, Gamble achieved 19 'apparent cures' in 1909, and treated almost 200 other patients between October 1910 and December 1912. Gamble became a well-known sleeping sickness expert in Britain after reporting these successes to the *Journal of Tropical Medicine* and, in 1913–14, the expert Sleeping Sickness Committee installed by the British Parliament. He also sent insects to the Imperial Bureau of Entomology in London.[206] Simultaneously, the Baptist missionaries capitalised on these successes to improve relations with both the Angolan population and the colonial state.

The main rationales undergirding Protestant medical work were religious and political. By offering professional healthcare, Protestant missions aimed to make Africans more receptive to the word of God. The destruction of 'pagan' healing traditions was seen as an important step in this conversion process, as

---

[202] See the reports in *Bulletin de la Congrégation du Saint-Esprit* 21 (1901–2), 718 and 726; 23 (1905–6), 195–7; 24 (1907–8), 392–8 and 25 (1909–10), 581–2. On this congregation, see also Chapter 6.

[203] For Protestant medical missionaries in general, see Hardiman, 'Introduction'. For Angola, see Soremekun, *History*, 115–9 and Tucker (ed.), *Angola*, 97–102.

[204] For the general history of the BMS in Congo and Angola, see Stanley, *History*, 122–40, 336–64, 439–70 and Grenfell, *History of the Baptist Church*.

[205] Compare with Leal, 'Memórias d'África', 113–8. On Gamble, see 'Obituary Mercier Gamble'.

[206] Gamble, 'English Translation'; Gamble, 'Sleeping Sickness'; Sleeping Sickness Committee, *Minutes of Evidence*, 187–92. For Gamble's entomological work, see, for instance, *Bulletin of Entomological Research* 3 (1912–1913), 225, 340 and 419 and Gamble, 'List of Blood-Sucking Arthropods'.

these lay at the core of 'traditional' belief systems.[207] BMS missionaries thus used the prolonged sleeping sickness treatment, with patients coming to the mission station twice a week for many months, to spread the gospel, holding 'evangelistic services' at each occasion.[208] Protestant missionaries in Angola also used medical work to appease widespread anxieties and resistance among Portuguese state officials about the 'intrusion' of foreign Protestants.[209] Indeed, although Portuguese colonial administrations would frequently hinder Protestant mission work in their colonies in the late nineteenth and twentieth centuries, they were generally sympathetic towards medical work carried out by the BMS. It was with financial support from the Portuguese government that, in the early 1910s, the BMS was able to establish a medical infrastructure in São Salvador that was exemplary for the times and the region. Initially, it comprised a dispensary for outpatients, a surgery and a pharmacy. In 1913, a laboratory, a general hospital and a special hospital for the segregation of sleeping sickness patients outside town were added. The Portuguese government contributed by allowing the prefabricated hospital to enter Angola free of charge and granting a plot of land for the isolation hospital, privileges normally reserved for Portuguese mission societies only. At Gamble's request, the Portuguese government even supplied atoxyl for free.[210] Gamble had to stay in Britain in 1914, but his successors further extended sleeping sickness and other medical work in São Salvador.[211]

Conclusion

In many fundamental aspects, the varied medical engagements with sleeping sickness in Angola between the 1890s and 1918 ran parallel to responses in other European empires: Portuguese doctors actively participated in the microbiological search for the aetiology of the disease, tested experimental drugs, largely ignored African knowledge and implemented a series of disease control measures tackling the vector, the parasite or human-fly contact. They were part and parcel of a European epistemic community of sleeping sickness experts, who communicated with each other through personal letters and visits, conferences and publications. However, this and the preceding chapter have also

---

[207] Moorshead, *Appeal*, esp. 49–115.
[208] Medical Mission Auxiliary of the Baptist Missionary Society, *Challenge of Pain*, 29.
[209] See Chapter 6.
[210] Reverend Graham to Governor-General of Angola, 5 October 1911, ANA, Cx. 3374; Reverend Graham to British Consul in Luanda, 23 January 1912, BMSA, A 124; Reverend Graham to Governor-General of Angola (with annexes), 1 August 1912, ANA, Cx. 2946; Conselho Colonial, 'Consulta 19/1913', 14 February 1913, AHU, Conselho Colonial, Livro 1913, 59–60; Ministério das Colónias, 'Decreto 128', 10 September 1913, *DG Série I* (1913), 3445–6; 'Medical Work at San Salvador (1914)'.
[211] See, for instance, 'Medical Work (1920)', 85 and Chapter 5.

teased out various particularities of Portuguese dealings with sleeping sickness.

Some relate to what Sarah Ehlers has analysed as the particular racialised and racialising views, practices and effects of early 'European' sleeping sickness research. It appears that Portuguese doctors had serious doubts about the 'racial' character of the disease long before Manson's 'proof' of European victims (see Chapter 1) and showed a greater propensity to emulate 'native' surgical methods than their British, French, German or Belgian colleagues. The research practices of Ayres Kopke, and before that of the first Portuguese commission, also differed from the supposedly 'European' standard. At minimum, they contradict Ehlers's claims that African cases were described in much less detail than those of European patients and that (African) sleeping sickness patients remained 'extremely rare', even 'exotic' in Europe.[212] This does not mean that Portuguese doctors had a fundamentally different attitude towards race: the particularities of Portuguese drug therapy research, for instance, were mainly due to Kopke's personal ambitions and a lack of good research facilities in Angola and Príncipe. Moreover, emulating vernacular surgical methods, just like some of the other 'unconventional' views and practices described in this chapter, such as the use of testicular liquids or the persistent rejection of the trypanosoma theory by high-ranking doctors such as Garcia, was probably not exceptional. More than most other works about sleeping sickness, this chapter concentrates on local medical officers. They may have been more inclined to openly admit diverging views and practices than the small group of microbiologically educated experts in tropical medicine.

Another important particularity was the successful eradication campaign on Príncipe between 1911 and 1914, replicated a few years later in Benguela. These unlikely and, in the case of Príncipe, unprecedented successes were achieved through campaigns that focused on vector eradication, through massive bush clearing, game killing and fly-trapping. This 'ecological' approach, which was based on entomological and environmental knowledge of tsetse flies, prevailed over drug treatment and the avoidance of human-fly contact, which only played a lesser role. Such radical ecological measures were intensively discussed in German and British East Africa in the 1910s as well, but it was only in the 1920s and 1930s that similar tsetse eradication policies were implemented, with modifications, in British territories, most notably in Tanganyika by Charles Swynnerton. Although they were sometimes adopted in West and Central Africa as well, they were most typical of sleeping sickness campaigns against *morsitans* flies and *T. b. rhodesiense* in East and Southeast

---

[212] Compare with Ehlers, *Europa und die Schlafkrankheit*, 84–105 (quotes 85 and 96).

Africa.[213] Overall, the inclusion of the Portuguese colonies reveals that early 'European' responses were more varied than hitherto accounted for.

Moreover, Portuguese dealings with sleeping sickness also varied much between the colonies: they can hardly be framed as a 'national style', a concept posited by Michael Worboys in 1994. According to Worboys, British, Belgian and German authorities preferred different approaches, either ecological (fly eradication), spatial (avoidance of human-fly contact) or medical (parasite destruction), in their East African colonies before 1914, because of different 'form[s] and content[s] of expert advice' and different 'colonial structures and policies of the respective imperial powers'.[214] Tying in with earlier critique, the comparative analysis of Portuguese responses to sleeping sickness provides further evidence against this idea, as it highlights the crucial role of local conditions in shaping sleeping sickness approaches.[215]

While in Príncipe and around Benguela, small areas of great economic importance, the ecological approach prevailed, the same expert who had devised eradication plans there, Correia Mendes, deemed them unapplicable to northern Angola, because of differences in scale and environment. Here, campaigns focused on reducing human-fly contact through local resettlement, bush clearing and some medication. Drug therapy was also the main approach of British medical missionary Mercier Gamble in São Salvador, despite his connections with British entomologists and experts in tropical medicine.

In Guinea, Portugal's Cinderella colony in Africa, sleeping sickness was virtually neglected until the mid-1920s. From the 1880s onwards, and sporadically earlier, doctors reported dozens of people showing the clinical symptoms of sleeping sickness, but due to the little interest the government showed for the issue, the small number of European doctors and the lack of microscopes in most districts, it was not until 1925 that the first provenly endogenous case of sleeping sickness was confirmed. Only in the second half of the 1930s would the number of diagnosed cases rise spectacularly and trigger a stronger response, which focused on drug treatment.[216]

In Mozambique, finally, the imminent 'invasion' of sleeping sickness from neighbouring colonies aroused great concern among health authorities even before the first autochthonous cases were confirmed in 1912.[217] Accordingly, measures initially focused on preventing the disease from entering the colony,

---

[213] Ibid., 170–83 and Tilley, *Africa*, 186–200. On the East-West divide, see Neill, *Networks*, 103–64, esp. 108 and 164.

[214] Worboys, 'Comparative History', quotes 89 and 99.

[215] For earlier critique, see Neill, *Networks*, 108, 134; Hoppe, *Lords of the Fly*, 12; Isobe, *Medizin und Kolonialgesellschaft*; Bell, *Frontiers of Medicine*, 127–8.

[216] Havik, 'Public Health and Tropical Modernity'. See also Barreto, *Sobre a doença do sono*.

[217] Braga, 'Afrique orientale portugaise'; Sant'Anna, 'Tripanosomíase humana'.

by restricting and monitoring cross-border movement, and establishing medical inspection posts in endangered areas.[218] This spatial approach, which also included the relocation of villages, was after the First World War complemented with vector control policies such as the agronomic re-occupation of territories invaded by tsetse flies. These strategies were largely conditioned by the epidemiological specificities of sleeping sickness in Mozambique. Identified in the early 1910s as *rhodesiense*, the disease in Mozambique rarely took epidemic forms, mainly attacked animals that also served as a reservoir and was less responsive to trypanocidal drugs. In the 1920s and 1930s, the number of cases in humans remained limited and did not provoke depopulation anxieties as it had in Angola and Príncipe.[219] In Mozambique, animal trypanosomiasis was generally considered the bigger problem for the social and economic life of both the Africans and Europeans living there.[220]

In conclusion, it is impossible to speak of a 'national' Portuguese style. Even though policies were to a considerable extent designed and supervised by the same experts, most notably Ayres Kopke, Annibal Correia Mendes, Bernardo Bruto da Costa and Firmino Sant'Anna, approaches in São Tomé and Príncipe, Angola, Guinea and Mozambique substantially differed, even before 1918. They ranged from denial and inaction (Guinea) to eradication (Príncipe and Benguela); from border control (São Tomé and Mozambique) to complex integrated responses with a focus on vector control (Príncipe) or the avoidance of human-fly contact in combination with drug treatment (northern Angola). These differences resulted from the complex interplay between varying local circumstances such as epidemiological patterns, practical possibilities of control and economic and political considerations. After the First World War, differences between Portuguese colonies grew greater still, reinforced by the different transimperial networks in which Portuguese doctors from these regions were integrated: while vector control measures were increasingly adopted in Mozambique, as in the rest of East and Southeast Africa, disease control in Angola leant towards the massive use of trypanocidal drugs, as in neighbouring Belgian Congo and French Equatorial Africa. Here, drugs, used both in preventive and curative ways, would become the centrepiece of eradication hopes and strategies.[221]

---

[218] Sant'Anna, *Relatório Zambezia*; Lapa and Sousa, *Serviço de defesa*.
[219] Rebêlo, *Doença do sono*, 21–2; Martins, 'Doença do sono', 50–3.
[220] See Direito, 'Terror dos homens'.   [221] See Chapter 3.

3 Introducing Social Medicine: Inter-Imperial Learning and the *Assistência Médica aos Indígenas* in the Interwar Period

In the 1920s, the colonial health services in Angola intensified the campaign against sleeping sickness. In 1923, two anti-sleeping sickness missions were sent to the Congo (1923–6) and Zaire (1923–4) districts.[1] Most importantly, in 1926, the fight against this paradigmatic disease became part of a more comprehensive and well-funded scheme of *Assistência Médica aos Indígenas* (AMI) or 'Native Medical Assistance'. The basic concept and terminology of this scheme, which aimed to provide basic healthcare to 'native' populations through an expanding network of small hospitals and maternity clinics, with the help of medically trained African auxiliaries, reached back to the late 1890s, when it was first put into practice in French Madagascar. Later, it was adopted in French Indochina, AOF and AEF as well, but coverage remained very limited before the 1920s.[2] In Angola, Governor-General Norton de Matos had tried to set up an AMI scheme in 1914, but failed due to lack of personnel and money.[3] Beyond anti-sleeping sickness and anti-smallpox campaigns, biomedical healthcare had remained limited to Europeans and Africans living in or close to the biggest towns.[4] This only began to change in 1926, when the newly established AMI services started to provide basic healthcare to Angolan populations in some rural areas.

This chapter examines the history of this AMI programme in interwar Angola from a transimperial perspective. While some of its core aspects will be explored further in Chapters 4 and 5, this chapter analyses the rationales and defining moments that led to its establishment, its general structures and objectives as well as the structural constraints that, after a successful start, eventually limited its expansion in the 1930s. It also looks at how the anti-sleeping sickness campaign was entangled with this new health scheme.

---

[1] Almeida, 'Relatório Congo'; Rebêlo, 'Relatório Zaire 1923–1924'.

[2] Paillard, 'Recherches démographiques', 23–9; Cooper, *Public Health*, 19, 47–85; Headrick, *Colonialism, Health and Illness*, 51–4 and, for coverage, 60–2.

[3] Norton de Matos, 'Portaria 406', 27 March 1914, *BOA* (1914), 302–3. For its failure, see Mora, 'Prefácio', 15–7.

[4] See, for instance, Alberto de Queiroz, 'Serviço de saúde de Angola', 28 May 1917, 17–18, AHU, MU, DGAPC 3449.

The chapter thereby argues that, in the interwar years, the history of both the AMI scheme and anti-sleeping sickness measures were profoundly shaped by processes of inter-imperial comparison and exchange. These could take on the form of (explicit or implicit) inter-imperial borrowing, collaboration and competition.

To understand the health reforms in interwar Angola, it is hence imperative to analyse new ideas and practices regarding 'native health' in other colonies and new international organisations such as the League of Nations Health Organisation (LNHO) and the Rockefeller Foundation (RF), and to look at how they were received by Portuguese actors in Angola. The chapter pays particular attention to the ideas and actions of António Damas Mora (1879–1949), the powerful long-term director of the Angolan health services and main architect of the colony's interwar AMI reforms. His eagerness to learn from and collaborate with other colonial powers, which he often believed to be more advanced than the Portuguese, were crucial for the development of AMI services in Angola.

First, the chapter looks at the changing conditions for empire in the interwar years. It argues that, aside from economic and demographic considerations (see Chapter 4), mounting international critique of Portugal's colonial policies in the mid-1920s was decisive in convincing decision-makers in Lisbon to invest in 'native' healthcare. It then turns to the establishment of the AMI programme and analyses how it was shaped by new ideals of social medicine and selective processes of inter-imperial comparison and borrowing. Subsequently, it analyses new developments in the core of the AMI programme, the fight against sleeping sickness, that reveal the limits of inter-imperial learning. Doctors used the programme's infrastructure to set up a massive yet contested preventive campaign with the trypanocidal drug atoxyl. The chapter argues that, against the backdrop of inter-imperial competition, some doctors emphasised the scheme's comparative advantages and hence the superiority of the 'Portuguese method', while others criticised its deviation from European norms. The final section explores the financial and political limits of the AMI programme more generally. It shows that the austerity measures imposed by the emerging *Estado Novo* and which clipped the programme's wings in the early 1930s were also a result of the comparative weakness of health provisions for the European population in Angola and the metropole. The conclusion wraps up different modalities of inter-imperial learning.

International Pressure and Portuguese Anxieties

The establishment of the *Assistência Médica aos Indígenas* in Angola in the second half of the 1920s was largely made possible by financial support from central government in Lisbon. In July 1926, only two months after a military coup had overthrown the First Republic and installed a military dictatorship that would gradually merge into the *Estado Novo*, the newly designated High Commissioner for Angola, António Vicente Ferreira, had obtained a loan of 7 million escudos 'for sanitation work and the fight against sleeping sickness'. This was part of a larger loan of 125 million escudos, with which the new government wanted to tackle the deep financial and economic crisis in Angola, which many attributed to financial mismanagement under the previous High Commissioner Norton de Matos (1921–3).[5] The 'health loan' was officially a reaction to persistent fears of population decline and its humanitarian and economic consequences.[6] Yet, perhaps even more importantly, the loan also responded to mounting international criticism of Portugal's colonisation methods in the mid-1920s and deepening anxieties in Portugal that such accusations could lead to the loss of some of the country's colonies.[7]

In June 1925, the Committee on African Welfare, a group of well-connected American philanthropists, had presented a report to the Temporary Slavery Commission of the League of Nations on labour conditions in Portuguese Angola and Mozambique, written on their behalf by the American professor in sociology Edward Ross.[8] The 'Ross Report' was hardly discussed on the diplomatic stage in Geneva, but its sharp criticism of Portugal's native policy, including the dearth of healthcare provisions, had a huge impact on Portuguese politics and public opinion at the time. It prompted official refutations yet also heightened fears about the future of the Portuguese colonial project.[9]

The explanation for this strong reaction is threefold. First, the report revived long-standing and recurrent accusations of Portugal's harsh colonial labour policies on the part of foreign – mainly British – diplomats, abolitionists and human rights activists. These accusations had culminated in an international scandal and economic boycott of São Tomé and Príncipe cocoa in the 1900s and early 1910s. They abated somewhat thereafter, but were never completely gone.[10] Second, fresh accusations of exploitation and indifference more than ever undermined the legitimacy of Portuguese colonial rule, now that the civilising mission had resurged after the First World War as '*mise en valeur*' (Sarraut) and 'dual mandate' (Lugard), key concepts of colonial ideology that wanted the economic exploitation of the colonies to go hand-in-hand with the 'development' of their human resources.[11] Finally, the report coincided with

---

[5] Ministério das Colónias, 'Decreto 12.022', 30 July 1926, *DG Série I* (1926), 922–4 (quote 923). For the controversies surrounding Angola's financial crisis, see Freudenthal, 'Angola', 288–90.
[6] On interwar demographic anxieties, see Chapter 4.
[7] For a similar argument, see Shapiro, *Medicine*, 232–9.   [8] Ross, *Report*.
[9] Jerónimo, *Civilising Mission*, 158–94.   [10] Ibid., 38–76, 134–56. See also Chapters 2 and 6.
[11] Sarraut, *Mise en valeur*; Lugard, *Dual Mandate*. On this ideological shift, see Hodge, *Triumph of the Expert*, 117–25.

the imminent entry of Germany to the League of Nations and its Permanent Mandates Commission, an event that also caused grave concern among other colonial powers.[12] Indeed, many Portuguese colonialists feared that an empowered Germany might capitalise on the image of Portugal as a 'bad coloniser' and, with the support of other colonial powers, try to win a mandate on a portion of the Portuguese colonies in order to satisfy its colonial revisionism.[13] These anxieties were not completely irrational. In 1898 and 1913, Germany and the United Kingdom had already negotiated secret treaties in which they partitioned the Portuguese colonies.[14]

Portugal was not the only colonial power that reacted to the German threat by increasing its investment in African healthcare. In response to persistent German criticism of French health politics in Africa, and in an attempt to forestall Germany's use of the health argument against France on the international diplomatic stage in Geneva, the French Colonial Ministry spectacularly increased health expenditure in its mandated territories Cameroon and Togo formerly under German colonial rule. Nowhere in the French Empire did health budgets increase so much in 1925–7. It was under these conditions that, for example, a well-funded permanent sleeping sickness mission was established in Cameroon.[15]

Portugal's new willingness to invest in African healthcare around 1926 must also be seen as a result of the country's growing scientific marginalisation in the international fight against sleeping sickness – and the political costs this entailed. While Portuguese scientists had conducted important research in the early 1900s, and even eradicated sleeping sickness on the island of Príncipe in the 1910s, their failure to provide the international community with detailed maps on the distribution of tsetse flies and the disease or to contribute to international drug therapy research had increasingly prejudiced the country's position in the international debate during and after the First World War.[16] In fact, the LNHO Expert Committee on Sleeping Sickness, which was established in 1922, did not have a Portuguese member, nor did the first report of that committee contain relevant information on the Portuguese colonies, since

---

[12] Callahan, *Mandates and Empires*, 122–56; Wempe, *Revenants*, 157–93; Vanthemsche, *La Belgique et le Congo*, 123.
[13] See, for instance, the Portuguese press articles collected by the Permanent Mandates Commission, 'The League of Nations, The Mandates System and the Portuguese Colonies', 5 January 1926, League of Nations Publications, CPM 352.
[14] See Tschapek, *Bausteine*.
[15] Lachenal, 'Médecine, comparaisons et échanges', 34–6; Tantchou, *Épidémie et politique*, 73–8. For mutual French and German accusations of inadequate colonial health policies, see also Neill, *Networks*, 182–204.
[16] See Chapter 2.

Portugal had failed to provide any.[17] Only after the intervention of the eminent Portuguese hygienist and recently appointed member to the League's Health Committee, Ricardo Jorge, was some summary information included in a second report.[18] Yet the ensuing International Conference on Sleeping Sickness, held in London in 1925 under the auspices of the League, reiterated Portugal's marginalisation with regard to this important question. According to the Expert Committee chairman Andrew Balfour, Portugal did not take a great interest in sleeping sickness, unlike the British, French and Belgians. Nor did Balfour mention any Portuguese research institution or propose a Portuguese member for the international research mission under discussion.[19]

It is telling that Ayres Kopke, Portugal's foremost sleeping sickness expert and delegate to the London conference, admitted that the country's marginalisation was in large measure due to its own shortcomings. In his report to the Colonial Ministry, Kopke bemoaned the fact that both research and health measures had been largely insufficient in the Portuguese colonies. He feared that if Angola, Mozambique and Guinea did not immediately intensify their fight against sleeping sickness, notably in the border areas, neighbouring colonies would start to interfere on the basis of the recommendations formulated at the London conference. Hence, immediate action was, he claimed, not only a humanitarian and economic, but also a political necessity.[20]

The Portuguese government did not ignore this alarming message, which coincided with the Ross controversy. In accordance with Kopke's recommendations, the Colonial Ministry prompted the affected colonies to establish and/or intensify their campaigns against the disease. The effects were immediate: in 1926, a study mission was organised in Guinea, and in 1927 a long-planned study mission finally departed for Mozambique, headed by Ayres Kopke himself.[21] Furthermore, the Portuguese government now viewed the absence of a Portuguese member in the LNHO sponsored research mission to Entebbe (Uganda) as highly prejudicial to the country's prestige and vested interests in Africa. 'Now that they unjustly accuse us of not fulfilling all of our duties as colonisers towards the native populations', the Minister of Foreign Affairs

---

[17] Expert Committee, 'Interim Report on Tuberculosis and Sleeping-Sickness in Equatorial Africa', 26 May 1923, 114–5, LON, R 854, 12B/24848/26254. For this expert committee, see Borowy, *Coming to Terms*, 109–10, 255–61.

[18] Expert Committee on Sleeping Sickness, 'Further report on Tuberculosis and Sleeping Sickness in Equatorial Africa', April 1925, 60–3, LON, R 855, 12B/43613/26254. See also the correspondence between Andrew Balfour, Norman White and Ludwik Rajchman (February–April 1924) in LON, R 854, 12B/26381x/26254, Jacket 2 and between Balfour, Rajchman and Jorge (April–August 1924) in LON, R 854, 12B/35529/26254.

[19] LNHO, 'Minutes of the International Conference on Sleeping-Sickness', London, 19–22 May 1925, 4, LON, R 855, 12B/44260/26254.

[20] Kopke, 'Conferência internacional', 515–7.

[21] Barreto, *Sobre a doença do sono*; Kopke, 'Estudos Moçambique'.

wrote to the Minister of Colonies, 'it is not in any way suitable that we are not represented in this mission, in which there are delegates from all nations that have colonies in Central Africa and even from Germany which does not have any'.[22] Upon Kopke's recommendation, the government added Máximo Prates, the director of the medical laboratory in Lourenço Marques, to the mission's international team.[23] With regard to Angola specifically, the reaction would even be stronger.

These circumstances help to explain why the Portuguese government officially dedicated such a large loan to the fight against sleeping sickness. Due to mounting international critique and scientific isolation, it had become a political necessity for Portugal as a colonial nation to intensify its efforts in this domain. Moreover, after 25 years of alarm and anxiety, public opinion in Angola finally demanded strong action against the disease, which 'still haunted almost everybody's mind', as health director António Damas Mora later put it.[24] However, Damas Mora was not convinced that absolute priority should be given to sleeping sickness. He believed that, 'though the noisiest of all diseases north of the Cuanza river', it was no longer epidemic. He also emphasised that it occurred almost exclusively in the northern, forested areas, while the rest of Angola was a 'country of savannah' and thus inhospitable to the tsetse fly. Based on a broader understanding of Africans' health needs, but without ignoring public pressure and international obligations, Angola's health services used the money to set up a system that integrated anti-sleeping sickness efforts into a more comprehensive programme of *Assistência Médica aos Indígenas*.[25]

Staging Inter-Imperial Learning

By the time the loan was approved in July 1926, leading doctors in Angola had already gathered many ideas about how to set up such a healthcare programme. A crucial role was played by António Damas Mora. In 1921, he had been appointed director of the Angolan health services (1921–4) and asked to finally organise the *Assistência Médica aos Indígenas* by Norton de Matos, who had

---

[22] Vasco Borges to Minister of Colonies, 30 January 1926, AHD-MNE, 3. Piso, Armário 28, Maço 65, Pasta 2.

[23] Kopke to Augusto Vasconcellos, 12 January 1926, AHD-MNE, 3. Piso, Armário 28, Maço 65, Pasta 2. See also Vasconcellos to Drummond, 12 February 1926, and further correspondence in LON, R 856, 12B/45430/26254.

[24] Mora, 'Assistance Médicale Indigène (1928)', 1334 (quote).

[25] Primeiro Congresso de Medicina Tropical da África Ocidental, 'Acta da 6a Sessão', 44; 'Conferência sanitária luso-belga', 379, 381 and 383 (first quote); Damas Mora to Ricardo Jorge, 9 May 1928, reprinted in Mora, *António Damas Mora*, 94–6 (second quote 96).

returned to Angola as High Commissioner with wide-reaching prerogatives.[26] By that time, Damas Mora was already a senior medical officer with extensive experience as a colonial doctor, hygienist and public health administrator. After graduating from the Lisbon Medical School, he had served on the island of Príncipe (1902–10), taking an active part in the local fight against sleeping sickness. Later, he had been sent to Timor (1914–19), where he reorganised the health services and established a rudimentary form of rural 'native medical assistance', and served as Interim Director of the Colonial Ministry's Health Department (1920–1). With an interruption between 1924 and 1926, he would remain in charge of the Angolan health services until 1934, ending his career as director of the health services in Macau (1935–6) and the Institute of Tropical Medicine in Lisbon (1936–9).[27] More important for the AMI reforms than his intra-imperial mobility was his ability to compare with and learn from other colonial powers.

Two moments of inter-imperial learning in the 1920s were of particular importance for the basic coordinates of the AMI project in Angola.[28] A first crucial moment was the First West African Conference on Tropical Medicine, which took place in Luanda from 16 to 23 July 1923. Organised by António Damas Mora, in close collaboration with his homologues in the Belgian Congo and the AEF, this first inter-imperial medical conference in tropical Africa itself, though largely neglected by historiography, had a large impact on the health services in Angola and on medical cooperation in Africa *tout court*. Gathering no fewer than 76 often high-ranking participants from British, French, Belgian, South African and Portuguese health services in Africa and medical institutions in Europe, the conference offered an unprecedented stage for the exchange of ideas and experiences on practical issues of African healthcare. Indeed, rather than discussing scientific questions of pathology or surgery, as they did at medical conferences in Europe, the organisers had deliberately placed the AMI at the centre of debate.[29] The first two sessions were almost entirely devoted to comparing systems of 'native' healthcare in various African colonies and analysing problems of establishment and expansion. In many other sessions – most revolving around common diseases in tropical Africa – discussion of prevention and treatment possibilities prevailed

[26] See, retrospectively, Mora, 'Serviços de Saúde em Angola (1928)', 89. On the system of High Commissioners, see Marques, 'Introdução', 24.

[27] AHU, Processo Individual de António Damas Mora. On his time in Príncipe, see also Chapter 2; on Timor see Mora, *Serviço de saúde em Timor*. See also the recent biography by his great-nephew Mora, *António Damas Mora*.

[28] For a more detailed analysis, see Coghe, 'Inter-Imperial Learning', 140–6.

[29] Damas Mora to Trolli, 4 February 1922 and Jérôme Rodhain, 'Avis et considérations', 11 March 1922, MAEAA, GG 16792. See also Mora, 'Raison d'être', 50–1.

over more technical debates.[30] Moreover, inter-imperial learning was not confined to the conference itself. Numerous leisure activities, including a 10-day trip across southern Angola after the conference, as well as the journeys to and from Luanda, offered ample opportunities for informal discussions.[31]

While the exchange of knowledge on health schemes and ways to fight particular tropical diseases was considered beneficial for all participating colonies, this also reflected the particular needs of Angola's health services. As Damas Mora emphasised in his opening speech, Angola was about to establish its own African healthcare scheme and was thus eager to learn from more advanced colonies.[32] An ambitious reform of the Angolan health services had already been decreed, with a huge increase in the number of doctors and nurses as one of its salient features, but the issue of how to bring Western biomedicine to the 'native' populations was still pending.[33]

The conference was widely considered a huge success.[34] However, it did not trigger the results Damas Mora had hoped for, at least not immediately. Due to Angola's mounting financial problems and the more or less forced resignation of Norton de Matos at the beginning of 1924, the project of establishing a comprehensive and costly system of African healthcare lacked political support.[35] Damas Mora stepped down and returned to Lisbon, where he edited approximately 2,200 pages of conference proceedings for the *Revista Médica de Angola*, the colony's first medical journal, which he had himself founded in 1921.[36]

The second moment was, in 1926, the participation of António Damas Mora, at the time still employed at the Colonial Ministry in Lisbon, and João Augusto Ornelas, a senior medical officer in Angola, in a study tour through French and British West Africa sponsored by the LNHO and the International Health Board of the Rockefeller Foundation. Both institutions supported the idea of closer collaboration and mutual learning between national health services and organised study tours and other forms of interchange between expert elites. During this West African study tour, which started in Dakar on

---

[30] See the conference proceedings, published in *Revista Médica de Angola* 4.1–5 (1923).

[31] The importance of these informal exchanges has been highlighted by Mertens and Lachenal, 'History', 1268–9. See also the extensive journey reports of some of the participants: Brumpt and Joyeux, *Voyage médical*, 4–14; Heckenroth, Leger and Nogue, 'Afrique Occidentale Française', 11–7; Vassal and Vassal, *Français, Belges et Portugais*.

[32] Mora, 'Raison d'être', 56–8.

[33] António Damas Mora, 'Circular aos médicos de Angola de 12 de Maio de 1921', *Jornal do Comércio (Luanda)*, 18 June 1921; Norton de Matos, 'Decreto n. 74', 17 November 1921, *BOA* (1921), 306–18.

[34] See, for instance, the very positive accounts in Brumpt and Joyeux, *Voyage médical*, 3–4, 12; Heckenroth, Leger, and Nogue, 'Afrique Occidentale Française', 19, 36–7, 76; Vassal and Vassal, *Français, Belges et Portugais*, 103–21.

[35] See Freudenthal, 'Angola', 288–90.

[36] AHU, Processo Individual de António Damas Mora.

20 March 1926 and ended in Freetown on 18 May, Damas Mora, Ornelas and ten other health administrators, one from Guatemala and the rest from other colonial powers in Africa, focused on studying and comparing questions of African healthcare and epidemiological control. They paid particular attention to maternity clinics, infant healthcare and venereal disease.[37] At the final conference in Freetown, the participants also discussed the establishment of an epidemiological bureau in West Africa, modelled upon the recently opened path-breaking Far Eastern Health Bureau in Singapore, in order to further foster and institutionalise exchange between colonial nations in the region.[38]

The study tour did not directly lead to an increase in official multilateral collaboration, however. Because of conflicting views on the scope and usefulness of such a bureau between the colonial nations involved (Damas Mora had probably been its most fervent supporter), the LNHO in Geneva eventually decided against it.[39] Moreover, the practical organisation of the interchange had been so arduous that it remained the only one in interwar Africa. Nevertheless, the impact of the tour on Angola's health system proved huge. In public lectures, newspaper contributions and medical journal articles, Damas Mora reported extensively on the innovative processes in African healthcare that he had observed in French and British West Africa, recommending that many of them be adopted in the Portuguese colonies, notably Angola. 'We need to confront and solve the sanitary problems of Angola along the same lines as the other colonizing nations,' he argued.[40] Moreover, his reform plans convinced the new High Commissioner for Angola, António Vicente Ferreira (1926–8), who reinstalled Damas Mora at the head of the Angolan health services, thus giving him the chance to put these reforms into practice.[41]

Of course, inter-imperial learning neither ended in 1926 nor was it confined to António Damas Mora. It was a continuous and complex process that involved many actors, including Portuguese doctors who read foreign medical reports or met with foreign colleagues in border areas, as I demonstrate below.

---

[37] [Louis Destouches], 'Rapport sur l'échange de personnel sanitaire en Afrique Occidentale', [July 1926], LON, R 955, 12B/52774/41908.

[38] W. D. Inness, 'Report of the visit of the League of Nations Study Tour to Sierra Leone', 29 May 1926, 7, LON, R 955, 12B/5681/41908; Lasnet to Rajchman, 27 May 1926, LON, R 955, 12B/50934/41908. On the Eastern Bureau, see Tworek, 'Communicable Disease'.

[39] Coghe, 'Inter-Imperial Learning', 144–5.

[40] Mimoso Moreira, 'O problema da Assistência ao Indígena na África ocidental. Entrevista com o Sr. Dr. Damas Mora', O Comércio de Angola, 7 August 1926 (quote). See also António Damas Mora, 'Missão sanitária da S.D.N.', O Século, 3 July 1926; 'Modernos processos de colonização em África', A Província de Angola, 29 September 1926; Mora, 'Assistência Médica ao Indígena (1926)'.

[41] Vicente Ferreira to Minister of Colonies, August 1926, ANTT, Processo individual de António Damas Mora (Proc. 90760 Pt. 1, Cx. 5620).

Yet, as director of the Angolan health services, Damas Mora continued to play a crucial role in shaping and debating inter-imperial learning on health issues at the highest level until the end of his term in 1934.[42] With his active support, Angola and the Belgian Congo concluded a far-reaching sanitary convention in July 1927, which not only stipulated the exchange of epidemiological data on a large group of diseases, but also the creation of bilateral study groups, joint medical missions and regular conferences between hygienists from both colonies.[43] Not all of these provisions were implemented, but at least three bilateral conferences took place in Luanda and Léopoldville between 1928 and 1930 and reports on the sanitary situation in border areas were, despite some irregularities, exchanged until the late 1950s.[44] Furthermore, in 1929, Damas Mora was nominated for the LNHO expert committee on sleeping sickness and, almost simultaneously, commissioned by LNHO director Rajchman to write a report about the problems of the *assistance médicale indigène* in tropical Africa.[45] While these nominations reflected the prestige Damas Mora had gained in Geneva, they also gave him the opportunity to further explore and compare the health policies of colonial powers in Africa. Six months of research at the LNHO headquarters in Geneva and in the colonial ministries in Brussels, Paris and Lisbon led to a voluminous report on health and medicine in the 'intertropical' colonies of West and Central Africa.[46] The report tackled a wide range of issues, from the demographic and economic rationales of African healthcare over the problems of budget and personnel to the outlines of a system of public hygiene suited to tropical Africa. It ended with 27 recommendations imbued with inter-imperial learning and calling for the mutual adoption of 'best practices'.[47] Finally, Damas Mora would also represent Angola in the first 'pan-African' medical conference held in Cape Town under the patronage of the LNHO in 1932.[48]

---

[42] For further detail, see Coghe, *Population Politics (2014)*, 176–84.

[43] The ratified text is included in *DG Série I* (1928), 409–13.

[44] MAEAA, H 4465 (Folder 926, 928–30) and 4466 (Folder 930). See also 'Conferência sanitária luso-belga'.

[45] Damas Mora to Rajchman, 18 September 1929 and Rajchman to Damas Mora, 25 September 1929, LON, R 5855, 8A/15008/687.

[46] The report was received in Geneva in March 1930 (see LON, R 5855, 8A/15008/687), but is lacking in the League of Nations Archives. Copies of various sections of the report can be found in the aforementioned folder, together with the correspondence between Damas Mora and the Health Committee. For two different résumés of the report, see António Damas Mora, 'L'état actuel de l'assistance médicale indigène dans certaines colonies et pays sous mandat de l'Afrique Équatoriale. Résumé du rapport présenté au Comité d'Hygiène', 28 February 1930, AHD-MNE, 3. Piso, Armário 28, Maço 65 and Mora, 'Estado actual'.

[47] Mora, 'État actuel'. This résumé reportedly contains parts of all chapters as well as the entire conclusions.

[48] 'A actuação do delegado de Angola na Conferência Médica do Cabo', *A Província de Angola*, 2 January 1933; Borowy, *Coming to Terms*, 226–30.

These opportunities allowed Damas Mora to further compare colonial health policies in Africa and to identify and adopt best practices. The 1923 conference in Luanda and 1926 study tour, however, were, as the next section will show and Damas Mora himself repeatedly asserted, milestones in his hygienist thinking and determining experiences for the conception of the Angolan AMI scheme.[49]

Implementing Inter-Imperial Learning: AMI and Social Medicine

Obviously, not all the innovations Damas Mora and Ornelas had observed in West Africa were immediately and randomly implemented in Angola. Most of them were still in their infancy in French and British West Africa itself and, above all, emulation was a selective process, for both fundamental and practical reasons. Thus, Damas Mora considered the 'typical' British way of providing healthcare in West Africa inappropriate for Angola, because it was, in his opinion, marked by an unsuitable *laissez-faire* attitude. It assumed that Africans would seek European healthcare of their own accord and focused on improving overall economic and social conditions. In Damas Mora's opinion, the 'Latin' (French, Belgian and Portuguese) approach, which sought to impose Western biomedicine upon the African population, was 'better adapted to the native psychology' and hence more effective at the current stage of the civilising process.[50]

Damas Mora was particularly impressed by how the French in the AOF were addressing the demographic question. Not only were they tackling the fundamental (and interrelated) problems of infant mortality and maternal health through the establishment of 'maternities' (specialised maternity hospitals), crèches and midwife training programmes, they had made the reconstitution and multiplication of the 'native' population the top priority of all departments. It was imperative for Angola to emulate this policy, Damas Mora claimed. As in the AOF, 'all services and not only the Health Services should be geared towards this and prioritise this problem over all others'.[51]

---

[49] See, explicitly, Mora, 'Assistência Médica ao Indígena (1926)', 353 and Mora, 'Prefácio', 19–20.

[50] Mora, 'Assistência Médica ao Indígena (1926)', 354 (quote). See also António Damas Mora, 'Rapport au sujet des services sanitaires de Dakar', 6 June 1926, 21–8, LON, R 955, 12B/58594/41908.

[51] Mora, 'Assistência Médica ao Indígena (1926)', 357, 393–4 and 396; Mora, 'Rapport Dakar', 14 and 34–7; Moreira, 'Problema'; Mora, 'Missão sanitária' (quote).

What Damas Mora described here were core features of the AOF's new AMI orientation. At the initiative of Alexandre Lasnet, one of France's leading colonial hygienists, the Governors-General Merlin and Carde had started to reshape African healthcare from individual, curative treatment to a system of collective and preventive healthcare in the 1920s.[52] New to colonial Africa, this policy shift followed a thrust towards 'social medicine' that had its origins in late nineteenth-century Europe, when hygienists began to promote a new understanding of health that was critical of the predominantly clinical approach to diseases. Influenced by social science, it stressed the social causes of both disease and health and advocated preventive measures to protect the health of the individual and social body.[53] To a large extent, social medicine remained a utopian vision a 'dream, inaccessible and constantly reiterated, of European hygienists'.[54] Yet, in the 1920s and 1930s, ideals of social medicine gained partial acceptance because they were actively promoted, mainly in Europe and Asia, by a powerful international community of public health experts associated with the LNHO and the Rockefeller Foundation, such as LNHO director Ludwik Rajchman.[55]

These ideals also underwrote the reforms that, from November 1926, established the AMI service in Angola. Because of international requirements, official expectations and public pressure, the fight against sleeping sickness was at the heart of these AMI reforms. However, also in the light of Damas Mora's doubts about the unique importance of this disease, the reforms had from the outset a broader scope and more far-reaching goals, which Damas Mora set out in Portugal's leading medical journal *A Medicina Contemporânea*.[56] In three stages, the reforms intended to bring the entire African population under medical surveillance and to make the transition from individual, therapeutic (or 'curative') treatment to a system of collective and preventive healthcare, in other words, social hygiene.[57] As the latter required the collaboration of many government services, the *Comissão de Assistência aos Indígenas* (CAI), the administrative body that took managerial decisions and administered the special fund created with the loan, was presided over by the High Commissioner and comprised the directors of all relevant

---

[52] Cooper, *Public Health*, 74–6.
[53] On the concept and its different definitions, see Porter and Porter, 'What Was Social Medicine?'; Borowy, 'International Social Medicine', 13–4. See also Porter, 'Introduction' and Weindling, 'Social Medicine'.
[54] Lachenal, 'Le médecin qui voulut être roi', 123.
[55] Weindling, 'Social Medicine'; Borowy, 'International Social Medicine'.
[56] Mora, 'Assistência Médica ao Indígena (1926)'.
[57] See Ibid., 355; Mora, 'Assistência Médica aos Indígenas (1927)', 2 and especially Mora, 'Serviços de Saúde em Angola (1928)', 91–4.

departments: Health, Finance, Public Works, Native Affairs and later Agriculture and Religious Missions as well.[58]

In a first stage, as codified in the ground-breaking laws of December 1926 and March 1928, those parts of northern Angola where sleeping sickness was deemed endemic were divided in four zones (Congo-Zaire, Cuanza, Lunda and Benguela), which were further subdivided into a total of 12 and later 15 sectors (see Map 3.1). Within each sector, a gradually expanding network of health centres (*postos sanitários*) and 'village-infirmaries' (*sanzalas-enfermarias*) was established. Each of the zones and sectors was directed by a doctor, while a European or 'native' nurse was placed in charge of the health centres. To reach the population, medical staff did not wait for the sick to come to them, but actively sought out patients within the area they had been assigned. With the help of the administrative authorities, the inhabitants of small groups of villages were told to gather at fixed points within walking distance once or twice a month. At these concentrations (*concentrações*), as they were called, the villagers were examined and received basic treatments, including injections with atoxyl against sleeping sickness and smallpox vaccinations. More complicated cases were sent to the nearest health centre, where they could be accommodated on a voluntary basis in the annexed *sanzala-enfermaria*, with or without family members (see Figure 3.1). While attending concentrations was compulsory and disobedience punishable with forced labour, treatment was free.[59] During the concentrations, the villagers were also counted and registered. This continuous population survey generated a wealth of demographic data and new insights into the composition and evolution of Angola's 'native' population, as shown in Chapter 4.

This scheme of sanitary occupation integrated many features of sleeping sickness campaigns organised throughout colonial Africa. Its territorial design emulated the system of 'prophylactic sectors' that had already been probed by Eugène Jamot in the AEF and French-mandated Cameroon and by Jacques Schwetz in the Belgian Congo. Several communications on this matter were presented at the 1923 Conference in Luanda.[60] The Angolan AMI scheme, however, differed from these predecessors in two important points. First, the duties and responsibilities of the medical staff in the AMI zones and sectors

[58] Vicente Ferreira, 'Diploma Legislativo 452', 20 November 1926, *BOA* (1926), 604–7. See also the member lists in each issue of the *Boletim da Assistência Médica aos Indígenas e da luta contra a moléstia do sono* (1927–9), the services' official Bulletin.
[59] Vicente Ferreira, 'Diploma Legislativo 463', 9 December 1926, *BOA* (1926), 647–52; Vicente Ferreira, 'Diploma Legislativo 744', 24 March 1928, *BOA* (1928), 112–5. For a good overview of how this system was functioning by 1930, see Waldemar Gomes Teixeira, 'Relatório da Zona Sanitária do Cuanza (1930)', June 1931, 5–13, AHU, MU, AGC 2336.
[60] For the AEF, see Headrick, *Colonialism, Health and Illness*, 345–56; for Cameroon, see Letonturier, Tanon and Jamot, 'Maladie du sommeil'; for the Belgian Congo Schwetz, 'Compte-rendu', 152.

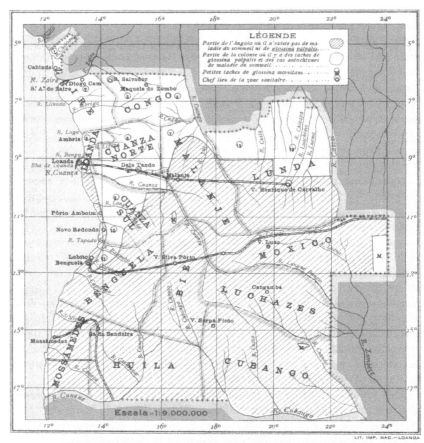

Division sanitaire approximative de l'Angola au point
de vue de la lutte contre la maladie du sommeil :

a) Zone sanitaire de Congo-Zaire :

Secteur de Mayombe
»   » Zaire-Sud
»   » Ouest Congo
»   » Est Congo

b) Zone sanitaire de Cuanza :

Secteur de Ambris Dande
»   » Golungo Dembos
»   » Malanje

Secteur de Cazengo Cambambe
»   » Sud Cuanza
»   » Seles

c) Zone sanitaire de Benguela :

Secteur de Benguela

d) Zone sanitaire de Lunda :

Secteur de Ouest Lunda
»   » Est Lunda

Map 3.1 AMI and sleeping sickness sectors in Angola, 1927–8. Printed on
the front page of the first issue of the *Boletim mensal da luta contra a
propagação da moléstia do sôno e da assistência médica ao indígena* (1927),
this map was composed in French to enhance its international circulation and
sent to the LNHO in 1928.
Source: United Nations Archives at Geneva, LON, S. 1740
Image courtesy of United Nations Archives at Geneva

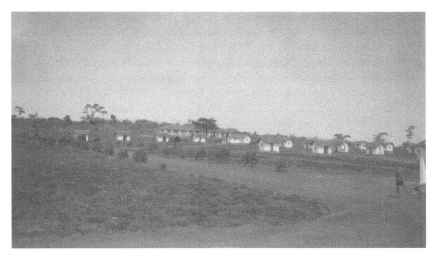

Figure 3.1 *Sanzala-enfermaria* in N'dalatando, the capital of the AMI Cuanza Zone, ca. 1929. The picture shows the small houses built to accommodate the sleeping sick and their families. By 1929, seven *sanzalas-enfermarias* were functioning in the Cuanza zone.[61]
Source: ANTT, Agência Geral do Ultramar, Angola, cx. 5, n.º 4447, PT/TT/AGU/001/004447. See also Ornelas and Mesquita, *Relatório da missão médica*, 164
Image courtesy of ANTT

were not confined to sleeping sickness. Damas Mora had used the 'tool' of prophylactic sleeping sickness sectors to plan and execute a broader programme of rural 'native healthcare', which also included smallpox vaccination, the treatment and prevention of venereal and intestinal diseases, maternal and infant welfare provisions and the propagation of new concepts of hygiene.[62] Soon, Damas Mora and other AMI doctors would claim that this scheme of 'integral' *Assistência Médica aos Indígenas* had been a Portuguese innovation and that this 'Portuguese method', as they termed it, had been adopted only at a later stage by the health services in the Belgian Congo, AEF and Cameroon.[63] Second, the establishment of permanent health centres within

---

[61] Ornelas and Mesquita, *Relatório da missão médica*, 70.

[62] See Vicente Ferreira, 'Diploma Legislativo 463', art. 21 and, for their practical implementation, for instance, Neves and Sousa, 'Assistência Médica aos Indígenas'; Silva, *Serviço de Assistência Congo (1930)*. See also Chapters 4 and 5.

[63] 'Conferência sanitária luso-belga', 381 and 383; Camoesas, 'Organização AMI', 140; Mora, *Luta*, 157; 'Assistência Médica ao Indígena: um diploma', *A Província de Angola*, 9 April 1929.

each sector ensured that Portuguese territorial presence was far more concrete and stable than previously in the French and Belgian 'prophylactic sectors'. After visiting northern Angola in October 1928, Giovanni Trolli, the director of the health services in the Belgian Congo, praised the Portuguese system as a combination of the Belgian mobile missions against sleeping sickness and the rural dispensaries that existed in Eastern Congo.[64]

Confined to northern Angola, the AMI zones and sectors only covered a small part of the colony and, with 400,000 registered Africans by 1930, only about 10 per cent of its estimated population.[65] In order to extend, in a second stage, 'native' healthcare to other regions without overstretching its resources, the CAI also made use of mobile missions *(missões volantes)*. In 1927–8 alone, at least four were dispatched into areas where sleeping sickness occurred rarely, if ever. Small teams of doctors and nurses inspected these areas for several months, vaccinating people against smallpox, treating them for various diseases and conducting anthropological and demographic studies.[66] By early 1928, Damas Mora viewed these mobile services as the future of the *Assistência Médica aos Indígenas* in sparsely populated areas.[67]

Profoundly influenced by his observations in West Africa and ideas of social medicine, Damas Mora considered the first two stages of his AMI project not as a goal in and of themselves, but as preliminary steps in the paradigmatic shift towards social medicine. If one truly wished to tackle the demographic and sanitary issues of Angola at the roots, he reasoned, there was no alternative but to realise the radical shift laid out in the third stage, the stage of collective and preventive hygiene. Here, expensive individual, curative medicine would cease to be a state matter and would instead become a private issue (i.e. a paid service) between doctor and patient. The state health services, on their part, would concentrate on their ultimate goal: caring for the healthy. To realise this Copernican turn, he stated, it would be necessary to actively enter into the lives of the 'natives' and change, through propaganda and education, their habits of hygiene, including practices connected with nutrition, housing and childbirth.[68] Expecting resistance from both the target population and conservative colleagues and administrators, Damas Mora acknowledged that this transition would be long and difficult.[69] Key steps were, in his opinion, the

---

[64] Trolli, 'Impression', 403.

[65] For registration numbers, see Silva, *Serviço de assistência Congo (1930)*, 45 and Teixeira, 'Relatório Cuanza (1930)', 16–17.

[66] For an example, see Silva, 'Relatório missão volante'.

[67] Vicente Ferreira, 'Diploma Legislativo 744', preamble point 4 and art. 6; Mora, 'Serviços de Saúde em Angola (1928)', 92–3.

[68] Mora, 'Assistência Médica aos Indígenas (1927)', 2–3; Mora, 'Serviços de saúde em Angola (1928)', 88 and 93–4.

[69] Ibid., 94.

establishment of maternal and infant welfare services (discussed in Chapter 5) and hygienic model villages.

Damas Mora had particularly high hopes of the latter. Inspired by his experiences during the West African interchange and his AMI work in Timor, he began to advocate for model villages as the most sustainable way to implement preventive and collective healthcare and to regenerate the Angolan population. Under the vigilant eye of medical and administrative authorities, these new villages would be located in healthy environments, with access to clean water and hygienic housing. Though resettlement was voluntary, only married and monogamous couples that medical examinations had proven to be free of communicable and other grave diseases would be admitted. Alcohol would be strictly prohibited and each village would have a 'native' nurse and a midwife trained at the nearest hospital, who would secure basic healthcare and disseminate new health concepts. To enhance its attractiveness for the Angolan population, the scheme also offered economic incentives and special privileges. Each couple would receive a land allocation large enough to nourish a family; all villagers would have access to education and agricultural aid; and fathers would be exempted from compulsory long-distance labour recruitment and military conscription. This burden would fall exclusively on men aged 18–22, who would thus constitute the large, vigorous and growing labour reservoir needed for the colonial economy.[70]

Damas Mora's plans for model villages, which he set out in newspaper interviews, journal articles and medical reports from 1926 onwards, epitomised his hygienic thinking. They reflected ideas about rural hygiene that were increasingly pushed by RF and LNHO in the 1920s and 1930s, mostly in Europe and Asia, as well as some eugenicist thinking that was often part of social medicine.[71] Above all, his plans understood hygiene in a very broad sense, as they connected solving sanitary and demographic problems to economic and social reforms such as agricultural production and labour recruitment. If model villages were fashioned according to his proposals, they would indeed improve what would later be conceptualised as the 'social determinants of health', such as living environment, housing, nutrition, income, education and access to infant and general healthcare.[72] Accordingly, Damas Mora was convinced that the success of the project hinged on the same kind of interdepartmental collaboration he had previously observed and praised in the AOF.

---

[70] References to this project can be found in António Damas Mora, 'Missão sanitária da S.D.N.', *O Século*, 3 July 1926; Mora, 'Assistance Médicale Indigène (1928)', 1336–7; Mora, 'Services de l'assistance', 16–7; Mora, 'Serviços de saúde em Angola (1928)', 93; 'Uma entrevista com o sr. dr. Antonio Damas Mora', *A Província de Angola*, 1 January 1929; Mora, 'État actuel', 40–1. The most elaborate sketch is Mora, 'Notas sobre um estatuto'.

[71] Borowy, *Coming to Terms*, 325–60; Packard, *History of Global Health*, 66–88.

[72] On this concept, see Cook, Bhattacharya and Hardy (eds.), *History*.

If all services, notably Health, Public Works, Agriculture, Native Affairs and the Territorial Administration, worked together, the project would embody the solution to all sanitary problems and prompt sustained population growth.[73]

Staffing the AMI Services

On a practical level, the expansion of the AMI system was only possible with a growing medical staff. For decades, the shortage of qualified medical personnel had been the subject of relentless complaints and one of the main hindrances to the expansion of European biomedicine. After the First World War, structural reforms had attempted to facilitate the recruitment of colonial doctors. In 1919, after many years of discussion, the Angolan health services were eventually separated from the army and given a civil organisation with administrative autonomy. This meant that newly recruited doctors and nurses were no longer in military service.[74] In 1921, further administrative reform considerably raised their salaries.[75] Due to these reforms and a growing health budget, the number of government doctors in Angola doubled from 25 to 51 between 1921 and 1923.[76]

By 1926, however, these reforms were not deemed sufficient to staff the AMI services. As in other colonies in tropical Africa, doctors who came to Angola competed for the best posts within the colony and most were reluctant to accept positions in the AMI sectors, where they could expect hard work, little comfort and very few lucrative private patients. To remedy this situation, the *Comissão de Assistência Indígena* offered high bonuses as compensation for the lack of private patients – a measure that was controversial, but praised as very effective by Giovanni Trolli.[77]

To further fill the ranks, the AMI service also tapped intra-imperial migrations and networks. It employed several doctors, pharmacists and nurses who had been deported to Angola because of their opposition to the military regime and/or participation in the pro-republican 'Reviralho' revolts that had erupted in Portugal after the 1926 coup.[78] The most famous of these was the former Minister of Education João Camoesas. Camoesas had initially been banished

---

[73] For more details, see Coghe, 'Reordering Colonial Society', 16–24.

[74] Governo Geral de Angola, 'Portaria 55-B', 1 March 1919, *BOA* (1919), 13–22 and Mora, 'Organisations sanitaires', 178. Compare with Leitão, *Serviço de saúde*, 34–6.

[75] Compare the tables in Norton de Matos, 'Decreto 74', 17 November 1921, *BOA Série I* (1921), 306–18 with those in Ministério das Colónias, 'Decreto 5.727 sobre a reorganização dos serviços de saúde das colónias', 10 May 1919, *DG Série I* (1919), 1143–5.

[76] Mora, 'Organisations sanitaires', 181; Matos, *Província de Angola*, 86–7.

[77] Vicente Ferreira, 'Diploma Legislativo 463', art. 8–10; Mora, 'Estado actual', 34–5; Trolli, 'Impression', 404.

[78] See the list in Martins, 'Relatório Inspecção Hospital Central', 177–8. On the revolts, see Farinha, *Reviralho*.

to São Tomé, but Damas Mora, who admired Camoesas's work as a social hygienist in Lisbon, relocated him to Angola and won him over to the AMI project. In 1928, Camoesas assumed the direction of the AMI services' monthly *Boletim* and wrote several influential reports and articles on public health in Angola.[79]

In 1927–8, the AMI services also hired seven young graduates from the Medical School of Goa, capitalising on the long-standing ties between the school and Portugal's African colonies.[80] Since its foundation in 1842, dozens of graduates had filled the ranks of the medical staff in Angola, Mozambique, and Guinea. Given the limited career chances of its graduates in Portugal and Goa itself, the school had increasingly specialised in tropical diseases and promoted its doctors as ideal intermediaries for Portugal's African medical mission. However, they mostly remained in subordinate positions, due to a mixture of racial discrimination and a refusal to fully recognise non-metropolitan degrees.[81] This was still the case in the late 1920s. Although the new Goan recruits were valued and given significant responsibilities within the AMI services – some were even appointed head of sector or, like Bruno de Mesquita, director of the central laboratory of the Cuanza zone (see Figure 3.2) – they were only employed as 'auxiliary doctors', with temporary contracts and low salaries.[82]

This intra-imperial recruitment scheme bore striking similarities to British, French and Belgians employing colonial subjects and non-national doctors in their sleeping sickness and AMI services in the 1920s: subordinate Syrian doctors in the Anglo-Egyptian Sudan, Russian *hygiénistes adjoints* in the AEF and Italian doctors *hors cadre* and other foreign *médecins compléments* in the Belgian Congo. Underwritten by racial prejudice and ideas of European superiority, all these schemes aimed to expand colonial health services without overstretching limited budgets.[83]

However, the Portuguese did not follow the French and the British when they established medical schools for Africans in some of their colonies, most notably in Dakar (Senegal, 1918), Makerere (Uganda, 1923–4), Khartoum

---

[79] See the correspondence in AHU, MU, GM 2832; Mora, *Publicações médicas*, 18–9. On Camoesas' career, see Bandeira, 'Camoesas'.

[80] Mora, 'Serviços de Saúde em Angola (1928)', 88. For short biographies of some of these doctors, see Costa, 'Médicos da Escola de Goa', n. 58, 14–6.

[81] Bastos, 'Doctors for the Empire'; Bastos, 'Ensino da medicina', 33–5. For Goan doctors in Angola, see 'Livro Mestre do Quadro de Saúde de Angola, 1858–1913', AHU, SEMU, DGAPC 895 and Costa, 'Médicos da Escola de Goa', n. 58, 3–10. For the better-studied cases of Mozambique and Guinea, see Bastos, 'Medical Hybridisms', 774–7 and Havik, 'Bóticas e beberagens', 254.

[82] 'Médicos da Escola da Índia'.

[83] Bell, *Frontiers of Medicine*, 40–8; Headrick, *Colonialism, Health and Illness*, 229, 244, 364; Trolli, *Rapport Hygiène Publique (1928)*, 4.

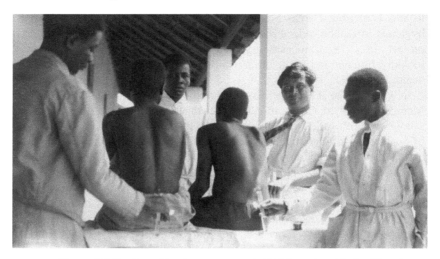

Figure 3.2 Session of lumbar punctures in N'dalatando with the (Goan)
director of the laboratory, Bruno de Mesquita (2nd right), and 'native' nurses,
ca. 1929.
Source: ANTT, Agência Geral do Ultramar, Angola, cx. 5, n.º 4455, PT/TT/AGU/001/
004455. See also Ornelas and Mesquita, *Relatório da missão médica*, 95
Image courtesy of ANTT

(Sudan, 1924) or Yaba (Nigeria, 1930), thus producing further cheap and
subordinate *aide-médecins* or *native medical assistants*.[84] This question was
also hotly debated in Angola. Quoting Jérôme Rodhain, the health director in
the Belgian Congo, Damas Mora in 1923 acknowledged that it was impossible
to indefinitely increase the number of European doctors and hence imperative
to 'assist the natives with natives'. However, disagreeing with Norton de
Matos and the Goan doctor Germano Correia, he eventually concluded that,
just like in the AEF and the Belgian Congo, neither social conditions nor
preparatory education were advanced enough in Angola for such a school.[85]
Only in 1962, a year after the outbreak of the anti-colonial revolt, would
university courses, including medicine, be established in Angola, and even
then, most students were white.[86]

[84] See Blanchard, 'Formation'; Iliffe, *East African Doctors*, 60–91; Lyons, 'Power to Heal'; Bell,
Frontiers of Medicine, 48–50 and Patton, *Physicians*, 33.
[85] Compare Correia, 'Processos práticos', 194–200; Mora, 'Raison d'être', 55 with Mora,
'Assistência Médica ao Indígena (1926)', 393–4 (quote) and especially António Damas
Mora, 'Serviços de Saúde e Higiene. Considerações finais', *A Província de Angola*,
27 June 1934.
[86] Carvalho, Kajibanga and Heimer, 'Angola'.

Overall, the new recruitment strategies bore fruit. By the end of 1928, the number of government doctors in Angola had further increased to 95, 36 of whom worked in the AMI zones and sectors.[87] Although this number was still very small for a population estimated at several millions, Angola compared very favourably with its neighbours.[88] In 1929, French Equatorial Africa employed only 51 doctors for roughly 3 million African inhabitants and the Belgian Congo about 120 for a population estimated at approximately three times that of Angola.[89] These and other statistics reveal that Angola had one of the best government doctor-to-population ratios in West and Central Africa in the late 1920s.[90] Moreover hygienists like Damas Mora and João Camoesas had come to believe that the transition to preventive healthcare would substantially diminish the need for European doctors. Whereas a 'clinical' doctor could only assure individual treatment to 3,000 people, a well-trained and well-equipped mobile hygienist would be able to assist 50,000–100,000 people, they assumed. Forty to 60 hygienists would thus be enough to cover Angola's entire 'native' population. Social medicine, they claimed, would solve the interrelated problems of recruitment and the increasing strain the health services placed on the colony's budgets.[91]

Another part of the solution was seen in the increasing use of cheap African nurses. Until the First World War, most nurses were recruited in Portugal, but in the late 1910s, courses for 'native nurses' (*enfermeiros indígenas*) became firmly established at the Nursing School of the Central Hospital in Luanda.[92] Nurses were probably also trained ad hoc in the AMI sectors. Colonial doctors highlighted their potential for the AMI services. Compared to European nurses, Firmino Sant'Anna stated, they were not only 'more resistant to the climate [and] less demanding with regard to salaries', but also 'of [particular] benefit to the service of native assistance, given the fact that they speak the same language [as the locals] and hence can influence the mind of the natives so that these follow the concepts of hygiene to which they are naturally opposed'.[93] The praises of African nurses as interpreters and cultural brokers who facilitated the acceptance of Western biomedicine were occasionally sung

---

[87] Compare Mora, 'Organisations sanitaires', 181 with 'Conferência sanitária luso-belga', 380.

[88] On population estimates, see Chapter 4.

[89] Headrick, *Colonialism, Health and Illness*, 228, 407; Trolli, *Rapport Hygiène Publique (1929)*, 6.

[90] See the comparative numbers in Headrick, *Colonialism, Health and Illness*, 407 and Mora, 'État actuel', 34.

[91] Mimoso Moreira, 'Assistência médica aos indígenas', *A Província de Angola*, 10 January 1930; Mora, 'État actuel', 10–1, 20–1.

[92] Castro, 'Preparação e aperfeiçoamento', 2871–4.

[93] Sant'Anna, 'Problema da assistência', 164.

in medical reports from the AMI sectors.[94] However, their position within the AMI services was, again partly due to racial prejudice, complicated and ambivalent.

On the one hand, it is questionable to what extent African nurses embraced the role assigned to them by European doctors. As Walima Kalusa has argued, to consider African nurses merely agents of medical imperialism reifies the writings of European doctors and does not attend to the spaces of agency these auxiliary workers carved out for themselves.[95] On the other hand, European doctors acknowledged and feared that very agency. Many programmatic treatises and medical reports emphasised that African nurses were only valuable in subordinate positions, under the strict control of European doctors or nurses. It was commonly believed that they were good at mastering basic techniques such as injections, but that it was far more difficult to instil them with a stable sense of morality. It was often suggested that many would abuse their power and even turn to extortion if they were left to manage a local health station on their own.[96] It was also feared that, in their 'traditional' environment, they would gradually strip away the basic principles of Western biomedicine that for them had only been a 'thin layer of varnish' and return to their 'ancient practices of fetishism and charlatanism'.[97] However, the shortage of European staff often left African nurses in command of AMI health stations all the same.[98]

Moreover, 'native' nurses in the interwar years formed a distinct group (*quadro*) within the medical staff, with fewer career opportunities and much lower pay than their white colleagues, even if many of them were now recruited from the growing settler population in Angola itself and trained on the same course as Africans.[99] In the 1930s, some senior African nurses protested against this discrimination in newspaper articles and petitions to the Governor-General and even the Minister of Colonies. They also pointed to the contradictory use of the term 'native nurses', arguing that the general laws in the colony would consider many of them to be non-native because of their education and Europeanised customs.[100] Only in 1945 did the creation of

[94] See, for instance, Gama, 'Missão volante', 64; 'A obra da assistência ao indígena no Congo', *A Província de Angola*, 16 March 1929.

[95] Kalusa, 'Language'. See also Lyons, 'Power to Heal', 212; 219–22.

[96] See, for instance, Almeida, 'Relatório Congo', 42–3; Mora, 'Assistência Médica ao Indígena (1926)', 394; Costa, 'Relatório Cuanza Norte', 34. See also Lyons, 'Power to Heal', 210–3.

[97] Sant'Anna, 'Problema da assistência', 164–5 (quotes).

[98] See, for instance, Mora, *Luta*, 65–6, 193–6, 219.

[99] Norton de Matos, 'Decreto 74', 17 November 1921, *BOA Série I* (1921), 306–18, art. 19, 34 and 44.

[100] See, for instance, Luis Abel Traça, 'Enfermeiros indígenas', *A Província de Angola*, 7 June 1932; 'Os enfermeiros nativos'; 'O caso dos enfermeiros nativos'. See also Conselho do Império Colonial, 'Parecer 53 (2a Secção)', 28 October 1940, AHU, CIC, Livro de Pareceres 1940.

non-racialised *quadros* of nurses and assistant nurses eliminate this discrimination, at least legally.[101] Despite these conflicts and ambivalences, the number of African nurses in government service grew from 76 in 1923 to 166 in 1938, of which 93 were fully trained and 73 (paid) trainees. Their number was now higher than that of European nurses (115 in 1923 and 110 in 1938) and most of them (108) worked in the AMI sectors.[102]

Eradicating Sleeping Sickness: Preventive Mass Atoxylisation, National Prestige and the Limits of Inter-Imperial Learning

The Copernican turn towards prevention would also permeate the Portuguese approach to sleeping sickness in Angola, which, as I have already indicated, was the (initial) cornerstone of the AMI programme. The shift from curing the sick to protecting the healthy was already palpable in French and Belgian anti-sleeping sickness efforts. Here, doctors adopted Koch's approach of 'treatment as prevention' or 'therapeutic prophylaxis', which consisted in 'sterilising' the blood of all infected individuals with atoxyl (or newer drugs like tryparsamide) to make them non-infectious and hence protect the healthy. Following Koch, they believed that, just like physical isolation, this would interrupt the human-fly infection cycle and thus help to contain and possibly even eradicate the disease.[103] In Angola, the approach was preventive in a still more direct sense, as atoxylisation was not confined to the infected part of the population, but extended to all healthy individuals.

Preventive mass atoxylisation was introduced right from the start of the AMI programme in December 1926 by Dr Alfredo Gomes da Costa, the first director of the Cuanza zone.[104] It consisted of two steps. First, on the basis of a clinical diagnosis, which mainly consisted in palpating the – in the case of sleeping sickness, often (but not always) enlarged – cervical lymph nodes, the people at the concentrations were divided into two groups: healthy and sick including suspected sick. Second, all individuals suspected of having sleeping sickness were given a series of curative injections of atoxyl (often in combination with emetics) or newer drugs, while all those considered healthy received a differently dosed and spaced series of preventive atoxyl injections. The standard *prophylactic* procedure was a series of 10 (later six) injections of 0.5 g. of atoxyl every two weeks. In the Congo zone, where concentrations

---

[101] Ministério das Colónias, 'Decreto 34.417 que reorganiza os serviços de saúde do Império Colonial Português', 21 February 1945, *DG Série I* (1945), 95–111.

[102] Compare the figures in Mora, 'Organisations sanitaires', 181 and *Boletim Sanitário de Angola* 1 (1937–8), 27 and 57.

[103] Lachenal, 'Genealogy', 76–80; Tousignant, 'Trypanosomes', esp. 631; Headrick, *Colonialism, Health and Illness*, 311–84; Mertens, *Chemical Compounds*, 74–5, 84–5, 95–7, 197–234. See also Chapter 2.

[104] Costa, 'Relatório Cuanza Norte', 31–3.

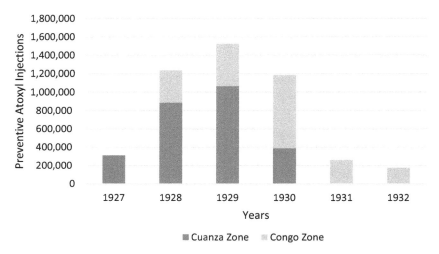

Figure 3.3 Number of preventive atoxyl injections in Angola, 1926–32.
Sources: Ornelas and Mesquita, *Relatório da missão médica*, 67–9; Teixeira, 'Relatório Cuanza (1930)', 58; Silva, *Serviço de assistência Congo (1930)*, 46; Mora, 'Prefácio', 24; 28; Mora, *Luta*, passim

could usually only be held once a month, doctors resorted to monthly injections of 1 g. The series were repeated at increasing intervals of three, four and six months, so as not to exceed the total dose of atoxyl considered safe.[105]

In the late 1920s, preventive mass atoxylisation became the most salient, but also most contested feature of Angola's anti-sleeping sickness programme. By the end of 1927, Gomes da Costa's team had already administered some 300,000 preventive injections.[106] From 1928 onwards, the measure was also adopted in parts of the Congo zone and the total number of annual registered preventive injections rose to more than a million between 1928 and 1930, before the method was gradually abandoned in the early 1930s (see Figure 3.3). Although overlooked by historiography, this was, with almost 5 million preventive injections administered between 1926 and 1932 to a (registered) population of about 400,000 Angolans, the first scheme of mass chemoprophylaxis against sleeping sickness in tropical Africa. After the Second World War, the same idea would be implemented on an even larger scale in various parts of West and Central Africa with another trypanocidal drug, pentamidine.[107]

---

[105] Good descriptions of this method can be found in 'Conferência sanitária luso-belga', 381; Ornelas and Mesquita, *Relatório da missão médica*, 78–9; Teixeira, 'Relatório Cuanza (1930)', 57–8, 63–4; Silva, *Serviço de assistência Congo (1930)*, 17–8.

[106] Mora, 'Assistência Médica aos Indígenas (1927)', 6.

[107] Lachenal, *Médicament* and Coghe, 'Sleeping Sickness Control', 79–88. See also Epilogue.

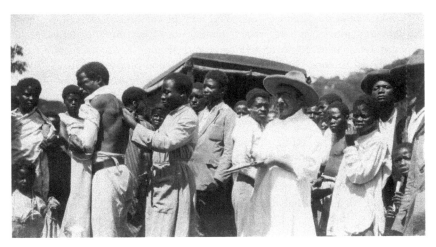

Figure 3.4 'Prophylactic session' in the Cazengo region, ca. 1929. African nurse injecting drugs, most probably atoxyl.
Source: ANTT, Agência Geral do Ultramar, Angola, cx. 5, n.º 4458, PT/TT/AGU/001/ 004458. See also Ornelas and Mesquita, *Relatório da missão médica*, 87
Image courtesy of ANTT

Preventive mass atoxylisation capitalised on the well-known advantages of atoxyl that had made it the preferred drug for 'treatment as prevention' campaigns after the First World War. Not only could atoxyl be used to break the fly-human transmission cycle as it destroyed the trypanosomes in the blood, but it was also suitable for massive use in the field: it was cheap and easy to administer in that European doctors entrusted African nurses with the subcutaneous injections, usually between the shoulder blades (see Figure 3.4).[108] By injecting healthy people on a massive scale, however, the scheme ignored the equally well-known disadvantages of the drug: the often severe side effects and the arsenic resistance caused by its long-term use. The rapid decomposition of the drug in the human body also required a high frequency of injections, which was prone to trigger popular resistance and almost impossible to achieve under field conditions. With the exception of German doctors, who had applied preventive mass atoxylisation in some heavily infested parts of Cameroon in 1913–14, these disadvantages had thus far prevented colonial health services from setting up campaigns of mass chemoprophylaxis with atoxyl.[109]

---

[108] See, for instance, Headrick, *Colonialism, Health and Illness*, 319–20, 330–1.
[109] See Sicé, *Trypanosomiase humaine*, 270. For the Germans, see Isobe, *Medizin und Kolonialgesellschaft*, 255–6. See also Chapter 2.

Doubts about the adequacy of atoxyl and the method of clinical diagnosis explain the reluctance with which Gomes da Costa initially defended his scheme. He considered preventive mass atoxylisation as an emergency measure designed to cope with extremely high infection rates of up to 27–30 per cent in some areas of the Cuanza zone. Given the choice 'between the mad empiricism of mass atoxylisation and the disappearance and degeneration [of the population] we observed in the native villages, we opted for the former', he noted in his first annual report.[110] Yet, as infection rates in atoxylised areas were reported to be falling quickly,[111] leading doctors like António Damas Mora began to see preventive mass atoxylisation as more than an ad hoc solution. They stressed the scientific basis of what they now considered a promising new method. In their opinion, continuous atoxylisation interrupted the transmission cycle between flies and humans in a twofold way, rendering the bodies of infected people non-infectious and protecting the healthy for up to six months after the last injection.[112] They also rationalised the reliance on clinical diagnosis, which had actually been a consequence of the shortage of both microscopes and well-trained (African) microscopists, arguing that microscopic diagnosis was a time-consuming and untrustworthy method that left many positive cases undiagnosed.[113]

Although there was no experimental evidence for long-term individual protection, let alone a detailed scientific explication of how it worked, this was not a surprising claim. With its 'double protection' of the healthy, preventive mass atoxylisation seemed to fulfil the ultimate dream of prevention fostered by interwar social hygienists like Damas Mora. It fitted perfectly within his general healthcare strategy for Angola. Atoxyl's harmful side effects were downplayed and did not constitute sufficient reason to end preventive atoxylisation in Angola, just like it continued to be used in 'therapeutic prophylaxis' campaigns in other colonies, revealing to what extent the necessity and legitimacy of such a shift had pervaded interwar colonial medicine.[114] With regard to 'native' Africans, most colonial doctors agreed to subordinate individual health risks to the greater good of collective health and security.

Some Portuguese doctors even became convinced that preventive mass atoxylisation could eradicate the disease and hence was superior to the

---

[110] Costa, 'Relatório Cuanza Norte', 32–3 (here also quotes). See also Alfredo Gomes da Costa, 'Combate à doença do sono', *Portugal. Órgão do Nacionalismo Português em Angola* (hereafter *Portugal*), 22 February 1930.

[111] See, for instance, Ornelas and Mesquita, *Relatório da missão médica*, 78–9; Teixeira, 'Relatório Cuanza (1930)', 61.

[112] Mora, *Luta*, 62–4, 186.

[113] Santos, 'Relatório Congo-Oeste (1927)', 173; Silva, *Serviço de Assistência Congo (1930)*, 18.

[114] See, for instance, Costa, 'Relatório Cuanza Norte', 33. One doctor later admitted frequent 'toxic accidents' with atoxyl. See Albuquerque, 'Combate', 173. On the downplaying of atoxyl accidents, see also Headrick, *Colonialism, Health and Illness*, 330–1.

methods of other colonial powers. Thus Joaquim Pires dos Santos, the doctor in charge of the Western Congo sector between 1927 and 1929 and member of a medical research mission to Catete in 1930–1, wrote that eradication efforts in other colonies had thus far all failed because doctors had been too cautious. By restricting injections to microscopically diagnosed cases only, they had – given the slowness and inaccuracy of such diagnosis – left many infected people untreated. Only the combination of curative injections for all suspects and prophylactic injections for all others could eliminate trypanosomes from their human reservoirs and break the transmission cycle, he claimed.[115] Driven by the same conviction, Damas Mora triumphantly wrote to LNHO director Rajchman in March 1929 that 'where preventive atoxylisation is systematic-ally applied, cases of sleeping sickness fully disappear. It is,' he emphasised, 'the victory of the system of preventive mass atoxylisation over that of the periodic scrutiny of a region and the treatment of the diseased only, as it is practised in the Belgian Congo and elsewhere'.[116] Later, he would characterise preventive mass atoxylisation as the 'Portuguese method'.[117]

Damas Mora's enthusiasm for mass atoxylisation was also closely linked with his and other doctors' growing insight that sleeping sickness incidence in Angola was – still or again – far higher than expected. Initially, the surveys of 1927, with 'only' 3,805 new verified cases, confirmed his long-standing intuition that 'the problem of sleeping sickness in Angola' had lost 'the acute dimensions it had possessed twenty years ago'. This led him to predict, in both the Portuguese and Belgian medical press, a maximum of 5,000 cases in the whole colony, 'a small percentage for a population of 3.6 million inhabit-ants'.[118] Over the course of 1928, however, surveys covered more and more of the Congo-Zaire zone, where they revealed local infection rates of up to 75 per cent and more than 17,000 new cases, totalling 18,966 for Angola as a whole. It was in 'this still quite densely populated area' now 'threatened by a sleeping sickness *débacle* similar to the one that [had] decimated the population of Cuanza-Norte' that the new prophylactic measures had to show what they were worth, Damas Mora claimed.[119]

While mass atoxylisation was said to be extremely effective in crushing infection rates, hopes of eradication were not met. Due to internal dissent,

---

[115] See Pires dos Santos in Amaral, *Relatório Catete (1930–31)*, 71–89; 'Assistência Médica aos Indígenas – Sector Congo Oeste'. For similar hopes, see Silva, *Serviço de Assistência Congo (1930)*, 18–20.

[116] Damas Mora to Rajchman, 12 March 1929, LON, R 5854, 8A/8999/687.

[117] Mora, *Luta*, 62 and 233.

[118] Mora, 'Assistance Médicale Indigène (1928)', 1334 (quotes). Similarly, Mora, 'Services de l'assistance', 15.

[119] Mora, 'Dos Serviços de Assistência aos Indígenas', 28 (quotes); Neves and Sousa, 'Assistência Médica aos Indígenas', 438; Mora, *Luta*, 148, 231.

preventive mass atoxylisation was abandoned in the early 1930s. Within the Angolan health services, mass atoxylisation had never met with unanimous enthusiasm: aware of diverging practices and debates in other colonies, doctors opposed the 'unscientific' character of the diagnostic method and the choice of atoxyl. Some, such as Waldemar Gomes Teixeira and Luís Pinto da Fonseca, did not apply the scheme in their sectors.[120] Indeed, by the late 1920s, leading Belgian doctors had ceased to defend clinical diagnosis and joined the French in their preference for laboratorial diagnosis (microscopic examination of blood, lymph fluid and cerebrospinal fluid), even if this was not always possible in practice.[121] Moreover, both French and Belgian colonial doctors had grown very critical of atoxyl. While this drug continued to be used in the field, they focused their hopes for sleeping sickness control on new drugs: they had declared tryparsamide their new drug of choice for therapeutic prophylaxis and begun to test direct prophylaxis with 'Bayer 205' or suramin.[122] As trials with suramin seemed to provide a preventive effect at the individual level, the delegates at the Second International Conference on Sleeping Sickness in Paris in 1928 recommended suramin, and not atoxyl, for the protection of healthy individuals.[123] In the 1930s and during the Second World War, the Belgians applied mass preventive bayerisation in some highly infected areas.[124]

Resistance to mass preventive atoxylisation gained momentum in 1929, when a new High Commissioner critical of the costs of mass health campaigns was installed and Damas Mora temporarily went back to Europe.[125] In May 1929, the new head of the Cuanza zone, João Augusto Ornelas, issued a circular letter announcing the end of the first 'empirical' phase of the anti-sleeping sickness campaign (the phase of 'assault'), and the start of the 'scientific' second phase, characterised by generalised laboratorial analysis and the restriction of atoxyl injections to suspected or verified cases only.[126] Simultaneously, a long anonymous article with the same claim and some of the same phrases appeared in Angola's leading newspaper *A Província de Angola*, probably also by Ornelas.[127] Many doctors in the Cuanza zone supported this 'scientific turn': at the first *journées médicales* held in Dalatando a few months

---

[120] See Waldemar Gomes Teixeira, 'Doença do sono,' *Portugal*, 26 February 1930.
[121] Mertens, *Chemical Compounds*, 212, 229–30, 237–9.
[122] Abbatucci, 'Révolution thérapeutique'; Trolli, 'Traitement', esp. 333. See also Mertens, *Chemical Compounds*, 141–59.
[123] Ibid., 135–7; Headrick, *Colonialism, Health and Illness*, 327–9; League of Nations Health Organisation, *Report (1928)*, 9–10.
[124] Mertens, *Chemical Compounds*, 137, 188; Lachenal, *Médicament*, 44–5.
[125] See later in this chapter.
[126] See Ornelas and Mesquita, *Relatório da missão médica*, 74–8.
[127] 'A luta contra a doença do sono nos sectores de profilaxia da Zona Sanitária do Cuanza,' *A Província de Angola*, 25, 26, 29 April and 3, 7 May 1929.

later, the participants adopted a corresponding motion.[128] These decisions, however, were apparently overruled, as both mass atoxylisation and protests against it continued.

Mass atoxylisation was only phased out some months later, in the wake of a violent dispute involving various leading AMI doctors writing in the new nationalist Luanda newspaper *Portugal*. This dispute not only illustrates how actors on both sides used international comparisons to bolster their 'scientific' claims, but the course and outcome of the debate also reveal how far the mass atoxylisation scheme had become entangled with ideas of national prestige and representation. Indeed, just like its rise, the fall of the preventive mass atoxylisation scheme cannot be understood through scientific arguments alone: how the actors framed the scheme within a context of inter-imperial comparison and competition was decisive.

The instigator of the debate was Eurico de Almeida, the young and much-praised director of the medical laboratory of the Cuanza zone.[129] In January 1930, in the absence of Damas Mora, he represented Angola in the second bilateral meeting with the health services of the Belgian Congo, which was anticipated by the 1927 Luso-Belgian Sanitary Convention.[130] Upon his return from Léopoldville, Almeida published a series of articles in the new Luanda-based newspaper *Portugal* in which he argued that the French-Belgian way of dealing with sleeping sickness compared very favourably with the Angolan scheme, since it was based on microscopic diagnosis, differential treatments according to disease stages and more cautious use of trypanocidal drugs. In Almeida's opinion, this scheme not only allowed for a more adequate treatment of the sick, but the restricted use of atoxyl also greatly diminished the costs of the campaign and the risk of arseno-resistant trypanosomes. It was imperative, he concluded, that Angola adhered to the superior and cheaper methods of their scientifically acclaimed neighbours.[131]

Almeida's call for a scientific turn was not new and echoed Ornelas' earlier appeal, but his public criticism of the Angolan scheme as inferior raised a storm of nationalist protest, which ultimately delegitimised his claim. In public responses in this and other Angolan newspapers, fellow doctors replied that the superiority of the French-Belgian method had not yet been proven or that this method was not as uniform and universally applied as Almeida asserted.[132]

[128] See Eurico de Almeida, 'Doença do sono', *Portugal*, 25 February 1930.
[129] See for instance the laudatory preface by Dr Carlos de Almeida, one of his later opponents, in Almeida, *Laboratório*.
[130] 'Relações luso-belgas', *Portugal*, 18 January 1930.
[131] His articles appeared in *Portugal* on 15, 17, 25, 26, 28 February and 7 and 10 March 1930.
[132] Costa, 'Combate'; Waldemar Gomes Teixeira, 'Doença do sono,' *Portugal*, 26 February 1930; Avelino Manuel da Silva, 'Doença do sono: uma carta', *A Província de Angola*, 8 and 9 May 1930.

They also defended the accomplishments of mass atoxylisation and, more generally, highlighted Portugal's historical achievements in the fight against sleeping sickness. The problem was that Almeida had gone public. Waldemar Gomes Teixeira, for instance, who opposed clinical diagnosis and preventive atoxylisation from the outset, now publicly defended the scheme, concluding his article by paraphrasing Salazar: 'In the struggle against sleeping sickness, the knowledge and competence of our doctors are not less valuable than those of our neighbours, and they are sufficient to fight the scourge.'[133] Carlos de Almeida, the former head of the Congo sleeping sickness mission, even exhorted Damas Mora to dismiss his 'denationalised' colleague who had, first in Léopoldville and then in the Angolan press, diminished the prestige of the Angolan health services.[134]

Upon Damas Mora's return to Angola, Eurico de Almeida was indeed forced to leave the Angolan health services. He was transferred to São Tomé and later to Guinea. Interestingly, however, Damas Mora presented this to his Belgian counterpart Trolli as prompted by Almeida's criticism of the medical infrastructure and lack of cleanliness in Léopoldville, and not his persistent calls for inter-imperial borrowing.[135] The newspaper debate shows that conditions for inter-imperial learning had changed. While Damas Mora had been very successful in buttressing his reform plans with overt international comparisons in the mid-1920s, this was apparently no longer accepted in 1930, a time when the emerging *Estado Novo* was pushing the idea of Portugal's imperial greatness and, partly due to the world economic crisis, nationalism and inter-imperial competition grew fiercer again.[136]

The importance of national prestige was also obvious in the official explanation given when the scheme was phased out shortly afterwards. This happened first in the Cuanza zone, where in July 1930 its new director Waldemar Teixeira decreed the general use of laboratorial diagnosis and limited preventive mass atoxylisation to heavily infested areas only, and then in 1931–2 in the Congo zone as well. Significantly, the doctors in charge did not legitimise their decision with a fundamental critique of the method, as Almeida had done, but by pointing to its success. Mass atoxylisation, they asserted, had reduced infection rates to such an extent that it had made itself superfluous.[137] This was clearly a polished version of the truth: in his

---

[133] Waldemar Gomes Teixeira, 'Doença do sono'.

[134] Carlos de Almeida, 'Carta aberta', *A Província de Angola*, 4 April 1930.

[135] Speech by Damas Mora and Compte-Rendu de la 3ième Conférence médicale luso-belge tenue à Léopoldville, both 17 September 1930, MAEAA, H 4465, Folder 929. For Almeida's critique of health conditions in Léopoldville, see 'Combate à doença do sono', *Portugal*, 15 and 17 February 1930.

[136] See Introduction.

[137] For the Cuanza zone, see 'Circular Letter 434' in Teixeira, 'Relatório Cuanza (1930)', 55–7. For the Congo zone, see Silva, *Serviço de assistência Congo (1931)*, 28 and the accounts by Damas Mora and Simões do Amaral in Mora, *Luta*, 210–3, 220.

(unpublished) report, Waldemar Teixeira cast serious doubts on the efficiency of the scheme. He claimed that, due to the long pauses between each series of injections, preventive atoxylisation had, at best, protected the population for only three months per year. Moreover, he did not trust the official statistics and suspected the real number of new infections to be considerably higher. If there had been a decline, in his opinion this was due to the treatment of diagnosed victims rather than the systematic atoxylisation of the whole population.[138]

The Boundaries of the *Assistência Médica aos Indígenas*

The gradual abandonment of preventive mass atoxylisation resulted from internal dissent within the medical services. It reflected the diverging views among doctors of how, against the background of inter-imperial comparison and exchange, the scheme either increased or diminished Portugal's national prestige. It also coincided with a broader and politically motivated attack against the AMI programme as a whole, which in 1929–30 arrested its rapid expansion.

While the AMI reforms had enjoyed the continuous support of High Commissioner Vicente Ferreira (1926–8), his successor Filomeno da Câmara (1929–30) felt that the programme was too ambitious and too expensive for Angola and on the verge of financial collapse due to financial mismanagement.[139] In vain, AMI proponents insisted that the expenses were commensurate with the colony's resources and that they would be more than compensated for by the manifold 'political, administrative, economic, social and biological advantages' the programme would produce.[140] Under Filomeno da Câmara, the entire AMI programme suffered severe financial and organisational cuts: through several consecutive decrees, the CAI was abolished; the yearly budget of the AMI services more than halved; the bonus system for AMI doctors curtailed; the integral approach officially replaced by an almost exclusive focus on sleeping sickness; and several zones, sectors and mobile missions abolished.[141]

In part, these counter-reforms were undergirded by personal and political motives. An anonymous newspaper article later suggested that Filomeno da Câmara's 'attack' on the AMI services was driven by a 'desire for revenge' against Damas Mora, 'his personal friend since their extended collaboration in

---

[138] Teixeira, 'Relatório Cuanza (1930)', 61–5.
[139] See especially the long preamble in Alto Comissariado da República em Angola, 'Diploma Legislativo 143', 17 August 1929, *BOA* (1929), 487–90.
[140] Camoesas, 'Organização AMI', 149 (quote). See also Amaral, *Relatório Catete (1930–31)*, 64–5; Mora, *Luta*, 162–3.
[141] Mora, *Luta*, 151–2, 161–3.

Timor, with whom he had fallen out shortly after his arrival in Luanda'.[142] Personal animosity between both men might indeed have aggravated the conflict. Damas Mora later explained his return to Europe in April 1929 by saying that the 'madman Filomeno' had refused to consult him on any health-related subject.[143] The fact that he re-embarked for Angola almost immediately upon the High Commissioner's dismissal a year later further corroborates the idea of a personal conflict.[144] In his absence, Filomeno da Câmara launched an investigation of parts of the health service, accusing Damas Mora and many other health officers of the embezzlement of public funds and goods, notably in order to pay for the services of political deportees.[145] All political deportees were eventually dismissed from the health services, also due to political differences. While most of them were left-wing republicans like Damas Mora, Filomeno da Câmara supported Mussolini and was also close to the Portuguese ultraconservative monarchist movement, the *integralismo lusitano*.[146]

However, after the forced departure of Filomeno da Câmara in March 1930 and despite the backing of the next Governors-General, Damas Mora did not manage to restore the organisational autonomy and ample funding of the AMI services.[147] This indicates that there were also structural problems. First, the measures taken by the last High Commissioner in Angola dovetailed with fundamental political and financial shifts. Filomeno da Câmara was the first 'man of confidence' of the nascent *Estado Novo* in Luanda and his measures were clearly in line with the overarching doctrine of financial austerity and balanced budgets that Minister of Finance (later Prime Minister) António de Oliveira Salazar had already begun to extend to the colonies.[148] In the early 1930s, balancing the colonial budgets – and especially that of notoriously indebted Angola – would be an absolute priority of the new regime in Lisbon, even if it further worsened the adverse effects of the world economic crisis.[149] Accordingly, Damas Mora's AMI plans and visions were also too expensive for Armindo Monteiro, Minister of Colonies from 1931 to 1935.

---

[142] 'Desfazendo mentiras', *A Província de Angola*, 2 June 1930.
[143] Mora, *Publicações Médicas*, 57; Damas Mora to Ricardo Jorge, 6 January 1931, reprinted in Mora, *António Damas Mora*, 98 (quote).
[144] See 'Dr. A. Damas Mora', *A Província de Angola*, 10 April 1930.
[145] 'A obra de moralizaçao. Inspecção aos Serviços de Saúde', *Portugal*, 8 March 1930. The inspection reports by Manuel Eduardo Martins have partly been published in *BOA Série II*, 8 March 1930, 161–84 and 14 March 1931, 147–51.
[146] Pimenta, *Angola*, 150–1.
[147] See the correspondence in 'Processo 4/3/1930', AHU, MU, DGAPC 3438 and Mora, *Luta*, 185–234.
[148] Leal, *Oliveira Salazar*, 30–40. On Filomeno da Câmara's short and turbulent term in office, see Pimenta, *Angola*, 149–56 and Torres, 'Angola' (quote).
[149] Havik, 'Tributos e impostos'. Further implications of Salazar's austerity policy are discussed in Chapter 6.

Empowered by the Colonial Act (1930), which had further curtailed the (financial) autonomy of the colonies and recentralised imperial decision-making in the Colonial Ministry in Lisbon, Monteiro thoroughly revised Angola's budget proposal for the financial year 1931–2. Instead of the scheduled 4.8 million Angolares (ags.), he only allowed the colony to spend 2.7 million for AMI services, 'a sum', Monteiro stated, 'which does not permit luxurious bonuses, but which allows an efficient establishment of services'.[150] Until the Second World and despite many complaints, the budget remained at less than half of what it had been in the late 1920s.[151]

Second, reservations against comprehensive healthcare for Angolan 'natives' were also linked to the situation of the 'white' European population in the colony. By the early 1930s, Angola had probably the largest European settler population in Central Africa, with estimates oscillating between a conservative 30,000 and a probably exaggerated 60,000.[152] For many of them, access to healthcare was complicated, because it was expensive (state medicine was only free of charge for civil servants) and doctors scarce.[153] The Angolan press asked why the state spent millions on free medical care and other provisions for the 'native' population, while some Europeans, including the families of deceased state employees, were forced to resort to private charity.[154] In the 1930s, the combined woes of the world economic crisis and Lisbon's budget restriction policy further worsened the economic and financial situation, thus exacerbating the issue of 'poor whites'.[155] In 1932, António Videira, an influential publicist and representative of settler interests, wrote in the *Província de Angola* that, in Luanda alone, hundreds of unemployed 'poor whites' were left almost uncared for, whereas there was enough money to fund charity work for African babies and mothers.[156] His article triggered a protracted correspondence with Damas Mora in the local press about the treatment of the 'native' population. What Videira and others criticised was not so much

---

[150] Ministério das Colónias, 'Decreto 20.071: Orçamento geral da receita e da despeza da colónia de Angola no ano económico de 1931–1932', 8 July 1931, *DG Série I* (1931), 1505–25, preamble (quote) and art. 46. On the Colonial Act, see also Havik, 'Tributos e impostos', 33–4.

[151] Costa, 'Assistência Médica ao Indígena', 61; *Anuário Estatístico de Angola (1939)*, 467.

[152] For the official estimate of nearly 60,000, see e.g. *Anuário Estatístico de Angola (1939)*, 21. In the light of the 1940 and 1950 censuses, the director of the statistical services would later criticise this estimate as too high, see Lemos, 'Introdução ao primeiro censo', 61–4 and Lemos, 'Censo da população de 1950', 16. For comparative numbers, see Clarence-Smith, 'Effects of the Great Depression', 190–1.

[153] Neves and Sousa, 'Assistência Médica aos Indígenas', 442.

[154] See, for instance, Eurico Lopes Cardoso, 'Montepio oficial de Angola', *A Província de Angola*, 10 May 1930 and Joaquim da Costa, 'Assistência indígena – assistência europeia', *A Província de Angola*, 14 May and 2 June 1930.

[155] Castelo, *Passagens para África*, 75–6, 86, 287–8; Clarence-Smith, *Third Portuguese Empire*, 178, 182; Clarence-Smith, 'Effects of the Great Depression'.

[156] On this charity work, see Chapter 5.

that the state cared about the 'natives', but the feeling that, notably through the AMI services, the colonial administration prioritised them over its own 'brothers in colour', thereby reversing the colonial order.[157] With the administrative recentralisation of the empire, the direct influence of the settler population on political decision-making in Angola had diminished, but their opinions and aspirations could not be completely ignored, especially given the government's fears of independence movements.[158]

Third and finally, resistance to continuous massive investments in 'native' healthcare must also be seen against the background of Portugal's public health system. It is telling that in 1929, Minister of Colonies Eduardo Marques pointed out that 'in Angola as well as in Mozambique, the medical and nursing services are much better than in many places in the metropole'.[159] In the late 1920s, Portugal's public health system was rudimentary. Relying on a centuries-old tradition of charity (beneficência), the state had kept its involvement to a minimum. In theory, there was a country-wide network of state-funded health officers (delegados de saúde), as in Angola. In practice, however, there was great geographical disparity between urban and rural spaces, and many rural areas were not adequately covered by health officers. Moreover, many of these health officers also worked as private practitioners, only giving free treatment to the poorest patients. Consequently, healthcare had remained largely in the hands of religious charities such as the Misericórdias, an institution that had spread all over mainland Portugal and its colonies since the sixteenth century, and more recent 'mutualities' (associações de socorros mútuos) and philanthropic institutions.[160]

Ideas of social medicine also circulated in Portugal, but they had not led to great improvements on the ground.[161] In a public lecture in 1923, Ricardo Jorge bitterly complained about Portugal's sanitary situation, which was not only discouraging but also internationally embarrassing: Portugal still did not have functioning prophylactic services against diseases such as tuberculosis, syphilis, rabies and smallpox, which continued to ravage the country.[162] A long-awaited reform of the health services was eventually promulgated in 1926, but public health would not be a priority for the Estado Novo before the

---

[157] António Videira, 'Providências imediatas', A Província de Angola, 19 August 1932 (here quote). Eight articles in total were published between 19 August and 9 September 1932 in the same journal. On António Videira, see Pimenta, Angola, 148, 169.

[158] Ibid., 160–4.

[159] 'As declarações do sr. Ministro das Colónias', A Província de Angola, 6–7 September 1929.

[160] Sobral, Lima, Sousa and Castro, 'Perante a pneumônica', 380–4; Sá and Lopes, História breve, esp. 103–19.

[161] Garnel, 'Consolidação'; Viegas, Frada and Miguel, Direcção-Geral da Saúde, 25–30.

[162] Jorge, 'A propósito de Pasteur', 205–9.

end of the Second World War.[163] While most European states began to invest large amounts of money and human capital in mass programmes of both curative and preventive medicine between the wars, successive Portuguese governments continued to underfinance the Health Department (*Direcção-Geral de Saúde*), thus preventing the extension of healthcare infrastructure, long overdue urban sanitation and the development of comprehensive prophylactic campaigns.[164]

Of course, there was no inextricable link between healthcare investment in Portugal and Angola, but with the recentralisation of the empire, both spheres became more closely bracketed in terms of governance. Further, when colonial experts like Eduardo Marques publicly declared that 'native' healthcare in the colonies was better than public health in Portugal, this subverted the hierarchy between metropole and colony. Angola's increasing dependence on a poor and, in public health issues, progressively underdeveloped metropole constituted a major difference from the British, French or Belgian colonies in West and Central Africa, although it is difficult to pin this down in numbers. In the 1930s, overall health expenditure in Angola stagnated around 11–13 million ags. annually, that is about 7–8 per cent of total expenditures and hence a rate comparable to other African colonies, while they for instance declined markedly in the Belgian Congo.[165] However, this says little about comparative health expenditure per capita. Moreover, while the Belgians set up a new, expensive and quickly expanding AMI scheme in 1930, the FORÉAMI (*Fonds Reine Elisabeth pour l'Assistance Médicale aux Indigènes*), the AMI services in northern Angola had lost momentum.[166] Certainly, after the approval in May 1932 of a reform plan, which conformed to the new financial framework of the Colonial Ministry, most of the abandoned sectors were reoccupied, medical surveillance reintroduced and the 'integral approach' revalorised.[167] However, lower budgets and fewer doctors than in the late 1920s did not allow the extension of the sector system to the rest of the colony.[168] Nor did the AMI services accomplish the Copernican revolution in the administration of healthcare from individual treatment to public hygiene. Improvements in official

---

[163] Saavedra, *Malária em Portugal*, 86, 92–100.

[164] See Garnel, 'Médicos e saúde pública', 236; Alves, 'Saúde e Fraternidade', 126–9; Faria, *Administração sanitária*, 350–4. For Europe, see Borowy and Gruner, 'Introduction'.

[165] Compare *Anuário Estatístico de Angola (1939)*, 467 with van Hoof, *Rapport 1939*, 5. For health expenditures in other colonies, see Headrick, *Colonialism, Health and Illness*, 406.

[166] Trolli, *Assistance Médicale aux Indigènes*.

[167] Governo Geral de Angola, 'Diploma Legislativo 351', 17 May 1932, *BOA* (1932), 160–2; Mora, *Luta*, 212–25. See also António Damas Mora, 'Assistência Médica aos Indígenas, em Angola', *A Província de Angola*, 6–8 August 1934.

[168] Costa, 'Assistência Médica ao Indígena'; Sarmento, 'História breve', 31. See also António Damas Mora, 'Serviços de Saúde e Higiene. Considerações finais', *A Província de Angola*, 27 June 1934.

maternal and infant healthcare remained modest (see Chapter 5) and Damas Mora's plans for polyvalent model villages were never put into a binding decree nor implemented on a grand scale. However, many of his ideas about such villages and the importance of rural hygiene, agricultural reform, and family recruitment continued to be debated over the next decades – and led to various reforms and, over and again, to local and less holistic realisations of model villages.[169]

Conclusion

This chapter has demonstrated the importance of inter-imperial learning for the AMI project in Angola. It has shown how national pride and competition between colonial empires intersected with practices of inter-imperial borrowing (and collaboration) in different and sometimes contradictory ways. While nationalist rivalry heightened colonial states' desire to learn from each other and to adopt 'best practices', it also induced them to try new methods and drugs. These were often claimed to be superior and framed as national innovations, even if they were just minor adaptations of existing models in other empires, and hence the result of inter-imperial exchange.[170] By 'nationalising' healthcare methods and trypanocidal drugs, colonial doctors aimed to showcase national ingenuity and special care for the African population before both audiences at home and colonial competitors. The way in which some Portuguese doctors would come to speak about the integral AMI approach and preventive mass atoxylisation as 'Portuguese methods' are two cases in point.

Processes of inter-imperial learning were not always so visible and explicit, however. Often, they were hidden by internal genealogies. This was, in many cases, not a random choice. Inter-imperial learning was an unequal exchange, governed by hierarchies of prestige that determined whether these borrowings were overt or hidden. For a Portuguese doctor like Damas Mora, acknowledging transimperial borrowing from bigger, richer and reputedly more advanced neighbours probably gave his claims additional authority – at least until the late 1920s, when, concurrent with the emergence of the *Estado Novo*, nationalist pride about Portugal's recent 'advances' in 'native' healthcare changed how doctors publicly perceived Portugal's position in the international hierarchy. Presumably, this 'authority bonus' was not available for colonial powers that wanted to learn from the Portuguese. This may explain why Damas Mora's counterpart in the Belgian Congo Giovanni Trolli presented an internal genealogy for FORÉAMI. Although it mirrored many aspects of the Angolan AMI

---

[169] Coghe, 'Reordering Colonial Society'.
[170] On the nationalisation of drugs, see particularly Mertens and Lachenal, 'History', 1262–70; Mertens, *Chemical Compounds*, 141–59, 188–90 and Lachenal, *Médicament*, 54–6.

system, which he had personally visited and publicly praised as 'the perfection in this field', Trolli did not acknowledge any foreign influence and instead stressed the originality of FORÉAMI's methods.[171] Arguably, due to the backward image of Portuguese colonialism, perhaps in combination with the crisis of the Angolan AMI scheme, citing Angola as a model would have weakened, rather than strengthened his argument. The way colonial actors perceived the position of their nation and rival nations on the hierarchical ladder of prestige not only determined whom they compared with and from whom they wanted to learn, but also conditioned the degree of overtness that accompanied inter-imperial borrowings.

---

[171] Trolli, 'Impression', 406 (quote); Trolli, *Assistance Médicale aux Indigènes*, 3–17. For a fuller presentation of this argument, see Coghe, 'Inter-Imperial Learning', 153–4.

4   Re-assessing Population Decline: Medical
     Demography and the Tensions
     of Statistical Knowledge

The establishment of the AMI services in 1926 not only changed colonial health paradigms in Angola: it also had a considerable impact on colonial knowledge and debates about the demography of Angola's 'native' population. Driven by persistent fears of depopulation and profound dissatisfaction with existing demographic data, medical doctors used the new AMI framework to probe novel methods of data gathering and analysis. This chapter illuminates the emergence, development and consequences of this 'medical demography', as I term the demographic endeavours of colonial doctors. It analyses how, during the interwar years, colonial practices of hygiene and demography became closely intertwined; how medical demography generated new insights into Angola's population dynamics; and how it played an important role in ongoing debates about the presumed decrease of the colony's 'native' population as well as the 'racial' specificities of African population trends.

Medical demography was by no means specifically Portuguese: it was a transimperial practice that can be observed in many colonies in Africa, particularly during the interwar years. However, despite the substantial paper trail, historiography has hardly engaged with it: both historical demographers in their attempts to reconstruct the demographic and socio-economic pasts of African societies, and cultural and postcolonial historians in their critical analyses of how censuses were conducted and used for bureaucratic control and racial or ethnic categorisation, have, with very few exceptions, overlooked doctors' demographic work.[1] Both strands of research have instead focused on administrative surveys and 'scientific' censuses, with historical demography

---

[1] On this historiography, see Introduction. The most notable exceptions are Headrick, *Colonialism, Health and Illness*, 95–153 and Sanderson, *Démographie coloniale congolaise*, who use the data produced by doctors to reconstruct fertility and mortality levels in the AEF and Belgian Congo respectively. However, they pay little attention to why and how doctors produced and used these data. See also Doyle, *Before HIV*, 244–60 for doctors' fertility studies in British Uganda in the 1950s.

also using demographic data gathered by missionaries and travellers.[2] The fact that some of the most significant efforts by colonial doctors to collect and analyse demographic data took place in the AMI sectors in French, Belgian and Portuguese Central Africa suggests that geographical and linguistic issues might be at the origins of this historiographical neglect, given the relative marginality of these regions and their colonial languages in African historiography.

In and of itself, the engagement of doctors with demography was not colonially specific. Before demography was institutionalised in Europe and North America as a discipline in its own right around the time of the Second World War (that is, when proper research institutes, journals and professional career paths were established), medical doctors were often at the forefront of demographic research.[3] Internationally, the International Congresses on Hygiene and Demography (1878–1912) and the collection and publication of vital statistics and other demographic data by the League of Nations Health Organisation (LNHO) epitomised the close connection that existed between the two fields since the late nineteenth century.[4] In Portugal, the Central Institute of Hygiene in Lisbon was in charge of publishing and analysing the country's official demographic data in the 1910s and 1920s.[5] Its director Ricardo Jorge was not only one of the country's most recognised hygienists, but also a leading expert in demography, just like his colleague António de Almeida Garrett in Porto.[6]

Yet the demographic work of colonial doctors in interwar Africa differed from that of their colleagues in Europe in various regards. Whereas doctors in Europe could base their studies on reasonably accurate pre-existing data from censuses or civil registries, doctors in colonial Africa usually still had to collect the data they wanted to analyse themselves, especially in rural areas, as censuses and civil registries were non-existent, incomplete or untrustworthy. Counting people in a very literal sense became an important part of their job. Analogous to a common distinction made in the history of anthropology, one could say that the 'colonial situation' turned doctors into 'field demographers', as opposed to 'armchair demographers' in Europe.[7] This also had implications for how they analysed their data. Since many of their demographic reports

---

[2] Regarding Angola, see, for instance, Heywood and Thornton, 'Demography'; Heywood and Thornton, 'African Fiscal Systems'.

[3] On the institutionalisation of demography, see Greenalgh, 'Social Construction', especially 30, 34–41 and Rosental, 'Wissenschaftlicher Internationalismus'.

[4] Rosental, 'Wissenschaftlicher Internationalismus', 257; Overath, 'Bevölkerungsforschung', 66–8; Borowy, *Coming to Terms*, 177–83.

[5] Sousa, *História da estatística*, 161–3.   [6] Baptista, 'Demografia em Portugal', 540–1.

[7] On this distinction and the shift from 'armchair' to fieldwork-based (social) anthropology in the 1920s, see for instance Kucklick, 'Personal Equations'.

were primarily written for practical purposes of medical control and policy-making rather than academic purposes, they did not always explicitly and intellectually engage with the issue of racial difference, which was central to debates among academics in Europe studying the demography of colonial populations.[8]

That does not mean that racial thinking was absent from their writings. Colonial doctors' demographic work in Angola both reflected and contributed to ideas and debates about racial difference in various ways.[9] Practised within the context of healthcare programmes that were explicitly aimed at halting 'native' population decline, medical demography was a priori underwritten by assumptions about different fertility and mortality patterns between Europeans and *indígenas* ('natives'); that is, those Africans still considered 'non-civilised'.[10] Tellingly, doctors' research into the demography of the colony's 'native' population was not paralleled by similar efforts to study the demographic behaviour of European settlers and/or racially mixed communities in Angola.[11] When, in the early 1940s, medical doctor Alexandre Sarmento began to publish articles on the evolution of the white population in Angola, his analyses were usually based on data from the 1940 census, not field research.[12] In the interwar years, demographic knowledge production was largely confined to the *indígena*, the 'non-white' and 'non-civilised' Other, whose difference was assumed on the basis of both biological and cultural traits.

Conversely, medical demography also shaped racial thinking. It contributed to the refashioning and entrenching of ideas about the different demographic regimes that existed between the *indígenas* in Angola and people in Europe on the one hand, and (to a lesser extent) between the colony's *indígenas* on the other. Hence, even when ideas about difference were not always fleshed out, interwar medical demography was clearly part of a broader colonial effort to study and categorise the different populations of the Portuguese Empire, an effort to which other disciplines such as physical anthropology were also – and more explicitly – contributing.[13]

This chapter explores how, in interwar Angola, doctors' demographic practices and assumptions intersected with ideas of population decline, racial

---

[8] See Ittmann, 'Colonial Office', 57–8, 64–5; Widmer, 'Imbalanced Sex Ratio', 547–8.
[9] For a broader view on the interaction between medical knowledge practices and ideas of racial difference, see Widmer and Lipphardt (eds.), *Health and Difference*.
[10] See Introduction.
[11] See the complaint in Correia, 'Luso-descendentes', 4–5. An exception is Silva Telles' demographic study on deported Europeans in Angola: Telles, *Transportação penal*, 38–56.
[12] See, for instance, Sarmento, 'Estudo da população'.
[13] See notably Roque, *Antropologia e Império*; Roque, *Headhunting and Colonialism*; Matos, *Côres do Império* and Santos, 'Birth'.

difference and African demographic regimes. First, it shows how the emergence of medical demography in Angola in the 1920s was conditioned by innovations in African healthcare, persistent anxieties about population decline and the inter-imperial transfer of demographic methods. It then demonstrates that, despite the often-well-known shortcomings of these methods, doctors did not refrain from producing demographic analyses that served their own purposes and had a significant impact on population debates in Angola. Not only did doctors suggest that ongoing healthcare investments had stopped population decline; they also claimed that, due to civilisational backwardness, Africans were governed by a demographic regime of high fertility and high infant mortality that was distinct from both Europe and low fertility zones in Africa.

The Emergence of Medical Demography

The rise of medical demography in Angola was inextricably linked to the establishment of the *Assistência Médica aos Indígenas* (AMI) in 1926 and its territorialised sector system in the northern part of the colony (see Chapter 3). The connection was twofold. Profoundly influenced by ideas of social medicine, leading proponents of the AMI programme like director of health services António Damas Mora emphasised the importance of demography. In their view, accurate data on demographic trends was key for identifying health problems, adapting the AMI programme to the needs of the population and monitoring its impact.[14] In the words of his colleague hygienist João Camoesas, the survey of the population was 'the fundamental basis of all socio-medical action'.[15] Conversely, the AMI programme also offered unprecedented opportunities for demographic study, as it brought doctors into a more regular and hierarchically structured contact with rural African populations.

The vivid interest doctors' demographic studies sparked in interwar Angola must also be understood against the backdrop of resurging fears of de- and under-population after the First World War, in Angola but also in similar ways in many other parts of colonial Africa and even the Pacific.[16] While the economic and political imperatives of the colonial *mise en valeur* required a healthy and growing 'native' population, many observers still believed that Angola's 'native' population was declining, or at best stagnating. Compared to

---

[14] Santos, 'Assistência Médica aos Indígenas', 52–4, 70; Costa, 'Relatório Cuanza Norte', 104 and Mora, 'Estado actual', 39–40.
[15] Camoesas, 'Organização AMI', 143.
[16] See, generally, Coghe and Widmer, 'Colonial Demography'. See also Sanderson, 'Congo belge'; Headrick, *Colonialism, Health and Illness*, 104–5.

the 1900s, epidemic and endemic diseases such as sleeping sickness, smallpox and malaria were still frequently cited as the main causes, together with emigration, but doctors and administrators also increasingly blamed natives' lack of hygiene and general ignorance, mal- and under-nutrition as well as exploitative colonial labour regimes. These conditions, they assumed, were responsible for a 'native' demographic regime characterised by low birth rates and high mortality, especially infant mortality.[17] However, reliable data on the mortality and natality of rural African populations were still virtually non-existent. Depopulation fears combined with a profound lack of knowledge made the production of more reliable demographic data urgent.

This was all the more important since, in the mid-1920s, the production of two new series of demographic data further heightened demographic anxieties. In 1913, the newly established Native Affairs Department had, under the direction of José de Oliveira Ferreira Diniz, begun to assemble colony-wide 'census' maps.[18] These were based on the population statistics that the administrators of the approximately 70 administrative units (the urban *concelhos*, the rural *circunscrições civis*, and the still military-ruled *capitanias-mores*) were obliged to produce every year to facilitate tax collection.[19] Just like earlier censuses, the Native Affairs surveys initially did not cover the entire territory of the colony, but as the administrative occupation of the interior advanced, more and more areas were incorporated.[20] When the first complete surveys were eventually published in the *Boletim Oficial de Angola* in 1928, they caused a stir, since the total population they charted was only around 2.5 million, and, until 1939, would continue to oscillate between 2.3 and 2.7 million, with an exceptional 2.9 million in 1933 (see Figure 4.3 later in this chapter).[21] Virtually all colonialists had expected the total population to be much larger, as geographers, explorers and missionaries in the late nineteenth and early twentieth centuries had published much higher estimates, ranging from 4 to 12 million.[22] Still in the mid-1920s, High Commissioner José Norton de Matos had assumed a total population of about 5 million.[23] These had not been random figures, but educated guesses, either based on the population density in sample areas or, as was the case for Norton de Matos, on the extrapolation of the number of registered male taxpayers.[24]

---

[17] Athayde, 'Perigo do despovoamento', 230, 237; Sant'Anna, 'Problema da assistência', 73–4; Matos, *Província de Angola*, 227–77.

[18] Diniz, *Negócios indígenas – relatório 1913*, 11–6.

[19] See, for instance Matos, *Regulamento*, 18, 52–4.

[20] Diniz, 'Contribuição'; Heywood and Thornton, 'Demography'.

[21] See for instance Neves and Sousa, 'Assistência Médica aos Indígenas', 434–5. For an overview, see Lemos, 'Introdução ao primeiro censo', 29–31.

[22] See, for instance, Vasconcelos, *Colonias portuguezas*, 162; Nascimento and Mattos, *Colonização de Angola*, 52; Athayde, 'Perigo do despovoamento', 229. See also Chapter 1.

[23] Matos, *Província de Angola*, 227.   [24] Muralha, *Terras de África*, 118.

The new figures from the Native Affairs Department, which in Ferreira Diniz's opinion were getting 'very close to the truth', seemed to corroborate the idea that the 'native' population had been and, possibly still was, declining.[25] Furthermore, they suggested a population density of only two inhabitants per square kilometre. This was less than half of what most observers, including Norton de Matos, had expected.[26] Portuguese colonialists also noted that this figure turned Angola into the least densely populated Portuguese colony and one of the least densely populated colonies in sub-Saharan Africa, even if some emphasised that density was still higher than in French Equatorial Africa, Namibia or Northern Rhodesia, and hence not so aberrant in a sparsely populated continent after all.[27] Yet against the backdrop of the interwar debates about optimum population density that Alison Bashford has incisively analysed, Portuguese colonialists interpreted low density as under-population and an obstacle to the future 'agricultural-industrial valorisation' of the colony.[28] It was in this vein that Damas Mora wrote in 1940 that, during his journey in West Africa in 1926, he had seen 'prosperity where density was greater than 10 inhabitants per square kilometre and a deficient situation where that density was lower than five'.[29]

The publication of the administrative censuses coincided with heated debate about labour scarcity in Angola's settler press. Since the early 1920s, European entrepreneurs, often backed by journalists and colonial officials, had, in numerous newspaper articles, expressed the fear that the African labour pool was not (or in the near future would not be) large enough to supply their demands.[30] In order to invalidate such complaints, which were also meant to pressure the colonial government into taking a more active part in the labour recruitment process, Norton de Matos and some of his successors commissioned surveys to determine the number of male adults of working age.[31] These surveys, however, did little to assuage fears of labour scarcity. On the contrary, even if the 559,192 available adult male workers in the first survey published in January 1925 by far exceeded official demand, it was also far below the 2.1 million Norton de Matos had assumed there were in 1921.[32]

---

[25] Diniz, 'Contribuição', 53.   [26] Matos, 'Síntese', 489.

[27] Mora, 'Estado actual', 17; *Anuário Estatístico de Angola* (1933), 5–6.

[28] Correia, 'Processos práticos', 180 (quote). Compare with Bashford, 'Population, Geopolitics' and *Global Population*, esp. 81–106.

[29] Mora, 'Mortalidade infantil', 563. For a more detailed account of these density debates, see Coghe, *Population Politics (2014)*, 169–70.

[30] See the debates in the *Jornal do Comércio*, *A Província de Angola* and *O Comércio de Angola* in the early and mid-1920s. For more details on this discussion, see ibid., 171–2 and Chapter 6.

[31] See, for instance, Alto Comissário da República José Norton de Matos, 'Portaria Provincial 148', 6 July 1923, *BOA Série I* (1923), 314–6 and Ferreira, *Situação de Angola*, 49–53. For later surveys, see Chapter 6.

[32] Compare Governador Interino Antero Tavares de Carvalho, 'Despacho', 16 January 1925, *BOA Série I* (1925), 46 with José Norton de Matos, 'Circular', 2 October 1921, *BOA Série I* (1921), 260.

Certainly, some, like former member of parliament and journalist Domingos da Cruz, stated that the real number had to be much higher, as many thousands had most likely evaded their taxes and hence had not been counted.[33] Yet others were more than happy to take the number at face value. One author asked, 'So, where is that surplus of labourers that only Mr Domingos da Cruz saw and nobody else can find?'[34]

While fuelling anxieties of de- and under-population, these two new sets of demographic data did not solve the particular knowledge problem for colonial hygienists. They neither trusted these new data nor considered them useful for their purposes. On the one hand, they complained that administrative censuses were erroneous and of little scientific value, because of various methodological and practical problems and above all the very rationale that underpinned them, that is the aim to measure the healthy adult male population for the sake of tax collection, labour recruitment and military conscription. Doctors claimed that many men hid from the administrator to avoid registration and that administrators often deliberately overestimated the age of male adolescents so that they could declare them recruitable and tax-paying adults. According to doctors, the focus on adult males also led to the undercounting or underestimation of the numbers of women and children. They accused administrators of not ensuring that all women and children were actually counted and of just deducing the number of women and children from the number of adult men through a mathematical calculation with a factor that, moreover, they criticised as too low.[35] On the basis of these criticisms, which are strikingly similar to those formulated by some Africanist historical demographers decades later, doctors legitimised their own censuses and explained why these came up with different numbers.[36] This was, for instance, the case of Venâncio da Silva, who had found fewer adult men, but 30–50 per cent more women and children during his medical census in two administrative posts in the Congo Zone in 1928, in comparison with the data of the administrator.[37]

On the other hand, doctors also criticised administrative censuses for only providing a static view of the population. As hygienists, they were more interested in population dynamics than total numbers; they wanted to know whether populations were growing or declining and to understand why that happened. Thus, they needed birth, death and migration rates and more specific

[33] Domingos da Cruz, 'A propósito do recenseamento indígena', A Província de Angola, 12 July 1925.

[34] 'Mão de Obra', O Comércio de Angola, 19 April 1926.

[35] See, for instance, Camoesas, 'Organização AMI', 143–4; Silva, Relatório do serviço permanente, 88–9; 92; Mora, 'Estado actual', 39. For a similar and very elaborate argument with regard to the Belgian Congo, see Schwetz, 'Contribution', 301–12.

[36] Compare with Heywood and Thornton, 'Demography', 243–4 and 250–1.

[37] 'Assistência Médica aos Indígenas – Zona do Congo (1929)', 298–9.

indices such as infant mortality rates, ratios of births per woman, sex ratios, age-group distributions and morbidity statistics indicating the incidence of certain diseases. Administrative reports and population maps generally did not contain such information, nor data that were sufficiently reliable for doctors to calculate these indices themselves.[38]

For these reasons, medical doctors began to use the framework of the new AMI programme to raise their own data. From a hygienist's perspective, the colonial administration would only begin to produce more reliable and useful data in the 1940s, when the first autonomous population census was conducted in 1940 and when the registration of births and deaths by the civil administration became obligatory for all Africans in 1942. Even then, however, these data sets would not end medical demography, as the civil registry did not work well, and the census did not provide enough dynamic data.[39]

The Methods of Medical Demography

AMI doctors in Angola used two different methods to measure the African population and their reproductive behaviour: a registration system and oral interviews. Registration was the norm in the AMI sectors of northern Angola, where the health services pursued the utopian vision of complete and continuous medical control. Here, the aim was nothing less than to register the entire population and its 'movements': births, deaths and in- and out-bound migration. To do so, the doctor and nurses in charge of a sector made use of the system of bi-weekly or monthly 'concentrations' (concentrações), established to monitor and treat sleeping sickness and other diseases (see Chapter 3). At these concentrations, people from the surrounding villages were not only examined and treated, but also registered, as can be seen in Figure 4.1. Registration was compulsory, nominative and double: each person was registered on a card (ficha sanitária), which he or she was supposed to keep, and also in the registry books kept by the medical authorities of the sector.[40] Doctors also recorded the deaths and migrations that were reported to them. Particular attention was paid to the registration of births. In order to keep track of newborns, doctors not only registered the births that were reported to them, but also took note of ostensibly pregnant women during the concentrations.

---

[38] Camoesas, 'Organização AMI', 143–4; Mora, 'Estado actual', 39.

[39] On the civil registry, see Morgado, 'Demografia do Ultramar português', 113–23. On the census, see later in this chapter.

[40] For a detailed description of this system, see 'Assistência Médica aos Indígenas – Zona do Congo (1929)', 296–7.

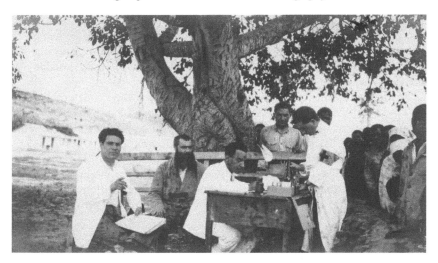

Figure 4.1 Medical registration of the population in the Quissama Subsector, ca. 1929.
Source: ANTT, Agência Geral do Ultramar, Angola, cx. 5, n.º 4471, PT/TT/AGU/001/ 004471. See also Ornelas and Mesquita, *Relatório da missão médica*, 22
Image courtesy of ANTT

They wrote down the probable moment of childbirth and exhorted expectant mothers to bring their babies to them once they had been born.[41]

This registration system, which constituted a kind of medical counterpart to the inexistent civil registry, was initiated in the Cuanza zone in 1927 and gradually extended to all zones and sectors in the following years. By the end of 1930, AMI services had registered almost 400,000 people, a number that would rise to almost 600,000 at the end of the decade.[42] Even though this registration scheme provided the raw material on which doctors would base many of their demographic studies and claims, its aim was not merely demographic. The *fichas* and books also contained information on diseases and treatments. Some doctors, like João Camoesas, wanted to further enhance the potential of this 'medical registry'. Camoesas, a renowned hygienist and former minister who had been exiled from Portugal to Angola for political reasons in 1928 (see Chapter 3), recommended that additional medical data and basic physiological information should be registered, ranging from height and weight to the so-called Pignet index (see Figure 4.2). This was an index that evaluated physical robustness by relating thorax circumference to height

---

[41] Ornelas and Mesquita, *Relatório da missão médica*, 24; Waldemar Gomes Teixeira, 'Relatório da Zona Sanitária do Cuanza (1930)', June 1931, AHU, MU, AGC 2336, 8, 15.

[42] Compare Teixeira, 'Relatório Cuanza *(1930)*', 16, 19; Silva, *Serviço de Assistência Congo (1930)*, 45 with *Boletim Sanitário de Angola* (1939), 63.

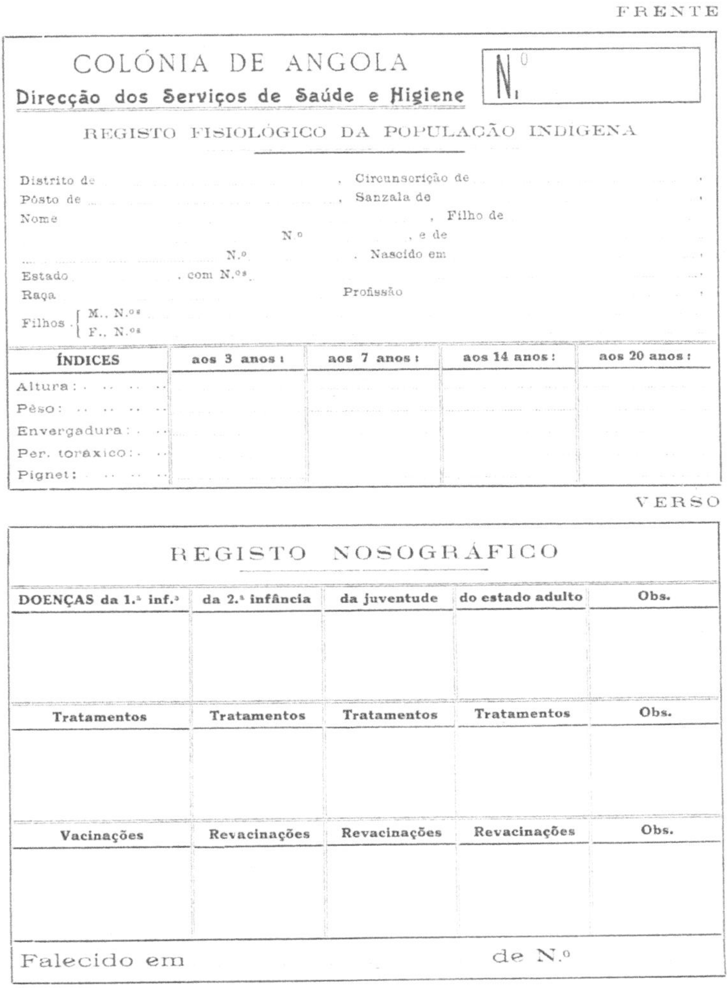

FRENTE

COLÓNIA DE ANGOLA   N.º
Direcção dos Serviços de Saúde e Higiene   N.

REGISTO FISIOLÓGICO DA POPULAÇÃO INDIGENA

Distrito de _____ , Circunscrição de _____
Pôsto de _____ , Sanzala de _____
Nome _____ , Filho de
_____ N.º _____ , e de
_____ N.º _____ , Nascido em _____
Estado _____ , com N.ºs _____
Raça _____ Profissão _____
Filhos . { M.. N.ºs F.. N.ºs

ÍNDICES	aos 3 anos :	aos 7 anos :	aos 14 anos :	aos 20 anos :
Altura :				
Pêso :				
Envergadura :				
Per. toráxico :				
Pignet :				

VERSO

REGISTO NOSOGRÁFICO

DOENÇAS da 1.ª inf.ª	da 2.ª infância	da juventude	do estado adulto	Obs.
Tratamentos	Tratamentos	Tratamentos	Tratamentos	Obs.
Vacinações	Revacinações	Revacinações	Revacinações	Obs.

Falecido em   de N.º

Figure 4.2 Demographic and medical registration card, late 1920s.
Source: Camoesas, 'Organização AMI', 153–4.
Images courtesy of Staatsbibliothek zu Berlin

and weight and that, in interwar Africa, was widely used by colonial companies and armies to evaluate the nutritional status and physical aptitude of (potential) workers and soldiers.[43] To facilitate the identification of individuals, he also proposed to introduce metal bracelets similar to those worn by

---

[43] Coghe, *Population Politics (2014)*, 333–4.

soldiers during the First World War. If well-organised, he claimed, such a medical registry would generate a huge amount of scientific data with which to study the vitality of the population, while simultaneously facilitating tax collection and rationalising labour recruitment.[44]

Some of Camoesas's ideas did not go unheeded. In 1930, the new head of the Cuanza zone, Waldemar Teixeira, adopted Camoesas's model of registration cards with minor changes for the area around Cazengo. Accordingly, he measured more than 5,000 people from both sexes and all ages and calculated their Pignet index. In a few hundred cases, he also determined the so-called Lefrou index, which was developed by the French colonial doctor Lefrou to adapt Pignet's Eurocentric formula to the 'particularities' of the African body. Yet, even according to this index, most adult males were considered too frail to be recruited.[45] However, it is important to note that, for Teixeira, this was only a scientific 'experiment' and that there is no evidence that his personalised data were used for labour recruitment.[46] Indeed, while Camoesas's recommendations reveal to what extent some interwar hygienists dreamt of a 'legible' population for the sake of medical and administrative governance, it is unlikely that doctors shared personalised demographic and medical data with administrators and other officials effectively, for the sake of tax collection, labour recruitment or military conscription. By giving up the independence of medical censuses, they would have compromised the trust of rural Angolans in the AMI operations and sapped the very basis on which AMI doctors thought to get more realistic demographic data than administrators.

In order to get a better grasp of the long-term biological reproduction levels of African populations, some doctors also resorted to a second method. During the concentrations, they questioned women in and beyond childbearing age about their reproductive life. In these oral interviews, mostly conducted with the help of an interpreter, doctors asked how many children they had given birth to, how many of them had died in early infancy or later and how often they had aborted or delivered stillborns. With this information, they calculated the total and age-specific number of children per woman, determined the level of infant mortality and mapped the incidence of abortions and stillbirths.

In contrast to the medical registry, interview-based fertility and infant mortality studies were sample studies. They encompassed small groups of a few hundred to a few thousand women, considered representative for a particular region or ethnic group in the colony. They were conducted in the AMI sectors, where they added historical depth to the registry data, but also during mobile medical missions in regions that were not yet under systematic

---

[44] Camoesas, 'Organização AMI'.   [45] Teixeira, 'Relatório Cuanza (1930)', 27–32.
[46] Ibid., 27 (quote).

medical control.[47] In these latter areas, interviews were the only means with which to obtain an approximate idea of fertility and infant mortality levels, and hence of population trends. Thus, even the two doctors attached to the *Brigada das Estradas* ('Roads Study Mission') dispatched to Central Angola in the early 1930s seized the opportunity to produce several studies of this kind. Both had previously worked in AMI sectors.[48] Interview-based fertility and infant mortality studies became a common feature of medical demography, demonstrating the particular importance the Angolan health services attached to these issues, but also the relative simplicity of the method.

It is important to note that neither the idea of a medical registry nor the technique of small-scale fertility and infant mortality studies originated among Portuguese doctors in Angola. Haunted by similar fears of low birth rates and high infant mortality, doctors in other African colonies had already introduced these novel forms of demographic inquiries. As early as 1909, German doctors began to conduct interview-based fertility and infant mortality studies among African populations in Cameroon, Togo and German East Africa.[49] After the First World War, Belgian, French and British doctors followed their example.[50] Moreover, this technique was used in other continents, as examples from French Indochina show.[51]

While fertility inquiries could be conducted virtually everywhere, medical population registries required a much higher level of control. In rural Africa, the medical sectors that were established to combat sleeping sickness, and later also other endemic diseases, constituted a particularly propitious environment. Such sectors were first established in French Equatorial Africa in 1917 and subsequently in French Cameroon, but it seems that they were first used for an encompassing population registry when the sector system was adopted in the Belgian Congo by Jacques Schwetz in the early 1920s.[52] It was also in the

---

[47] See, for instance, Teixeira, 'Relatório Cuanza (1930)', 15–26; Amaral, 'Natalidade e mortalidade', 172 and 'Missão volante da Lunda'. For a somewhat different method based on 'family tickets', see Amaral, *Relatório Catete (1930–31)*, 13–50.

[48] João Araújo de Freitas and Luís Pinto de Fonseca, 'Relatório dos médicos da Brigada de Estradas', 31 December 1930, 8–12, AHU, MU, DGAPC 407; Luís Pinto de Fonseca, 'Relatório do médico da Sub-Brigada Norte', 30 June 1931, 2–11, AHU, MU 585; João Araújo de Freitas, 'Relatório do médico da Sub-Brigada Sul', 31 October 1931, 5–11 and 29 February 1932, 2–5, AHU, MU, DGOPC 737.

[49] See, for instance, Külz, 'Pathologie', 33–5; Rodenwaldt, 'Beitrag'; Peiper, *Geburtenhäufigkeit*.

[50] For the Belgian Congo, see Schwetz, 'Contribution', 325–40; Mouchet, 'Natalité'; for French Africa, see Clapier, 'Enquête démographique'; Cazanove, 'Essai de démographie' and Bauvallet, 'Résultats'; for British Africa, see Kuczynski, *Cameroons and Togoland*, 272, 282–6 and 519–20.

[51] Chesneau, 'Natalité et mortalité infantile'.

[52] Compare Schwetz, 'Contribution', esp. 299–300 with the analysis of the French sectors in Headrick, *Colonialism, Health and Illness*, 345–56; Piot, 'Fonctionnement'; Jojot, 'Secteur de la prophylaxie'.

Belgian Congo that the FORÉAMI, a sector-based AMI programme established in the Bas-Congo region in 1930, would use medical registries to undertake what were probably the most extensive and detailed studies of medical demography in interwar Africa.[53]

Clearly, demographic techniques circulated across colonial and imperial boundaries and there is no doubt that inter-imperial learning was crucial for their introduction in interwar Angola. As shown in Chapter 3, the health services in Angola, and most notably its director António Damas Mora, were eager to emulate best practices in healthcare and hygiene from other colonies. This included demographic techniques: during the LNHO study tour in West Africa in 1926, Damas Mora attended a pioneering lecture in medical demography in French-mandated Togo.[54] And when he later wrote a lengthy report on 'Native Medical Assistance' in tropical Africa for the same LNHO in 1929–30, he encountered many further studies in medical demography on French, British and Belgian colonies.[55] Moreover, many of the demographic studies by doctors in Angola openly referred to similar studies in foreign colonies as examples and role models.[56] Inter-imperial learning thus filled a double gap: during the first decades of the twentieth century, Portuguese doctors had generally received little to no training in demography before going to the colonies, as it was not included in the curriculum of Portugal's medical faculties, nor in that of the School of Tropical Medicine in Lisbon.[57] Only in 1960 was a comprehensive manual on statistics and demography for Portuguese colonial doctors published.[58] Moreover, doctors in Angola could not benefit from intra-imperial transfers, since field studies in medical demography only appeared in other Portuguese colonies later on.[59]

The Tensions of Medical Demography

Medical demography did not automatically lead to a more accurate view of population trends. First of all, the practical implementation of medical

---

[53] See, for instance, Trolli, 'Contribution'; Trolli and Dupuy, *Contribution* and Sanderson, *Démographie coloniale congolaise*, 110–65. On FORÉAMI, see also Chapter 3 and Coghe, 'Between Colonial Medicine and Global Health'.

[54] See Dr Mercier, 'Conférence sur la démographie et les statistiques démographiques au Togo, faite en présence de la mission des médecins échangistes à Atakpame', 20 April 1926, LON, R 955, 12B/54511/41908.

[55] See, in one of his résumés of this report, Mora, 'Estado actual', 39–43. For a more elaborate analysis of this report, see Coghe, *Population Politics (2014)*, 180–1.

[56] Ornelas and Mesquita, *Relatório da missão médica*, 23–4; Teixeira, 'Relatório Cuanza (1930)', 13–14; Fonseca, 'Relatório Sub-Brigada Norte', 9.

[57] Some basic notions of demography may have been taught in the courses of public hygiene and epidemiology at these schools, however, personal communication by Rita Garnel, 2 September 2013. See also Garnel, 'Régia Escola'.

[58] Reis and Sarmento, *Manual*.   [59] See, for instance, Ribeiro, *Apontamentos*, 3–14.

registries and retrospective interviews in rural Angola challenged the boundaries of European medical power; its success depended on several intersecting negotiation processes between AMI staff and local actors. Furthermore, the interpretations doctors made of the collected data were often devoid of scientific rigor and used to serve a particular purpose.

The most basic problem was that, for both methods, the accuracy of the demographic data was fundamentally contingent upon the collaboration of the African population. Certainly, some doctors had great confidence in the reporting strategies of the Africans in their medical sector. Alfredo Gomes da Costa, the first director of the Cuanza zone, asserted that probably only 2 per cent of the population in the entire zone were not in regular contact with the medical staff.[60] Similarly, the young Goan doctor Eduardo Diniz da Gama claimed that, in his sector, only very few persons failed to attend the concentrations and that expectant mothers readily reported pregnancies to AMI personnel. These cases, he concluded, were duly registered and 'all pregnant women thus become responsible towards us for the foetus and, in the case of abortion, they come and tell us. On this point, some even say jokingly that the census of the [medical] assistance [services] is so complete that the blacks [*pretos*] are even registered when they are still in the belly of the mother.'[61] Many other doctors, however, were far more sceptical and expressed their frustration over the reporting strategies of 'their' Africans. While Africans reported deaths with relative ease 'because of the benefits associated with such a declaration' (that is, exemption from tax payments), it was commonly felt that they were much more reluctant to declare births.[62]

Even if their assessment of African reporting rates diverged, doctors were unanimous in their analysis of how to (further) improve these rates and thus the accuracy of their demographic data. They agreed that Africans' distrust of medical demography was the main cause of avoidance and underreporting and that, consequently, the cultivation of trust was the key to success. It was imperative, they stated, to convince Africans that registration was an autonomous operation for medical and demographic purposes only and that the data would not be used for the purposes of taxation, labour recruitment or conscription.[63] Trust was also important in another sense: because of the simultaneity of registration and medical treatment, the quality of the demographic data also depended much on the trust Western biomedicine inspired among the African population.

---

[60] Costa, 'Relatório Cuanza Norte', 104.   [61] Gama, 'Um ano de chefia', 541.

[62] Sousa, *Relatório Dande*, 16; Teixeira, 'Relatório Cuanza (1930)', 15; Mora, 'Mortalidade infantil', 575–6. For similar complaints concerning other colonies, see Bauvallet, 'Résultats', 604–5 and Lefrou, *Le Noir d'Afrique*, 300.

[63] Sousa, *Relatório Dande*, 16; Mora, 'Mortalidade infantil', 575. For a successful account of inspiring such trust, see Silva, 'Relatório missão volante', 221–2.

The success of medical demography and the AMI programme in general not only hinged on the persuasive power of the Portuguese doctors and nurses, but also on the collaboration of intermediaries, such as African nurses, local chiefs, missionaries and local administrators. These groups played a crucial role in mediating power and trust between Portuguese doctors and the African population.[64] Effective collaboration, however, was far from given. 'Native' nurses, for instance, were often praised by AMI doctors for their services as interpreters and active propagators of Western biomedicine, but there were also frequent complaints about them following their own agenda and sometimes even abusing local populations if they were given too much power and autonomy.[65] Local administrators, then, were needed to assure that all people appeared at the concentrations and to assist the AMI doctors in other matters. However, conflicts of interest or other tensions between doctors and administrators frequently thwarted efficient collaboration. Where doctors could not rely on local alliances to dissipate mistrust and, if necessary, to punish no-shows, concentrations often remained empty.[66]

Finally, compared to the medical registries, retrospective interviews with women allowed for even fewer possibilities to effectively control the numbers. Here, intelligence was fully dependent upon the informants' understanding of the questions and the accuracy of their memories, but also their goodwill in not under- or over-reporting childbearing practices.[67] Women could have had many motives to retroactively reshape their fertility, from mistrust of colonial intrusions to an unwillingness to admit childlessness in front of other women, given the high prestige that was assigned to motherhood and the grave dishonour associated with childlessness.[68]

The contingencies of medical demography created a dilemma for the AMI doctors involved. While most of them were, at least to some extent, aware that the demographic data they had themselves collected or received from subordinate doctors could not be entirely accurate, they also knew that it was almost impossible to overcome the biases in the production of such and that there were no better data available. Unless they wished to discard the very possibility of studying population dynamics in rural Angola, they had little other choice than to use their data.[69] Indeed, most doctors in Angola solved this dilemma by ignoring or downplaying the inaccuracy of their data. When it

---

[64] For positive examples, see Gama, 'Missão volante', 60–3.   [65] See Chapter 3.
[66] See, for instance, Costa, 'Relatório Cuanza Norte', 104; Jacinto de Sousa, 'Relatório da missão médica volante de assistência aos indígenas do Dande, 1928, 38 and 68–9, AHU, MU, AGC 2336; Freitas and Fonseca, 'Relatório (1930)', 6–7 and Freitas, 'Relatório Sub-Brigada Sul (1931)', 2 and 8.
[67] Teixeira, 'Relatório Cuanza (1930)', 24; Sousa, *Relatório Dande*, 16.
[68] Mora, 'Mortalidade infantil', 588. Similarly Cazanove, 'Essai de démographie', 36.
[69] For a particularly upfront confession, see Fonseca, 'Relatório Sub-Brigada Norte', 2 and 4.

came to interpreting them, they presented the numbers, percentages and indices as positivist truths and often even based bold claims on them.

This phenomenon was not confined to Portuguese doctors in Angola, but was a basic tension in medical demography and colonial demography in general. Already in 1937, Robert René Kuczynski, a prominent German-Jewish demographer who had started working on colonial populations after his emigration to London, criticised the 'appalling' extent to which 'the authors of colonial reports are tempted to draw far-reaching conclusions from the scanty population data at their disposal'.[70] In his detailed studies on demography in British, French and former German colonies, Kuczynski was very critical of most demographic methods that had thus far been used in colonial Africa. He also repeatedly pointed out the methodological shortcomings of the fertility and infant mortality studies conducted by colonial doctors.[71] For Kuczynski, the problem was not only how data were gathered, but the way in which colonial officials mis- or over-interpreted demographic indices because of their lack of basic statistical skills or, more or less willingly, in order to support their views.[72]

The interpretation of the birth and death rates registered in the AMI Cuanza zone is an illuminating example for this. In his annual report for 1930, Waldemar Teixeira drew attention to the fact that the registered birth and death rates had both increased between 1927 and 1930, from 8.4 to 40.81 per thousand and 11.4 to 29.58 per thousand respectively (see Table 4.1). While he admitted that this increase mainly resulted from better registration, he also interpreted the figures as proof of a distinct demographic shift. Under the impact of the AMI health programme, he claimed, population decline (still visible in the negative growth rates of 1927) had slowed in 1928 and reversed into population growth in 1929, a trend that was further consolidated in 1930.[73]

In Teixeira's opinion, two other indices corroborated his claim. First, there was the shifting age distribution: between 1927 and 1930, he wrote, the percentage of people aged 0 to 15 had increased from 35.45 to 43.57 per cent, thus changing the prospect for the future evolution of the population from 'stationary' to 'clearly progressive'.[74] With this interpretation, Teixeira followed a well-known scheme. In interwar Africa, comparing the distribution of age groups (0–15, adults, elderly people) in a given population with the standard millions (that is, the distribution found in the 'standard' population of

---

[70] Kuczynski, *Colonial Population*, xii.
[71] See, for instance, Kuczynski, *Cameroons and Togoland*, xiv, 42–3 and 138–42.
[72] Kuczynski, *Colonial Population*, xii–xiii.
[73] Teixeira, 'Relatório Cuanza (1930)', 14–15 and 18–9.
[74] Teixeira, 'Relatório Cuanza (1930)', 23.

Table 4.1. *Demographic indices in the Cuanza Zone, 1927–30*

Years	Birth rates (%)	Mortality rates (%)	Evolution of the population	
			Decline (%)	Growth (%)
1927	8.40	11.40	– 3.00	
1928	18.73	20.65	– 1.88	
1929	32.99	28.95		+ 4.04
1930	40.81	29.58		+ 11.23

Source: Waldemar Gomes Teixeira, 'Relatório da Zona Sanitária do Cuanza (1930)', June 1931, 19, AHU, MU, AGC 2336

either Sweden (census of 1890) or England and Wales (census of 1901)) had become a widely used method by colonial demographers to predict whether that population was regressive (decreasing), stagnating or progressive (increasing), even though Kuczynski later objected that population growth or decline could not be deduced from such broad age-group ratios.[75] Second, during the same time span, the sex ratio had fallen from 110 (men to 100 women) to 84. Thus the sex ratio in the Cuanza zone had both approached global standards and turned positive.[76] Indeed, many a colonial doctor and demographer interpreted a low sex ratio (that is, more women than men) as an indication of future population growth, arguing that women were more important than men for reproduction and that high sex ratios had been shown to be a symptom of racial degeneration and population decrease in some Pacific islands.[77]

Although he knew that the data for 1927 and 1928 were very fragmentary, Teixeira did not admit the possibility, at least not openly, that proportions were distorted or that the population had already been growing before the establishment of the AMI programme. His positivist analysis of the scanty data available was not an isolated case. A year earlier, his predecessor Augusto Ornelas analysed the birth and death rates in the Cuanza zone in very similar terms.[78] This alleged reversal from population decline to modest but continuous population growth, which would be confirmed by the medical registries in the Cuanza zone throughout the 1930s, also figured prominently in the

[75] Compare Cazanove, 'Essai de démographie', 26–30 and Trolli, 'Contribution', 276–9 with Kuczynski, *Colonial Population*, xii.
[76] Teixeira, 'Relatório Cuanza (1930)', 22.
[77] José Firmino Sant'Anna, '1.° Relatório da missão médica ao arquipélago de Cabo Verde em 1930', July 1931, 19–21 and 27, IHMT; Mora, 'Mortalidade infantil', 574. For the debate on the correlation between high sex ratios and population decline in the Pacific, see Widmer, 'Imbalanced Sex Ratio'.
[78] Ornelas and Mesquita, *Relatório da missão médica*, 22–3.

writings of other AMI doctors, including health director António Damas Mora.[79] Arguably, there was a clear rationale to their claims: by giving credence and publicity to these data and their interpretation in both internal reports and press articles, doctors aimed to legitimise the health investments and the particular methods of the AMI programme to the general government of the colony and the wider public.

The impact of these claims on the depopulation debate is more difficult to measure. They certainly did not completely dissipate depopulation fears in Angola. The AMI zones had often been considered the worst regions in terms of demographic evolution, but they only covered a small part of the colony. Moreover, depopulation anxieties were constantly reinforced by the increasingly pervasive idea that numerous Africans were emigrating to neighbouring colonies.[80] When, for instance, in 1930, a representative of Union Minière visited Angola to recruit labourers for its mines in Katanga, Damas Mora was disinclined to support this demand, given that, with the available statistics, it was still unclear whether the colony's total population was growing or diminishing.[81]

A few years later, however, he and others would be less reluctant to extrapolate the demographic effects of healthcare improvements. In the mid-1930s, the director of the colony's newly established Statistical Department Alberto de Lemos published new estimates for the whole of Angola, suggesting that the 'black' population had fallen from 5.38 million in 1846 to 2.83 million in 1927, after which it had begun to recover, reaching 3.15 million in 1934 (see Figure 4.3). While Lemos did not fully disclose the origin of his data – they seem to have been based on retrospective estimates, recalculations and, for 1933 and 1934, new surveys – his interpretation was straightforward: he attributed the reversal after 1927 mainly to the merits of the AMI programme.[82] A few years later, at the Colonial Congress in Lisbon in 1940, Damas Mora publicly endorsed this view. Although he maintained that most of the decline must have happened between the 1880s and 1900s and not 1920–7 as Lemos's figures suggested, he happily agreed that the healthcare investments had lived up to their promise and were a decisive factor in turning the demographic tide.[83] This interpretation was not unanimously shared, however. Addressing the same Congress, former Governor-General and High

---

[79] See, for instance, Gama, 'Um ano de chefia', 540–1; Amaral, *Relatório Catete (1930–31)*, 19–20; Mora, *Luta*, 216, 221 and António Damas Mora, 'Assistência Médica aos Indígenas, em Angola', *A Província de Angola*, 6–8 August 1934. For birth and death rates in the Cuanza zone in the 1930s, see Costa, 'Assistência Médica ao Indígena', 61–2 and *Boletim Sanitário de Angola* (1939), 65.

[80] See Chapter 6.

[81] 'Rapport de voyage en Angola', 1930, AR, I 254 (Union Minière), dossier 338.

[82] *Anuário estatístico de Angola* (1934), 21–3.   [83] Mora, 'Mortalidade infantil', 579–83.

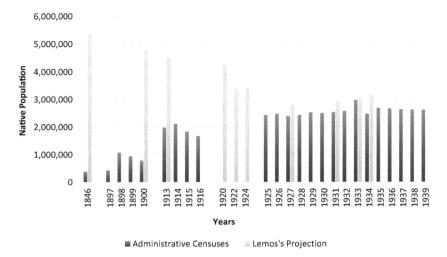

Figure 4.3 Evolution of the 'native'/'black' population in Angola, 1846–1939.[84]

Sources: See Table 1.1 and Diniz, *Negócios indígenas – relatório 1916*, 5; Lemos, 'Introdução ao primeiro censo', 30, 33; *Anuário estatístico de Angola* (1934), 21–3

Commissioner Norton de Matos, who had become a prolific and influential publicist, was full of praise for the sanitary reforms under Damas Mora, but much more sceptical about their demographic impact. Accusing the general shortcomings of Angola's native policy, most notably the high tax pressure and the recrudescence of forced labour practices after his departure in 1923, he did not believe that recent colonial efforts had been sufficient to halt and reverse the process of population decline.[85]

Measuring and Debating Fertility, Infant Mortality and Racial Difference

Medical demography also reshaped the debate on fertility and infant mortality in interwar Angola. Up to that point, both low fertility and high infant mortality had frequently been mentioned as major causes of population decline.[86] Now, on the basis of the birth rates and the average number of

---

[84] Compared to the administrative censuses, which enumerated the 'native' population, Lemos's figures of the 'black' population included 'assimilated' Africans and excluded 'native' *mestiços*. On the issue of *mestiços*, see Chapter 5.

[85] Matos, 'Síntese', 487–9, 498–9 and 523. On taxation and forced labour, see Chapter 6.

[86] See footnote 17.

children per woman calculated in medical sectors or during mobile missions, many doctors concluded that, in most parts of the colony, fertility was high, even much higher than in the metropole, and therefore could not be in itself a cause of depopulation. Questioning many thousands of women, doctors around 1930 registered averages of 3.8–5.7 live births among women beyond (or towards the end of) childbearing age in Northern and Central Angola, and in the sparsely populated northeastern Lunda district Alfredo de Rezende still calculated averages of 3.6–3.9.[87] A decade later, Antero Antunes do Amaral reported that he had personally registered birth rates between 44 and 58 per thousand and total rates of seven pregnancies per woman in the different sectors of the Cuanza zone where he worked during the 1930s, concluding that 'there [was] in fact no natality problem to resolve'.[88]

In the memoir he presented at the Colonial Congress in Lisbon in 1940, António Damas Mora argued along the same lines. Doctors' inquiries, he wrote, had shown consistently that Angolan women above the age of 50 had, on average, borne five to six children during their reproductive life. However, he also added that many women died before reaching that age and that averages were lower in 'regions where the native suffers from pronounced and permanent under-nutrition'.[89] The example he gave for this was the so-called 'Bushmen' in South Angola, often also designated as Khoisan or !Kung at the time.[90] Due to the 'permanent state of under-nutrition' and 'extreme misery' in which they lived, the 'Bushmen' had exceptionally low birth rates and were on the brink of extinction, Damas Mora stated.[91] More generally, his observation reflected the concern that he and other doctors had voiced throughout the interwar years of the adverse effects of under-nutrition and malnutrition on the health and reproductive life of many African populations.[92]

Regarding the 'Bushmen', Damas Mora also added racial factors to his socio-medical explanation for differential fertility. Endorsing the widespread idea, first formulated by anthropologists in the late nineteenth century, that the 'Bushmen' were the last remnants of an older race that had been pushed into inhospitable regions by the territorial expansion of Bantu peoples and Boers, he assumed that 'low fertility can also mean the senescence or ageing of a race'.[93] Maybe, he concluded, the demographic decline of the 'Bushmen' was,

---

[87] Teixeira, 'Relatório Cuanza (1930)', 25–6; Amaral, *Relatório Catete (1930–31)*, 26. For Central Angola, see the reports in footnote 48. For Lunda, 'Missão volante da Lunda', 310.

[88] Amaral, 'Natalidade e mortalidade', 172. Similarly, Sarmento, *Aspectos da natalidade*, 2.

[89] Mora, 'Mortalidade infantil', 573–4.

[90] On Portuguese conceptualisations and policies regarding the 'Bushmen', see Coghe, 'Reassessing Portuguese Exceptionalism'.

[91] Mora, 'Mortalidade infantil', 595–6.

[92] Coghe, *Population Politics (2014)*, 331–40. See also Freitas, 'Relatório Sub-Brigada Sul (1931)', 8–11.

[93] See Coghe, 'Reassessing Portuguese Exceptionalism', 185–8.

similar to that of the Australian 'aborigines', the result of their 'collective old age' and they would disappear just as the Tasmanians had in the nineteenth century. The 'natives' of the 'Bantu lineage', the overwhelming majority in Angola, by contrast, had kept the 'psychology of the primitive peoples concerning the advantage of having many children'.[94]

With this last remark, Damas Mora pitted the reproductive behaviour of Angola's 'native' populations against the decline of fertility that had been diagnosed in most European countries in the late nineteenth and early twentieth centuries and had provoked widespread anxieties of degeneration and depopulation.[95] Even in Portugal, where birth rates were among the highest in Europe and only began to fall markedly in the 1930s, some observers, most notably the influential gynaecologist and university professor Sebastião Cabral da Costa-Sacadura, warned already in the 1920s that neo-Malthusian practices of birth control such as 'voluntary restriction' and 'criminal abortion' were causing denatality and depopulation.[96] Damas Mora may also have been referring to the theory of deliberate racial suicide, which W. H. R. Rivers advanced two decades earlier to explain population decline in Melanesia. Rivers posited that Melanesians, with the exception of those who had become Christian, refused to have children because they had lost interest in life due to the destruction of their traditional customs and the hardships of colonial rule. To avoid procreation, they made wide use of contraceptive and abortive practices.[97] Echoing much older anxieties over the use of abortifacients by African slave women in the eighteenth- and nineteenth-century Atlantic World, this psychological explanation of population decline among 'native' populations became influential in the interwar period.[98] Nancy Rose Hunt has shown that, due to the '"global circulation" of such "ethnographic commonplaces of colonial intelligence"', tropes of 'racial suicide, dying races, empty villages and self-aborting women' also widely circulated among French and Belgian colonial officials in Central Africa.[99]

In Angola, stories of abortive practices as expressions of psychological resistance occasionally appeared as well, but they were rare and clearly politically unwanted. In his inspection report on the Dande region of 1928, Dr Jacinto de Sousa conveyed a rumour according to which African parents sometimes destroyed male foetuses 'to prevent [the possibility] that there

---

[94] Mora, 'Mortalidade infantil', 595–6.
[95] By way of example, see Tomlinson, 'The Disappearance of France'; Soloway, *Demography and Degeneration*. See also Introduction.
[96] See, for instance, Costa-Sacadura, *Despopulação em Portugal*. For more detail, see Coghe, *Population Politics (2014)*, 249–53.
[97] Rivers, 'Pyschological Factor'. See also Widmer, 'Of Field Encounters'.
[98] Compare with Schiebinger, 'Feminist History'.
[99] Hunt, 'Colonial Medical Anthropology', 252–4 (quotes 254).

would be *serviçais* for the Europeans'. While Sousa did not know whether to believe this rumour, the passage was censured in the version of the report later printed in Lisbon.[100] At least officially, most doctors in Angola appear to have assumed, like Damas Mora, that neo-Malthusian practices of birth control were rare, because of the high value Africans attached to motherhood and parenthood in general. 'When we ponder hygiene and demography', Augusto Ornelas stated, 'we recognise immediately [...] that the births of black children are always wanted, that Malthusian practices are not adopted, that criminal abortions do not exist and, finally, that births are very numerous'.[101] As proof of the innate pronatalism of Africans, doctors and other colonial officials referred to the social advantages of having many children and the consequences of childlessness in African societies. Such assumptions did not come out of thin air. Ethnographic work in Angola, which until the 1930s was mostly done by administrators and missionaries, suggested that in many so-called ethnic groups, childlessness was believed to be a curse and a dishonour for both African women and men – and that it was also a commonly accepted ground upon which they could obtain a divorce and, in the case of the husbands, compensation from the woman's family, often the restitution of the brideprice.[102]

Rather than an expression of psychological resistance, doctors in interwar Angola usually perceived spontaneous abortions, stillbirths and infertility as a physiological problem, as the consequence of under-nutrition and poverty or of particular illnesses such as sleeping sickness, malaria and venereal diseases. While doctors knew that tackling under-nutrition and poverty would necessitate long-term agricultural reforms and economic development, they were more optimistic about disease-induced fertility problems. These were considered temporary conditions that could and would be resolved by treating the disease that had caused them.[103] Treatment with trypanocidal drugs, for instance, was widely believed to remedy temporary fertility problems in men and women caused by sleeping sickness – and to be the main reason for the rapid recovery of the birth rates in the AMI sectors.[104]

---

[100] Compare Jacinto da Sousa, 'Relatório da missão médica volante de assistência aos indígenas do Dande', 1928, 14, AHU, MU, AGC 2336 with Sousa, *Relatório Dande*, 17.

[101] Ornelas, 'Obra de protecção', 525. Similarly, Silva, 'Pian', 1 and Amaral, 'Natalidade e mortalidade', 172.

[102] See especially Diniz, *Populações indígenas*, 22, 147, 234, 244–5, 274, 330, 361–2 and 454; Ivo Benjamin de Cerqueira, 'Organisação social indigena. Seu estado actual – usos e costumes', 1930, 17, AHU, MU, AGC 2336. See also Mora, 'Mortalidade infantil', 587–8.

[103] Neves and Sousa, 'Assistência Médica aos Indígenas', 439; Mora, 'Mortalidade infantil', 594–5.

[104] Sousa, *Relatório Dande*, 16; Mora, 'Mortalidade infantil', 594–5. Compare with Sicé, *Trypanosomiase humaine*, 76–7, 94–5 and contemporary evidence of reproductive problems in Ikede, Ehlassan and Akpavie, 'Reproductive Disorders'.

Doctors' optimism had also much to do with how they misconceived, ignored or willingly downplayed the incidence of venereal or sexually transmitted diseases (STDs) such as syphilis and gonorrhoea in Angola and their impact on birth rates. Certainly, concern over STDs initially intensified with the expansion of AMI services in the 1920s. Reports stressed the high incidence of syphilis and gonorrhoea in various regions, especially in the eastern and central districts of Moxico, Lunda, Malange and Bié (see Map 4.1), which was usually attributed to the belated military 'pacification' campaigns and the stationing of European and African soldiers in these regions.[105] In Moxico, a special anti-venereal service was set up in 1927.[106] However, whereas the spread of STDs triggered depopulation scares in several parts of colonial Africa in the first decades of the twentieth century (insofar as they were held responsible for high rates of miscarriage, stillbirth, neonatal death and infertile women), the colonial health services in Angola do not seem to have attached particular importance to them after the initial shock of the 1920s.[107] Cases were registered and treated, but no large-scale campaigns were set up. By the early 1940s, they had even disappeared from the list of the colony's most important endemic diseases and little research into STDs was done until the 1950s.[108]

There are various possible reasons for this apparent neglect. One explanation is that in eastern Angola, the region with the highest verified incidence of syphilis and gonorrhoea, doctors and healthcare infrastructure were still scarce. In Moxico, coverage had deteriorated in the early 1930s, after the AMI efforts of the late 1920s were cut back.[109] Therefore the health services may not have grasped the complete extent of the problem or preferred to ignore it, as they lacked the means to tackle it.[110] Conversely, AMI doctors were generally convinced that the incidence of syphilis was very low in the much better known and economically more important Cuanza and Congo districts.[111] Another explanation is that doctors like Damas Mora believed that syphilis was 'less damaging to black than to white people' and also caused fewer miscarriages in the tropics than in temperate climates.[112]

<hr/>

105 Silva, 'Relatório missão volante', 237; Distrito do Mochico, 'Relatório Sáude', 340–1; Gama, 'Missão volante', 66; 'Missão volante da Lunda', 310.
106 Mora, 'Services de l'assistance', 14.
107 See, for instance, Summers, 'Intimate Colonialism' and Vaughan, *Curing Their Ills*, 129–54.
108 Ribeiro, 'Notas'; Ribeiro, 'Investigação ciêntífica', 2814.
109 Neves and Sousa, 'Assistência Médica aos Indígenas', 438–9; António de Almeida, 'Relatório do Governador do Distrito do Moxico (1931)', February 1932, 21–3, AHU, GM 600.
110 See Frederico Leopoldino Rebêlo in António de Almeida, 'Relatório do Governo da Província do Bié (1938)', 117 and 121, AHU, MU, DGAC 543.
111 See, for instance, Ornelas and Mesquita, *Relatório da missão médica*, 157–8; Silva, *Serviço de Assistência Congo (1931)*, 18–9.
112 Mora, 'Mortalidade infantil', 607.

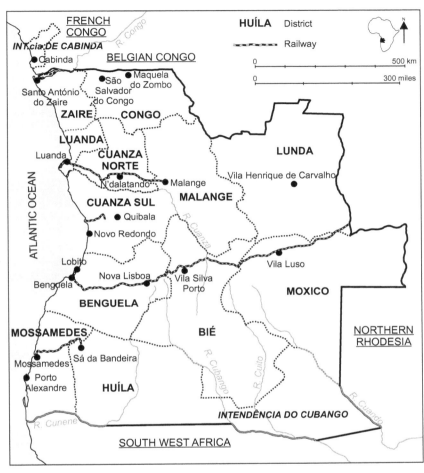

Map 4.1 Administrative divisions of Angola, including major towns, 1929. Angola was divided in 12 districts and two *intendências* (Cabinda and Cubango). In 1934, they were subsumed into five large provinces (Luanda, Malange, Benguela, Huíla and Bié).
Source: Redrawn from *Colónia de Angola. Esboço da carta escolar* (Luanda, 1929) http://purl.pt/8143/3/ with the kind permission of the National Library of Portugal

Both beliefs – in the low incidence of syphilis in northwestern Angola and its weaker effects on African women – might have been wrong. In the 1920s, it was still very difficult to distinguish venereal syphilis from yaws, as each disease was caused by almost identical bacteria and provoked very similar symptoms. Doctors might sometimes have mistaken syphilis for yaws, which they found to be very common in northwestern Angola – just as many doctors in early twentieth-century Africa mistook yaws for syphilis, thus triggering massive fears of miscarriage, stillbirth and infant mortality. This would explain why doctors like Venâncio da Silva associated yaws with repeated miscarriages, a typical consequence of venereal syphilis.[113] Finally, doctors in interwar Angola probably underestimated the incidence of gonorrhoea as well, a disease that can cause infertility in women. Official numbers remained low as Africans continued to be very reluctant to seek biomedical treatment before the advent of penicillin in the 1950s greatly enhanced the prospects of a rapid cure.[114]

Certainly, this positive view of Angolan women's fertility was not shared by all. While some doctors did call for stronger action against STDs, others wanted to fight the widespread social practices of birth spacing and polygamy, both held to limit births, to further increase fertility, as in the neighbouring Belgian Congo.[115] In 1931, the government eventually adopted a long-discussed pronatalist and anti-polygamist measure: it exempted men with four or more (still living) children from the same woman from paying the 'native tax' (*imposto indígena*).[116] And from the mid-1930s onwards, when the economy recovered and anxieties about labour scarcity resurged, administrators and (provincial) governors increasingly engaged in a controversial discussion about the effects of single male long-distance labour migration on birth rates. While some held that the demographic impact was negligible, arguing that most women would not wait long before having sexual relations and children with other men, others felt labour migration caused considerable *denatalidade* ('denatality'). In the words of Álvaro de Freitas Morna (Governor-General 1942–3), the 180,000 contract labourers who had spent one to two years away from home in 1943 equalled 100,000 unborn babies.[117]

Debates about polygamy and migration were never about birth rates alone, however. They also struck at the heart of colonial ideas about morality and the organisation of family and society, thus revealing a tension between the predominantly medical and demographic view on fertility by AMI doctors and the social and moral framework in which administrators were more likely to see it. Administrators thus blamed single male long-distance labour

---

[113] Compare Silva, 'Pian', 1–3 with Summers, 'Intimate Colonialism', 787–8; Headrick, *Colonialism, Health and Illness*, 37–8; Doyle, *Crisis and Decline*, 150–7, 221–3.

[114] Neves and Sousa, 'Assistência Médica aos Indígenas', 438–9; Barros, 'Gonorreias'.

[115] Sousa, 'Capital humano', 162. For the Belgian Congo, see Hunt, 'Bébé en Brousse'; Hunt, 'Noise', 472–5.

[116] Colónia de Angola, *Regulamento do recenseamento (1931)*, preamble and art. 2. For the discussion, see Diniz, *Populações indígenas*, 730 and Diniz, *Missão civilisadora*, 17. Compare also with Hunt, *Colonial Lexicon*, 4 for the Belgian Congo.

[117] Morna, *Angola*, 173. For this debate, see Coghe, *Population Politics (2014)*, 366–8. On the labour debate, see also Chapter 6.

migration, among many other things, for promoting promiscuity and prostitution among the women who stayed behind in the villages and for 'detribalising' the workers: that is, alienating them from their societies of origin and hence hampering their reintegration once they had fulfilled their contract. When, for instance, the governor of the Malange province in 1943 asked his administrators at their annual meeting about the effects of this migration, they all agreed that women's extramarital relations and the often ensuing divorces furthered the disintegration of the family, that 'small social and economic cell which we must care for', and hence native society as a whole. Their more or less unanimous condemnation of single male labour migration, hence, was less because of its supposed effects on the birth rate and more because they defended the Portuguese moral ideal of stable, faithful and monogamous relationships and the nuclear family as the most basic unit of society.[118]

This ideal, common to various European colonial regimes at the time, was particularly key to the conservative ideology of the *Estado Novo* in Portugal.[119] As debates about polygamy and labour migration show, it was, from the 1930s onwards, increasingly projected onto the African population in Angola as well. It was in this vein that, in his report of the meeting to the Governor-General, the governor of Malange concluded that wives should always accompany their husbands if they were recruited for long periods and distant regions. Rather than keeping the birth rate up, spousal accompaniment was to protect the integrity of the family, monogamy and women's morality.[120] Family migration, hence, was in Angola not only pursued by big companies such as Diamang in order to 'stabilise' the labour force in newly created villages nearby and to diminish recruitment costs.[121] It also corresponded with the increasingly conservative family ideals of the colonial state.

In summary, if leading AMI doctors believed in relatively high and growing birth rates, that was mainly because they extrapolated the statistical data from their own fertility inquiries and birth registrations, were convinced of the pronatalist stance of the Angolan populations and probably underestimated the reproductive problems caused by STDs. They were also less concerned about the social and moral context into which children were born. While they agreed that fertility could still be higher if certain obstacles were removed, they

---

[118] Manuel da Cruz Alvura, 'Relatório da Conferência dos Intendentes e Administradores da Província de Malange (2–8 December 1942) – Acta da Reunião', 9–13, AHU, MU, ISAU 1730; Idem, 'Relatório do Governador da Província de Malanje (1943), 14 (quote), AHU, MU, ISAU 1663.

[119] Pimentel, *Política feminina*, 32–54.

[120] Manuel da Cruz Alvura, 'Relatório da Conferência dos Intendentes e Administradores da Província de Malange (2–8 December 1942) – Relatório para o Governador Geral', 28 January 1943, 3–5, AHU, MU, ISAU 1730.

[121] See Coghe, 'Reordering Colonial Society', 38–43.

also agreed that it was not the main problem. For most doctors, Angola was clearly not part of what would later be termed the Central African Infertility Belt, a zone with particularly low birth rates stretching from Gabon to Uganda.[122]

Medical demography not only dismissed the notion of low fertility: it simultaneously consolidated the idea that the Angolan population suffered from appalling infant mortality rates and that this was *an* (if not *the main*) obstacle to sustained population growth. 'The percentage of children who die in infancy', one AMI doctor suggested in summarising the debate, was so enormous that 'although African women were usually extremely prolific, the population [was] either stable or decreasing instead of increasing'.[123] Damas Mora was one of the most tenacious and influential supporters of this view. 'There is, these days, no epidemic scourge that produces victims in a similar or even approximate proportion', he stressed in 1930.[124] Over the next decade, he would repeat this position many times and urge the colonial health services to reconcentrate their efforts on infant mortality.[125] Clearly, infant mortality had already been described as terribly high previously, but it was only in the late 1920s and 1930s that demographic statistics in medical reports turned this assumption into an apparently objective and irrefutable truth, frequently mentioning infant mortality rates of 50 per cent and more.[126]

Such appalling percentages, which circulated for other colonies as well, were usually the result of a particularly broad definition of infant mortality. Whereas in Europe infant mortality related to the number of deaths occurring in the first year of life, infant mortality rates in colonial Africa seem to have often included all deceased children up to the age of 15, and sometimes even miscarriages and stillbirths.[127] In part, this was the consequence of the method used and of ignorance with regard to statistical mathematics and definitions. Frequently, as the Belgian doctor Jérôme Rodhain noted at the time, doctors calculated infant mortality rates by simply inverting the total survival index, that is the number of children currently still alive, determined in fertility enquiries (100 per cent minus survival index), without discerning at what age the children had died.[128]

[122] Hunt, 'Colonial Medical Anthropology'. See also the Epilogue.
[123] Gomes, 'Reconhecimentos sanitários', 450.
[124] António Damas Mora, 'Um belo gesto das senhoras de Luanda', *A Província de Angola*, 1 August 1930.
[125] Mora, *Luta*, 233; Mora, 'Mortalidade infantil', 559.
[126] See, for instance, Freitas and Fonseca, 'Relatório (1930)', 9; Amaral, 'Natalidade e mortalidade', 173–4; Teixeira, 'Relatório Cuanza (1930)', 21.
[127] See, for instance, Prum, 'Observations', 18; Thiroux, 'Natalité et mortalité', 569; van Nitsen, *Contribution*, 50–3.
[128] For explicit examples, see António Damas Mora. 'Um belo gesto das senhoras de Luanda', *A Província de Angola*, 1 August 1930 and Alfredo de Rezende's calculations in 'Missão

Many medical reports in Angola also contained infant mortality rates calculated according to the international definition.[129] However, these more cautious figures, which usually varied between 20 and 35 per cent, were less prominently cited. This suggests that, beyond statistical incompetence, other issues were in play. Arguably, some leading colonial officials preferred to cite the much higher percentages because they served their agenda. Those who favoured stronger medical interventionism in infant welfare used the alarming figures to underscore the urgency of the situation and to bolster their demands for investment.[130] Conversely, high percentages also served those who wanted to criticise Portuguese health services as ineffective and Portuguese colonialism in general as backward and inhuman, like Henrique Galvão in 1947.[131] Finally, using maximalist infant mortality rates (0–15 years) also reflected a utilitarian reasoning: the resulting percentage quantified those who did not make it into productive and reproductive life. Significantly, these were sometimes termed '*déchét*' (waste), in other words, those who were lost to the colonial project.[132]

Medical demography, hence, reinforced the idea that infant mortality was much higher in tropical Africa than in Europe. In the Belgian Congo, leading doctors like Mouchet and Rodhain alongside Governor-General Ryckmans blamed this on the particularly high mortality during second infancy and adolescence, which they viewed as a distinctive pattern of Central African demography.[133] Damas Mora, who knew about such interpretations by Belgian (but also French and British) doctors, believed that they also applied to Angola. Mortality rates of children between 1 and 15 years, he wrote, were more or less equal to those of infants in their first year of life, thus adding up to total rates of 50–60 per cent. He thereby probably overstated mortality in the 1–15 age group, which AMI doctors in Angola usually calculated at only about half of that between 0 and 1 year.[134]

volante da Lunda'. For Rodhain's critique, see Rodhain, *Mortinatalité et mortalité infantile*, 6, 9 and 16.

[129] See Ornelas and Mesquita, *Relatório da missão médica*, 22; Teixeira, 'Relatório Cuanza (1930)', 21; Fonseca, 'Relatório Sub-Brigada Norte (1931)', 6–9; Amaral, *Relatório Catete* (1930–1), 37–8, 49–50; Amaral, 'Natalidade e mortalidade', 174.

[130] See, for instance, Manuel Pereira Figueira, 'Relatorio do Curador Geral dos Indígenas da Colonia de Angola para 1937', 15 May 1938, 11, AHU, MU, ISAU 2243; Morna, *Angola*, 174–81.

[131] Henrique Galvão, 'Exposição à Comissão de Colónias da Assembleia Nacional', 22 January 1947, 24, AHP, Section XXVIII, Box 48A, n. 10. On this report, see Chapter 6 and Epilogue.

[132] See Mouchet, 'Natalité'; Prum, 'Observations', 22.

[133] Mouchet, 'Natalité', 170, 173; Rodhain, *Mortinatalité et mortalité infantile*, 16–7; Ryckmans, 'Démographie Congolaise', 257.

[134] Mora, 'Mortalidade infantil', 615–6. Compare with the references in footnote 129.

Like their foreign colleagues, doctors in interwar Angola did not attribute this divergence to biological differences but the civilisational gap that separated the continents. Almost invariably they blamed high infant mortality primarily on the formidable backwardness and incompetence of African mothers, whom they described as full of prejudices and ignorant of the most basic principles of infant hygiene.[135] This racialist argument mirrored accusations previously levelled against working-class women in Europe.[136] The solutions would be similar: as in Europe, the first prudent measures of maternal and infant welfare in interwar Angola focused on reforming motherhood through education, before such cultural explanations began to be challenged by a broader debate on the social determinants of health.[137]

In conclusion, doctors built upon medical demography to claim that, with few exceptions, the 'native' population in Angola was subjected to a demographic regime that was distinct from that of Europe, in that both fertility and infant mortality were much higher. If, except for the Bushmen case, these differences were interpreted as culturally and socio-economically (rather than biologically) determined, that was partly because doctors knew that Europe itself had experienced such a demographic regime in the past and only moved away from it during its industrialisation over the last century. Difference, hence, was a matter of change over time. Although the classic version of the demographic transition theory would only be formulated in 1945 by the Princeton-based demographers Notestein and Kingsley, its basic idea that, with the advancement of civilisation, all societies would move from a regime of high fertility and (infant) mortality to one of low fertility and (infant) mortality, just like Europe had, was already palpable in interwar population research.[138] This is particularly true for infant mortality. By the interwar period, the level of infant mortality was already widely considered to indicate the 'material and moral condition of a nation', namely its level of civilisation.[139] Moreover, Portuguese doctors were in a particularly bad position to talk about these differences in terms of biological race if they did not want to discredit their own position. Despite anxieties about falling birth rates, Portugal's birth and infant mortality rates were both still clearly higher than

---

[135] Silva, *Serviço de Assistência Congo (1930)*, 9–10; Ornelas, 'Obra de protecção'.

[136] Compare with Lindner, 'Transfer', and, more specifically for Portugal, Garrett, *Como organizar a luta*.

[137] See Chapter 5.

[138] See Hodgson, 'Demography'; Szreter, 'Idea of Demographic Transition'. For Angola, see Mora, 'Mortalidade infantil', 589–94.

[139] Quote from Julia Lathrop, first director of the United States Children's Bureau, in 1921, in Rooke and Schnell, 'Uncramping Child Life', 179. Similarly Sousa, 'Necessidades e deficiências', 225.

most other European countries in the interwar period and doctors were very aware of this.[140]

Conclusion

In 1940, the first autonomous and complete population census was conducted in Angola. The initiative had been taken by Salazar and his government, the *Conselho dos Ministros*, in Lisbon. In the year of the big commemorations (that is, '800 years of independence' and '300 years of restoration' from Spain), Salazar wanted to survey the population of the whole colonial empire 'to present another testimony of Portugal's expansion in the world'.[141] In Angola, the huge logistical operation was coordinated by the colony's Statistical Department and its director Alberto de Lemos. Although the international scientific principles of simultaneity and universality could not be fully implemented in the colonial situation, as Lemos himself admitted, the census differed significantly from earlier administrative censuses: it had been decoupled from practical concerns such as tax registration and military conscription to become an autonomous instrument of knowledge. One of the most visible consequences was that with 3,665,829 'natives' (plus 44,083 'whites' and 28,035 people of 'mixed race'), the census figures exceeded earlier administrative counting exercises (2,615,400 in 1939) by more than a million – and the administrative survey in 1940 (2,993,658) with still almost 700,000 – thus also confirming medical doctors' longstanding distrust of the latter (compare with Figure 4.3).[142] Together with doctors' demographic data, the 1940 census results, published in 12 volumes between 1941 and 1947, would contribute to (further) dissipating anxieties of population decline.[143]

The role of the 1940 census in this reversal was not limited to the higher population figures it attested. Confidence in population growth was also based on the simple but large-scale fertility study it contained. Extending AMI doctors' methods to the whole colony, census agents had asked all 'native' women above the age of 14 years how many children they had borne and how many of them were still alive.[144] The results listed 3,035,587 children born to 875,115 mothers, or an average ratio of 3.46 births per woman. For women in

---

[140] Livi Bacci, *Century of Portuguese Fertility*. For contemporary voices, see Garrett, *Como organizar a luta*; Sousa, 'Necessidades e deficiências', 224.

[141] Presidência do Conselho, 'Decreto-lei 29.750', 14 July 1939, *DG Série I* (1939), 719–20.

[142] Compare Lemos, 'Introdução ao primeiro censo', 30 and 33 with Repartição de Estatística Geral da Colónia de Angola (ed.), *Censo geral da População* (1940), vol. I, 78–9. For the administrative census of 1940, see 'Mão de obra: elementos estatísticos' (1945), AHU, MU, ISAU 1661.

[143] See Epilogue.

[144] Repartição Técnica de Estatística Geral do Governo Geral de Angola, *Bases*, 64 and 68.

the highest age group (usually 50 and over), this ratio reached 4.7, with a peak of 5.5 in the Luanda province, where the AMI sectors were located – figures that seemed to confirm the optimism of doctors like Damas Mora and Antunes do Amaral.[145]

Certainly, these figures need to be handled with care. Beyond the inevitable inaccuracies in the registration process, fertility rates were greatly inflated, since they were not calculated on the basis of all adult women, but of mothers only. The more than 360,000 women older than 14 years (that is, 29.2 per cent of all 'adult' women (1,236,296)) who had not or not yet borne any children were not taken into account. They were only briefly and indirectly mentioned further on, where one can learn their region of origin and age.[146] Moreover, both the percentage of mothers among adult women and their fertility rates varied greatly according to region. While both figures were highest for the Luanda province, the eastern Bié province and particularly its Moxico district had the lowest scores, with only 59.5 per cent of mothers and a fertility rate of 2.3 children per mother – scores that correlate with the high incidence of STDs in the region.[147]

However, the low scores in Moxico and some other districts did not produce generalised fertility scares. On the contrary, in one of the rare published analyses of the 1940 census, Alexandre Sarmento, a medical doctor with a strong interest in physical anthropology and demography, conveniently used the inflated fertility rates to bolster his old argument about the absence of a natality problem in Angola (even though he wrongly assumed that 29 per cent of Angolan women were sterile). He also backed his argument with other indices deduced from the census data: a high average birth rate of 35.8 per thousand, the 'progressive' character of the population due to the existence of 40.3 per cent of children and a low sex ratio of 89.6. Overall, the demographic perspectives of Angola's 'native' population were looking good, he concluded.[148]

This notwithstanding, Sarmento also knew that the census was far from perfect and that it did not contain any trustworthy information on such important demographic phenomena as general mortality, infant mortality and stillbirth.[149] This also explains why the 'scientific' censuses, which would now be conducted every 10 years, did not entail the end of medical demography.

---

[145] Repartição de Estatística Geral da Colónia de Angola (ed.), *Censo geral da população* (1940) vol. xi–xii, 107–81 and 218.

[146] Ibid., 217.   [147] Ibid., 217–8.

[148] Sarmento, 'População indígena de Angola', 644–8. See also Sarmento, 'População infantil de Angola'.

[149] Sarmento, 'População indígena de Angola', 635, 649. On the quality of the 1940 census from the perspective of a historical demographer, see Heisel, 'Indigenous Populations' and Heisel, 'Demography'.

In northern Angola, AMI doctors continued until at least the mid-1950s to register the population and its movements independently of the civil registry by the administrative authorities, thereby recording natality and mortality rates almost twice as high as the latter.[150] Further, in the 1950s and early 1960s, medical doctors including Sarmento still conducted small-scale fertility and infant mortality studies in areas or among ethnic groups that elicited particular interest, such as the 'Bushmen'.[151] Certainly, they lost their virtual monopoly on these kinds of studies: encouraged by students of colonial demography at the Centre of Demographic Studies that had been created in Lisbon in 1944, some administrators in the Portuguese colonies began to conduct small-scale fertility and infant mortality studies as well.[152] Yet, overall, the persistence of such sample studies is illuminating. On the one hand, it reveals that demographic indices, especially with regard to fertility and infant mortality, continued to be seen as markers of racial and ethnic difference. On the other, it testifies to the continuous shortcomings of colonial censuses and civil registries and, as fertility studies relied on doctors and administrators, to the slow professionalisation of colonial demography.

---

[150] See the analysis in Morgado, *Aspectos*, esp. 16–24.
[151] See, for instance, Sarmento and Henriques, 'Alguns aspectos demográficos' and the studies in Ministério do Ultramar – Junta de Investigações do Ultramar (ed.), *Contribuição*, 17–45.
[152] See, for instance, Brito, 'Aspectos demográficos'.

5 Saving the Children: Infant Mortality and the Politics of Motherhood

In June 1931, approximately 200 delegates gathered in Geneva to attend the International Conference on the African Child. The first of its kind in Europe, the conference had been convened by the Save the Children International Union (SCIU), a philanthropic organisation with a strong Christian background. It brought together doctors, missionaries, social scientists and philanthropists, as well as high-ranking official representatives of colonial powers and international institutions like the League of Nations and the International Labour Office and even a few representatives of African associations. There were two Portuguese participants, one of whom was the Count of Penha Garcia, who also acted as vice-president of the conference and chaired one of the sessions. Being one of Portugal's foremost colonial experts and diplomats of the time, his presence was testimony to the importance the Portuguese government attached to the event.[1] For four days, the participants discussed issues considered key to the welfare of African children: the medical and socio-economic causes of and solutions to stillbirth and infant mortality, education, and working conditions for children and adolescents.[2]

The conference had been carefully prepared for several years. About 1,500 copies of a long and detailed questionnaire (with 168 questions) had been sent to colonial representatives all over Africa, many of them missionaries. On the basis of the 358 replies, 19 selected experts had prepared reports dealing with one of the questions on the agenda for a specific part of the continent, circulated in advance to guide the discussions during the conference.[3]

---

[1] By 1931, the Count of Penha Garcia, José Capello Franco Frazão, was director of the *Escola Superior Colonial* (ESC) in Lisbon (from 1926), president of the Geographical Society of Lisbon (from 1928), member of the Portuguese High Council of the Colonies (*Conselho Superior das Colónias*) and member of the Mandates Commission of the League of Nations (from 1928). For biographical information, see Vieira, *Conde de Penha Garcia*.

[2] See Save the Children International Union, *Proceedings* and the account given by the English novelist and social commentator Sharp, *African Child*. For a first analysis, see Marshall, 'Children's Rights'.

[3] Save the Children International Union, *Proceedings*, iii–viii; Marshall, 'Children's Rights', 283–5. Copies of the questionnaire and reports can be found in AEG, UISE, 92.4.2 and 92.4.10.

The Geneva conference was a product of growing attention to the issue of infant and child welfare from governments, municipalities and philanthropic organisations in Europe since the late nineteenth century. Gradually, attention had shifted from the 'abnormal' – that is, abandoned, dependent and delinquent – children to 'normal' working- and middle-class children, a process that occurred in tandem with the medicalisation of childhood.[4] In the twentieth century, infant and child welfare had also become an object of intense inter- and transnational debate and intervention. Founded in Geneva in 1920, the SCIU was one of several international child welfare organisations operating during the interwar period.[5] What was new to this context of international humanitarianism in 1931, however, was the focus on African children, traditionally the domain of Christian missions, and on socio-medical issues like infant mortality and health, which occupied two of the four sessions.[6]

The organisers explained this focus with humanitarian and demographic urgency. The president of the conference, Lord Noel-Buxton, emphatically stated in his opening speech that 'the whole future of Africa' depended on the welfare of the African child. Yet, although Africa 'share[d] with South America and Australia the characteristic of being underpopulated', there was 'no part of the world where the dissipation of human life [was] so great'.[7] Indeed, while rapporteurs and conference participants advanced a wide variety of statistics, causes and solutions, they all agreed that infant mortality rates in Africa were 'intolerably high'.[8] In his comments on the conference debates, the eminent British colonialist Lord Lugard concluded that 'not less than half the babies die' and that

to this must be added a very heavy percentage of stillbirths and miscarriages and of deaths in infancy subsequent to the first year. The number, therefore, which reaches maturity must, if these assumptions are correct, be a comparatively small percentage of the potential increase, and this in a continent which needs to be re-populated in order to recover from the tribal wars, the slave raids, and the epidemics of the past.[9]

For Lugard, as for Noel-Buxton, infant mortality in Africa was a humanitarian, demographic and economic problem.

The practical outcomes of the conference were limited. The resolutions were rather general and non-binding. With regard to stillbirth and infant mortality, they called for the further study of causes and remedies, such as nutrition, social diseases and African customs; for more collaboration and exchange between governments and private associations; and for the deployment of

---

[4] Rooke and Schnell, 'Uncramping Child Life', 177–8; Cooter, 'Introduction', 1 and 11.
[5] See Rooke and Schnell, 'Uncramping Child Life', 182–9; Bolzman, 'Advent of Child Rights'.
[6] Compare with Clarence-Smith, 'Redemption' and Stornig, 'Promoting Distant Children'.
[7] Save the Children International Union, *Proceedings*, 3–4 (quotes).   [8] Ibid., 17 (quote).
[9] Sharp, *African Child*, v–ix (quote vi).

more trained doctors, nurses and midwives in colonial Africa.[10] Furthermore, in the mid-1930s, the SCIU stopped its activities in Africa and the European movement for the protection of African children stalled, as humanitarian attention shifted to the Spanish Civil War and the Second World War. Only around 1950 would the SCIU resume its activities in Africa, now accompanied by other international agencies such as UNICEF.[11]

Yet the conference in Geneva was more than an ephemeral episode in the history of European humanitarianism and internationalism. The desire of the participants to combat infant mortality and stimulate population growth was deeply embedded in the colonial biopolitical agenda of the interwar period. It reflected an increasing awareness after the First World War that, in addition to epidemic and endemic diseases, infant mortality was *a*, if not *the*, main cause of de- and underpopulation in colonial Africa, as discussed in Chapter 4. The very organisation of the conference and the participation of so many high-ranking representatives testifies to the growing attention colonial governments, missionary societies, philanthropists, and international organisations devoted to this issue.

By 1931, concerns over high infant mortality, which were often intertwined with concerns over low fertility and maternal mortality, had already generated a range of maternal and infant welfare programmes in colonial Africa.[12] Often linked to similar initiatives in Europe, these programmes were part of a global development. As Nancy Rose Hunt has concluded, 'maternal and infant healthcare as a movement dedicated to saving the lives of mothers and babies' had become 'a global phenomenon by the interwar period'.[13] The shape and success of these programmes, however, also depended on local conditions and circumstances.

This chapter explores the colonial interventions aimed at curbing maternal and infant mortality in Angola in the 1920s–1940s. It analyses their specificities, but also how they connected to debates and policies in Europe, particularly in Portugal, and in other African colonies. The chapter particularly focuses on three kinds of interventions in this field: state efforts to establish maternity clinics for 'native' women and to educate 'native' midwives; philanthropic initiatives such as infant welfare dispensaries promoted by high-ranking Portuguese women in urban areas; and Protestant mission maternity work. The chapter argues that, though pursued by different groups of actors

---

[10] Save the Children International Union, *Proceedings*, 91–3.
[11] Marshall, 'Children's Rights', 275. On the beginnings of UNICEF in Africa, see Coghe, 'Between Colonial Medicine and Global Health'.
[12] See, for instance, Hunt, 'Bébé en Brousse'; Hunt, *Colonial Lexicon*; Summers, 'Intimate Colonialism'; Allman, 'Making Mothers'; Turrittin, 'Colonial Midwives'; van Tol, 'Mothers' and Lindner, 'Transfer'.
[13] Hunt, *Colonial Lexicon*, 239–40 (quote 239).

with partly diverging goals and rationales, all three schemes were underwritten by an utterly negative image of the competence of African mothers. Their main goal was to re-educate African women and to instil them with the veritable 'art of motherhood'. Their success, however, varied greatly and depended mainly upon the (more expensive) material and individual medical assistance they were prepared to offer. While African mothers remained rather critical of preventive approaches that implied changing their habits of dealing with pregnancy, newborns and infants, they often actively sought curative medicine in the form of medication, surgery and assistance with difficult births. Overall, their passive resistance and selective appropriation altered the orientation of maternal and infant welfare programmes.

Colonial Maternities and 'Native' Midwives

For leading medical doctors in Angola, part of the solution to the problem of infant mortality consisted in establishing so-called *maternidades* ('maternities'), specialised birth or maternity clinics. Damas Mora and Augusto Ornelas were full of praise for the maternities they had seen in the French and British colonies during the LNHO study tour and, in 1928, the *Comissão de Assistência Indígena* (CAI) decided to emulate this example and to construct three 'native' maternities (*maternidades indígenas*) for African women in Angola as well: a model maternity in Luanda and two more modest structures in Dalatando and São Salvador, the respective capitals of the Cuanza and Congo sanitary zones.[14] Filomeno da Câmara's attack on the *Assistência Médica aos Indígenas* (AMI) services in 1929–30, however, thwarted this project.[15] Denounced as too expensive and grandiose ('a fool's endeavour'), the construction of the model maternity in Luanda was halted, and the one in São Salvador was not even begun.[16] Before 1930, the only maternity to open its doors was the one in Dalatando.[17]

Despite these difficulties, Ornelas, Damas Mora and others did not give up their idea of creating a larger network of 'two to three dozen' maternities throughout the colony. But, even more than before, due to predictable constraints of budget and (European) personnel, they saw maternities as 'preventive' rather than 'curative'. Particularly in rural areas, their primary goal would not to be to hospitalise pregnant women and/or provide them with individual assistance before, during and after childbirth, as their colleague João Camoesas

---

[14] Mora, 'Estado actual', 46; Neves and Sousa, 'Assistência Médica aos Indígenas', 440. On study tour and CAI, see Chapter 3.

[15] See Chapter 3.

[16] 'Assistência indígena', *A Província de Angola*, 28 June 1930 (quote); Mora, 'Estado actual', 46.

[17] The inauguration took place during the First Medical Days of Dalatando in October 1929, see '1.ª Jornada Médica de Dalatando', *A Província de Angola*, 29 October 1929.

had previously recommended or as the French state maternity in Dakar intended, but to offer (much cheaper) medical and moral education. In state maternities, African mothers were to be taught the 'art of motherhood', namely the basic principles of infant welfare (*puericultura*).[18]

This preventive orientation was in accordance with the general ideas of social medicine and addressed what many doctors, administrators and missionaries believed to be the biggest problem: the backwardness and incompetence of African mothers. This trope of 'bad mothers', which is still today a powerful sociocultural explanation of high infant mortality in parts of Africa, readily emerged in the early days of European colonialism. It often obscured deteriorating economic conditions for women under colonial rule.[19] Prior to the end of the First World War, many colonial administrators in Angola had already warned of how 'native' customs and beliefs prejudiced maternal and infant health. The reports bundled by Secretary of Native Affairs José de Oliveira Ferreira Diniz in the voluminous *Populações Indígenas de Angola (1918)*, for instance, the first ethnographic overview of the colony, provided a varied, but mostly pessimistic view of African birth practices and maternal and infant healthcare. Administrators lamented that in most 'tribes' neither pregnant women nor infants received any special care. Moreover, while breastfeeding continued until the age of two or three (also linked to the social practice of birth spacing as the informant for the Cabinda people emphasised), infants were often given solid food, like manioc or maize flour, weeks or even days after they were born, thus causing grave digestive disorders. Along with polygamy and child marriage, Diniz concluded, these practices 'damaged and limited the population'.[20]

In the interwar years, social hygienists in Angola initially took the same line. 'The education of the mothers is of the greatest importance', Augusto Ornelas stated, 'because their atavistic ignorance, more than the lack of material resources of all kinds, is the main factor compromising the offspring of the people. The prejudices, the ignorance and the lack of knowledge about the basic laws of maternal and infant hygiene must be combated with the local resources that we have at our disposal.'[21]

According to this interpretation, African women had to be taught how to feed and clothe their babies correctly and how to protect them against diseases and the dangers of everyday life.[22] Therefore, it was imperative to replace

---

[18] Ornelas, 'Obra de protecção'; 'Assistência indígena', *A Província de Angola*, 28 June 1930. Compare with Camoesas, 'Organização AMI', 146; Le Dantec, 'Hygiène sociale', 347.
[19] See Cooper, 'Chronic Malnutrition'.
[20] See Diniz, *Populações indígenas*, passim and summary 567–70 (quote 568). For birth spacing, see ibid., 268 and Athayde, 'Perigo do despovoamento'. See also Hunt, 'Bébé en Brousse'.
[21] Ornelas, 'Obra de protecção', 523.
[22] See also Silva, *Serviço de Assistência Congo (1930)*, 9–10.

'backward' and 'harmful' customs with Western concepts of hygiene and child-rearing. More than direct medical intervention in childbirth, the dissemination of Western paediatric knowledge among Angolan women was considered key to reducing infant mortality. To achieve this, maternities would not only offer infant welfare courses for mothers, but also serve as training sites for Angolan midwives (*parteiras*).[23] Portuguese doctors envisioned that, duly educated, these certified midwives would disseminate Western notions of maternal and infant hygiene. They would be sent back to their region of origin, where they would assist in deliveries and teach other women their skill. This process would take many years, but eventually, each village would have its own midwife, its own 'great agent of hygienic transformation', Damas Mora hoped.[24]

This maternity scheme did not exclude individual consultations and, in problematic cases, hospitalisations, but the direct supervision of childbirth in maternities was not to be the rule. One explanation for this orientation was the prevailing ideology of preventive and collective healthcare and its promise to better allocate the scarce resources of money and personnel.[25] However, it also anticipated the non-cooperation of African women. During their first experiences with the maternity in Dalatando, doctors noticed that the vast majority of African women still preferred to give birth at home.[26] While some viewed this as a sign of backwardness, others were more accommodating. Rather than forcing them into maternities and exposing them to the psychological stress of being away from home and separated from their families, it would be better to let mothers give birth at home, under the supervision of a trained 'native' midwife, the director of the health services in 1944, Manuel Fonseca, maintained.[27]

This defence of home births was, in part, informed by the common ethnographic and medical belief that African women gave birth easily and that infections and other complications requiring hospital care were rare.[28] It is also worth remembering that until at least the late 1930s the majority of women in France or the UK gave birth at home.[29] Above all, Manuel

---

[23] Neves and Sousa, 'Assistência Médica aos Indígenas', 440; Ornelas, 'Obra de protecção'; 'Assistência indígena', *A Província de Angola*, 28 June 1930.

[24] Mora, 'Estado actual', 44 (here quote); 'Liga para protecção da infância de Angola', *A Província de Angola*, 5 August 1930. See also Mora, 'Mortalidade infantil', 622–3.

[25] See Chapter 3.

[26] Teixeira, Waldemar Gomes, 'Relatório da Zona Sanitária do Cuanza (1930)', June 1931, 73, AHU, MU, AGC 2336; Mora, 'Mortalidade infantil', 622.

[27] Manuel Ferreira Peixoto Fonseca, 'Algumas considerações sobre a actuação dos serviços de saúde en Angola', 17 October 1944, 5, AHU, MU, DGSA_RSH_004, Cx. 5.

[28] Ibid.; Mora, 'Mortalidade infantil', 607. The same idea is also present in many descriptions of birth practices in Diniz, *Populações indígenas*, e.g. 267 and 301.

[29] Thébaud, *Quand nos grand-mères*, 151–63; McIntosh, *Social History*, 64, 90.

Fonseca's justification of home births echoed the ideological position of the *Estado Novo* in mainland Portugal. Within the scope of a broader re-education programme aimed at transforming women into housewives, the *Estado Novo* actively campaigned for home births through women's organisations such as the *Obra das Mães pela Educação Nacional* and the *Mocidade Portuguesa Feminina*. In the opinion of the regime, maternity clinics violated the integrity and dignity of the family, the central pillar of Portuguese society. Women should give birth at home, within the intimacy of their families.[30]

Certainly, this discourse was contested by some leading doctors, like Sebastião Cabral da Costa-Sacadura.[31] It was in part due to their continuous activism that, after three decades of debate and postponements, the first modern state maternities were eventually opened in Lisbon in 1931 and 1932 and in Porto in 1938, paradoxically under the conservative regime of the *Estado Novo*.[32] However, over the coming decades the government did little to expand the number of maternities or to make maternity births affordable for all. By 1950, only 8 per cent of the births in Portugal occurred in hospitals or maternities, far fewer than in Western Europe, where numbers increased greatly during the 1920s–1940s and where a majority of women gave birth in hospital by the 1950s. According to a study in 1944, most home births in Portugal were not even attended by certified midwives, but only by so-called *curiosas* ('folk midwives').[33] Only after the demise of the *Estado Novo* in 1974 would hospital births become the norm in Portugal.[34]

The ideological and institutional situation in the metropole helps to explain why, in 1929, High Commissioner Filomeno da Câmara, an adept of the conservative doctrines of the emerging *Estado Novo*, thwarted the plans for a model maternity in Luanda; and why, over the next decades, only a few state maternities were established. Under the *Estado Novo*, metropole and colonies were more than ever governed under the same (in this case, conservative) doctrines, with a metropolitan government that, through its Colonial Ministry, also strictly controlled Angola's budgets.[35] Given the government's reluctance to establish maternity clinics in the metropole, it is highly unlikely that it would have supported expensive plans to give Angolan women easier access to medicalised childbirth than their Portuguese 'sisters' at home, thereby reversing imperial hierarchies. Arguably, the much quicker and stronger medicalisation of childbirth in the neighbouring Belgian Congo in the 1930s–

---

[30] Pimentel, *História das organizações femininas*, 54–73, 134–40, 148–54. See also Pimentel, *Política feminina*.
[31] See, for instance, Costa-Sacadura, *Maternidades*.   [32] Costa, 'Inaugurada a Maternidade'.
[33] Compare Pimentel, *História das organizações femininas*, 70 with Thébaud, *Quand nos grand-mères*, 151–63; McIntosh, *Social History*, 90.
[34] White and Schouten (eds.), *Normal Birth*.   [35] See Chapter 3.

1950s was closely linked to much more favourable ideologies and institutionalisation processes in its European metropole.[36]

Ideological reservations and the severe budgetary constraints imposed by the metropole, particularly between 1930 and 1945, led to strong tensions between discourse and practice in Portuguese policy towards maternal and infant healthcare in Angola. Clearly, many doctors and leading colonial officials favoured the multiplication of state maternities and 'native' midwife training programmes as a necessary measure to reduce infant mortality. In the 1930s and 1940s, Governors-General like António Lopes Mateus (1935–9) and Álvaro de Freitas Morna (1942–3), the Director of Native Affairs Manuel Pereira Figueira (1935–9) and long-standing and influential provincial governors like António de Almeida and Manuel da Cruz Alvura all voiced their support.[37] In contrast to these convictions, however, stood a practical imbroglio. Doctors and provincial governors struggled hard to establish even a single maternity. Mostly, the problem was money – money that did not arrive, or only very slowly, from Luanda and hence, indirectly, from Lisbon.[38] The story of the *maternidade indígena* in Luanda is even more disturbing. Interrupted in 1929 by High Commissioner Filomeno da Câmara, the construction of the maternity was only resumed in the late 1930s and, once finished, the government used the building to accommodate the troops that had arrived from Portugal in 1941. It was not until the arrival of the next Governor-General, Álvaro de Freitas Morna, that the *Maternidade Indígena Vieira Machado* finally served its original function.[39]

Freitas Morna proved to be a great supporter of maternal and infant welfare programmes during his short term as Governor-General (1942–3). In collaboration with the health services, he conceived an ambitious project to gradually equip each of the 66 *delegações de saúde* (health districts) in the colony with a standardised maternity. Each year, 10 new maternities would be constructed, each run by the local Portuguese health officer in tandem with a qualified Portuguese midwife. The basic principles of the project were similar to those

---

[36] Compare Hunt, *Colonial Lexicon*, 3–4 and 272–6 with Masuy-Stroobant and Humblet (eds.), *Mères et nourrissons*.

[37] See, for instance, António Lopes Mateus, 'Relatório e propostas do Conselho de Governadores de Angola', 11 May 1935, 33–5, AHU, MU, ISAU 1730; the annual reports of Manuel Pereira Figueira (1936 to 1938) in AHU, MU, ISAU 2243; António de Almeida, 'Relatório do Governo da Província de Bié (1935–36)', 31 December 1936, 82, AHU, MU, ISAU 1727 and further reports by provincial governors cited in next footnote 38.

[38] See, for instance, António de Almeida, 'Relatório do Governo da Província do Bié (1938)', 31 December 1938, Vol. I, 85, AHU, MU, DGAC 543; Manuel da Cruz Alvura, 'Relatório do Governo da Província de Malanje (1941– 1942)', 31 December 1942, 31–5, AHU, MU, ISAU 1663.2.

[39] Manuel Pereira Figueira, 'Relatório do Curador Geral dos Indígenas da Colonia de Angola (1937)', 15 May 1938, 11, AHU, MU, ISAU 2243; Morna, *Angola*, 176; Levy, 'Plano de assistência', 171.

outlined by the health services in the late 1920s. Aside from treating complicated cases of pregnancy and childbirth, the European staff were mainly responsible for training Angolan midwives, who would then spread Western concepts of childbirth and child-rearing.[40] Freitas Morna personally defended his project to Salazar, explaining that the gradual establishment of maternities and the annual training of 20 midwives in each would cost an estimated 3.7 million ags. a year, but that this would be 'blessed money, since it will save thousands of lives and Your Excellency can be sure that after 10 years we will have increased the population of Angola – its greatest value – by roughly 1,000,000 souls'.[41] Salazar's reaction is unknown, but after Freitas Morna was removed from office, following a conflict with Minister of Colonies Vieira Machado, his project was not implemented. By 1951, there were only 12 state-run maternities in Angola.[42]

Given their pivotal function as educational centres, the dearth of maternities contributed much to the colonial medical service's failure to train the dozens or hundreds of 'native' midwives it considered so essential in spreading modern ideas of maternal and infant welfare. Unlike Uganda, Nigeria, French West Africa or the Belgian Congo (colonies that launched more or less successful midwifery training programmes in the interwar period), the colonial health services in Angola had trained very few midwives before the 1940s.[43] According to medical officer Antero Antunes do Amaral, this was primarily the result of further institutional shortcomings, most notably the poor quality of the nursing schools and the lack of a special midwifery school in Angola.[44] Others, like Damas Mora, however, preferred to blame the mental and moral backwardness of African women. In a paper presented at the Third National Colonial Congress in Lisbon in 1930, he had argued that it was extremely difficult to find suitable candidates for midwifery training. Many, he complained, dropped out from 'laziness, thoughtlessness or pride'. Nevertheless, he was confident that, with 'patience and perseverance', health authorities would eventually achieve their aims.[45] Ten years later, however, this optimism had been replaced with overt and deeply racist frustration: 'In Angola', he lamented,

the attempts to transform native girls into good nurses have always failed until today. In four centuries of rule we have not managed to extract the diamond of intelligence and the spirit of sacrifice from the gangue of superstitions and the sexual obsession of native

---

[40] Morna, *Angola*, 179–81.
[41] Freitas Morna to Oliveira Salazar, 22 March 1943, 11–3 (quote 13), ANTT, AOS-CO-UL-8G, Pasta 6. Similarly, Morna, *Angola*, 181.
[42] Nunes, 'Aspectos', 2600.
[43] Compare with Summers, 'Intimate Colonialism'; van Tol, 'Mothers'; Turrittin, 'Colonial Midwives'; Barthélémy, 'Sages-femmes africaines' and Hunt, *Colonial Lexicon*.
[44] Amaral, 'Natalidade e mortalidade', 182.   [45] Mora, 'Estado actual', 44.

women. Native girls are full of self-love and distrust, and at the first indulgent remark, they disappear and do not come back.[46]

One of the solutions devised to address this issue of recruitment was to enrol older 'traditional' midwives *(matronas)* into the midwifery courses, until younger and better-educated women were found. Although doctors reckoned that these *matronas* would only be capable of rudimentary training and that their resistance to new principles would have to be overcome by material benefits, they saw various advantages. Educating and incorporating them into the machinery of the health services would not only reduce their 'harmful' influence, but also enhance Western biomedical techniques and concepts of hygiene with the prestige they brought to it. This strategy, also used as a temporary measure in other colonies, acknowledged that the successful intro-duction of novel practices hinged on the prestige of those who performed them, and that young girls, especially when childless, would have a very difficult time doing so without the support of *matronas*.[47]

Urban Philanthropy and the Intricacies of Race

The apparent failure of its maternity and midwife training schemes in the 1930s does not mean that the Portuguese colonial state did not intervene in maternal and infant welfare at all prior to the Second World War. In AMI sectors, doctors and nurses sought to transmit Western notions of infant feeding and hygiene during the regularly held concentrations, and were some-times called to assist in difficult births.[48] Yet, due to the lack of specialised institutions and female personnel – and the limited trust many African women presumably had in male birth helpers[49] – their influence in rural areas was necessarily restricted.

In the interwar years, state intervention proved more effective in supporting private initiatives in urban areas. Once again, Angola followed the example of other colonies. In the 1920s, high-ranking French, Belgian and British colonial women had founded philanthropic associations aimed at educating African mothers and improving the health of their children. As Barbara Bush has argued, such social welfare initiatives were at the core of European women's increased involvement in the imperial mission after the First World War, when

---

[46] Mora, 'Mortalidade infantil', 623.
[47] Mora, 'Assistência Médica ao Indígena (1926)', 394; Ornelas, 'Assistência maternal', 45–6; Levy, 'Plano de assistência', 174. Ornelas related that a doctor from the French Congo had recommended this scheme. On similar efforts in the British and French colonies, see Bell, *Frontiers of Medicine*, 198, 205–12; Barthélémy, *Femmes*, 202–7.
[48] Silva, *Serviço de Assistência Congo (1930)*, 5–6; Ornelas and Mesquita, *Relatório da missão médica*, 62.
[49] See Hunt, *Colonial Lexicon*, 8.

more women than before accompanied their husbands to colonial Africa or were recruited as doctors, nurses or teachers.[50] The existence of such charitable associations for African women and children was well known to the medical establishment in Angola, since Madame Nogue and Madame Vassal, the wives of leading French doctors, had presented the goals and activities of their respective associations in the AOF and AEF at the Congress of Tropical Medicine in Luanda in 1923.[51] However, no similar initiatives emerged in Angola during the 1920s. When, in the view of Damas Mora, this situation had reached embarrassing levels for the prestige of Portuguese colonialism – according to his own statements, he had been ashamed to confess the lack of such philanthropic associations in Angola to a SCIU representative during his stay in Geneva in 1929[52] – he publicly called upon the colony's female elite to fill this gap. 'When', he asked in an interview with the daily newspaper *A Província de Angola* in June 1930, 'will the ladies of Angola finally decide to participate with heart and soul in the blessed crusade of saving the black race'?[53]

Damas Mora's appeal did not go unheeded. Only one month later, women from Luanda's 'high society' started meeting and publicly debating the issue. Most were wives of high-ranking colonial officials, but among them figured also at least two female doctors, Berta de Morais Esteves and Adelaide Cabete.[54] A year later, in August 1931, the statute of the League for the Protection of the Children of Angola *(Liga de Protecção à Infância de Angola)* was officially approved.[55]

Although little is known about her exact engagement in the *Liga*, the participation of gynaecologist Adelaide Cabete (1867–1935) is noteworthy. Cabete, who came to Angola as a political exile in 1929, was one of the first female doctors and a leading feminist in early-twentieth century Portugal. Best known in historiography for her key role in Portugal's principal feminist associations, the *Liga Republicana das Mulheres Portuguesas* (1909–19) and the *Conselho Nacional das Mulheres Portuguesas* (1914–47), she was also an important proponent of new, hygienic concepts of childbirth and childrearing. Along with her interventions in public debates, she taught 'Hygiene

[50] Bush, 'Motherhood', 277–9. See also Hunt, 'Bébé en Brousse', 413–4.
[51] Vassal, 'Natalité'; Primeiro Congresso de Medicina Tropical da África Ocidental, 'Acta da 2.ª sessão', 8–9. For the Belgian Congo, see Hunt, 'Bébé en Brousse', 402–6.
[52] 'Liga para protecção da infância de Angola', *A Província de Angola*, 5 August 1930.
[53] 'Assistência indígena', *A Província de Angola*, 28 June 1930. See also Mora, 'Estado actual', 45–6.
[54] António Damas Mora, 'Um belo gesto das senhoras de Luanda', *A Província de Angola*, 1 August 1930; 'Liga para protecção da infância de Angola', *A Província de Angola*, 2, 5 and 19 August 1930.
[55] Govêrno Geral de Angola, 'Estatutos da Liga de Protecção à Infância de Angola', 22 August 1931, *BOA Série II* (1931), 581–3.

and Infant Welfare' (*Higiene e Puericultura*) for more than 15 years at the *Instituto Feminino de Educação e Trabalho*, a republican reform school for girls in Odivelas near Lisbon.[56] In Luanda, Cabete opened a doctor's surgery and wrote educative pieces on motherhood and hygiene for several local newspapers, until she returned to Lisbon in 1934.[57]

The *Liga de Protecção à Infância de Angola* was a private association, funded mainly through membership fees, donations and profits from sponsored cultural and sporting events. In addition, it received modest subsidies from the Native Affairs Department.[58] The *Liga* was an explicitly gendered association: although men could be members (*sócios*), only women could be elected to the directing bodies, which were presided over by the wife of the Governor-General. There were a few exceptions to this rule, however, that reveal the vivid interest some state departments took in the issue as well as their pervasive paternalism: the treasurer of the League was the Director of the Native Affairs Department, and on the technical council sat three government doctors, initially António Damas Mora, João Augusto Ornelas and Isaac Levy. The positions that exerted medical and fiscal control were hence all filled by men.[59]

The League's first and most important project, for which it had done much fundraising, consisted in the establishment of the *Gota de Leite para crianças pobres* ('Drop of milk for poor children') in Luanda in August 1931 (Figure 5.1). Modelled on similar institutions in both Europe and other African colonies, the *Gota de Leite* provided a wide range of services to infants and their mothers. As well as supplying milk and other nutritional supplements, it offered medical examinations and vaccinations of infants, and supervised their physical development through regular weighing and measuring appointments. In addition, the *Gota de Leite* distributed baby-clothes, soap, toys and money. These presents were of dual purpose: directly beneficial to infant health, they were also incentives for mothers to submit their minds and the bodies of their newborns to regular supervision.[60]

Such *Gouttes de Lait* had first emerged in France in the last decades of the nineteenth century. By the early twentieth century, they had spread to other European countries and become one of the hallmarks of the infant welfare movement, with their representatives meeting at several international

---

[56] See Esteves, 'Adelaide Cabete' and Lousada, *Adelaide Cabete*.

[57] Lousada, *Adelaide Cabete*, 30–1, 52–3 and 62.

[58] Govêrno Geral de Angola, 'Estatutos da Liga', art. 43; Manuel Vicente d'Almeida Neves, 'Relatório da Direcção dos Serviços e Negócios Indígenas e Curadoria Geral', 10 April 1933, AHU, MU, DGCO 595, Table 17. For an example of fundraising, see 'Iniciativa benemerita', *A Província de Angola*, 25 May 1931.

[59] Govêrno Geral de Angola, 'Estatutos da Liga', art. 10, 22 and 54.

[60] See, for instance, ibid., art. 25–9; 'Protecção à infância', *A Província de Angola*, 8 August 1931; 'A "Arvore de Natal" da Gota de Leite', *A Província de Angola*, 18 December 1931; Mora, 'Mortalidade infantil', 621.

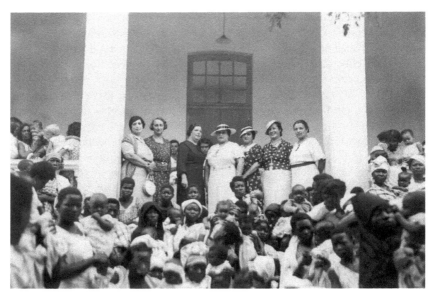

Figure 5.1 Infant welfare in Luanda, ca. 1935. The picture shows mostly
African mothers and children waiting and, in the middle, seven European
women, probably *zeladoras* of the *Gota de Leite*.
Source: ANTT, Agência Geral do Ultramar, Angola, cx. 6, n.º 4506, PT/TT/AGU/001/
004506
Image courtesy of ANTT

congresses to exchange experiences.[61] In Portugal, the first *lactário*, as they
were usually called there, was opened in 1903 by the newly founded
Associação Protectora da Primeira Infância in Lisbon. It was soon followed
by others, but compared to France or Belgium, the expansion of this kind of
maternal and infant welfare institution, which was either funded by private
associations or municipalities, remained modest. As the name suggests, the
initial and primary task of these institutions was to supply milk to infants
whose mothers were unable to breastfeed due to disease, malnutrition or work
schedules. Yet by the time this kind of institution was recreated in the colonies,
lactários in the metropoles had evolved into integrated centres for maternal
and infant welfare and healthcare, often called *dispensários de puericultura*.[62]

The *Gota de Leite* in Luanda was supervised by Isaac Levy, an experienced
paediatrician who led the paediatric ward in the Central Hospital of

---

[61] Hunt, 'Bébé en Brousse', 402–6; Ferguson, Weaver and Nicolson, 'Glasgow Corporation
Milk Depot'.
[62] Caldeira, *Assistência infantil*, 36–79; Garrett, *Como organizar a luta*, 12–3.

Luanda.[63] Most of the daily work, however, was carried out by European women: two female nurses from the same hospital and a group of voluntary *zeladoras* ('female overseers'), who distributed the milk, weighed and measured the children and, above all, instilled novel principles of infant hygiene in Angolan mothers. To reach more women, the latter were also supposed to make home visits.[64] Lacking medical training, they did not supervise births, but in many other respects their role resembled that which had been delineated for the qualified European or African nurse-midwives. In 1933, the *Gota* received the support of two 'visiting nurse-midwives' who had received three years of training in maternal and infant welfare in Lisbon.[65]

The number of supervised children increased rapidly, from 135 by the end of 1931 to more than 1,000 annually from 1933 onwards, with an average of about 350 new admissions annually (1931–8).[66] With the encouragement of João Augusto Ornelas, other *dispensários de puericultura* were founded in Benguela (1935) and Nova Lisboa (now Huambo) (1936), and, in the early 1940s, in a few more towns. Under the direction of female doctors like Augusta da Silva Ferreira (Benguela) and Hortência de Visitação Nunes (Nova Lisboa), these *dispensários* provided a similar range of services to the prototype in Luanda, including phototherapy sessions with ultraviolet light that were also popular in Europe as preventive measures against all kinds of diseases, notably rickets.[67] By this point, the movement had gained more active support from the colonial government. On the initiative of Manuel Pereira Figueira, the new director of the Native Affairs Department, the *Liga* was replaced in 1935 by the *Instituição de Assistência às Crianças Indígenas* (IACI) ('Institution for the Assistance of Native Children'). The IACI was still a private organisation under female direction, but since it had been recognised to be of 'public utility', it enjoyed more financial and practical state support. It also had a more comprehensive agenda: beyond providing material, nutritional and medical assistance for infants and their mothers, it also aimed to assist

[63] On Levy's career, see Manuel Ferreira Peixoto Fonseca, 'Isaac Salomão Levy – extracto da folha de serviço', 25 May 1945, AHU, MU, DGAPC 34.

[64] Isaac Levy, 'Questões de puericultura', *A Província de Angola*, 19 and 20 May 1931; 'Protecção à infância', *A Província de Angola*, 8 August 1931; 'A "Arvore de Natal" da Gota de Leite', *A Província de Angola*, 18 December 1931; Mora, 'Mortalidade infantil', 621.

[65] António Damas Mora, 'Higiene social e visitadoras de higiene', *A Província de Angola*, 27 June 1933.

[66] *Boletim Sanitário de Angola* 1 (1937–8), 69.

[67] Mora, 'Mortalidade infantil', 620–1; Augusta da Silva Ferreira, 'Dispensário de puericultura de Benguela', *O Intransigente*, 8 July 1936; Hortênsia Nunes, 'O dispensário de Nova Lisboa', *O Intransigente*, 21 September 1936. By 1943, there were six 'official' *dispensários de puericultura* and three private ones in Angola, see *Boletim Sanitário de Angola* 6 (1943), 10. For UV sessions, see also Ornelas, *Primeiro viver*.

pregnant women, build and maintain maternity clinics and establish crèches throughout the colony.[68]

In one important point, the *lactários* and dispensaries in Luanda, Benguela or Nova Lisboa were quite different from similar institutions elsewhere in colonial Africa: they included both African children and children of European and mixed descent. Although the statutes of the *Liga* and later the IACI did not mention 'white' or *mestiço* children, and the name IACI suggested that it would only assist 'native' children, it was the explicit goal of the *Gota de Leite* in Luanda to assist all poor children, regardless of 'race'.[69] This policy was adopted in the other dispensaries as well: of the 833 children registered with the *Dispensário de Puericultura de Benguela* in 1946, for example, 613 were listed as 'black', 66 as 'white' and 154 as '*mestiço*'.[70] In the British, French and Belgian colonies in sub-Saharan Africa, by contrast, infant welfare institutions appear to have been for African children only; or mechanisms of racial segregation were erected when European children were included, as occurred in the industrialised centres of Katanga.[71]

In Angola, members and supporters of the *Liga* had, from early on, spoken of the necessity of caring for poor European children too. 'In Luanda', Berta de Morais Esteves stated in an interview, 'we do not only have to assist native people. Because they are closer to our heart and more visible to us, it is still more upsetting to see these poor, innocent white children who have been swept far away from a favourable climate by the crimes of their parents.'[72] This was a clear reference to the children of the *degredados*, convicted criminals who had been deported from Portugal to Angola, often with their families. Until 1932, Angola served as Portugal's 'imperial prison': up to a few hundred convicts were sent to Angola every year and these *degredados* constituted a considerable percentage of the European population in the colony's cities, particularly Luanda.[73] They were generally decried as debauched individuals living in physical and moral misery. Their massive presence, which had been a thorn in the side of local government for many decades, explains at least in part the inclusion of white infants in urban philanthropy initiatives. Moreover, the economic crisis of the early 1930s had impoverished many Portuguese families in Angola and exacerbated the so-called problem of 'poor whites'. Their

---

[68] See Govêrno Geral de Angola, *Estatutos IACI*.

[69] 'Iniciativa benemérita. A gota de leite para crianças pobres', *A Província de Angola*, 2 May 1931. Compare with Govêrno Geral de Angola, 'Estatutos da Liga'; Govêrno Geral de Angola, *Estatutos IACI*.

[70] Passos, 'Contribuição', 402.

[71] Compare with Allman, 'Making Mothers'; Hugon, 'Redéfinition'; van Tol, 'Mothers' and, for Katanga, Hunt, 'Bébé en Brousse', 415–6.

[72] 'Liga de Protecção da Infância de Angola', *A Província de Angola*, 19 August 1930.

[73] Coates, *Convict Labor*, 4 (quote) and 55–117. See also Bender, *Angola under the Portuguese*, 59–94, esp. 86–93.

misery endangered the image of Portuguese superiority and, while the government repatriated a few hundred in the first half of the 1930s, there was intensifying public pressure to provide better healthcare for them.[74]

The strong representation of *mestiço* children in the Benguela dispensary, then, points to both their numerical importance and precarious position in colonial Angola. On the one hand, it reflects that the number of people who were officially identified as *mestiços* in Angola was, in absolute numbers, high compared to other colonies in sub-Saharan Africa, particularly in urban areas. The census of 1940 listed 28,035 *mestiços* (0.7 per cent of the total population) of which 1,215 were in the city of Benguela (6.9 per cent of Benguela's population) and 6,191 in Luanda (10.0 per cent of Luanda's population), against ca. 3,500 *métis* (or 0.02 per cent) in the whole AOF in 1938 or up to 5,000 (or 0.05 per cent) around the same time in the Belgian Congo.[75] These numbers, however, do not necessarily indicate any special Portuguese propensity to 'racial mixing', a long-standing accusation against the Portuguese, and as the *Estado Novo* would start claiming in the 1950s (see Introduction and Chapter 1). Gerald Bender has argued that the number and percentage of *mestiços* in Angola was not exceptional for African colonies when compared to the high number of whites and considering the imbalance in the male-female ratio across the white population.[76] Moreover, definitions of *mestiço* (and their official number) varied greatly between actors and over time, as they oscillated between somatic, race-biological and cultural criteria, partly depending on political purposes. With regard to the 1940 census, census director Alberto de Lemos, himself considered *mestiço*, thus assumed that many had declared themselves *mestiços* but should actually be considered 'white', since racial mixing had occurred generations earlier, effectively leaving little somatic or cultural traces. They had only done so, he argued, because the census instructions gave a narrow biological definition and promised anonymity. Conversely, many of those categorised as 'civilised blacks' (*pretos civilizados*) were, biologically speaking, *mestiços* according to Lemos.[77] Former High Commissioner Vicente Ferreira, by contrast, expressed the view that the real number of *mestiços* was still much higher since, in the absence of anthropological control, many had, depending on their somatic features, falsely declared themselves to be either 'white' or 'black'.[78] It is important to note

[74] See Chapter 3 and Castelo, *Passagens para África*, 277–8.
[75] Repartição de Estatística Geral da Colónia de Angola (ed.), *Censo geral da população* (1940), vol. I, 64, 78–9, 86–7. Compare with White, *Children of the French Empire*, 2; Jeurissen, 'Ambitions', 501–2. See also Saada, *Empire's Children*, 40 for equally low numbers in other French colonies.
[76] Bender, *Angola under the Portuguese*, 45–54. Similarly Neto, 'Ideologias', 351.
[77] Lemos, 'Introdução ao primeiro censo', 63–4. See also Neto, 'Ideologias', 353.
[78] Ferreira, 'Colonização étnica', 196–7.

here that, although *mestiços* were a statistical category, they were not a legal category, as they were either considered Portuguese and/or European (*civilizado*) or 'native' (*não-civilizado*), according to their 'civilisational level'. The 1940 census thus counted 23,244 'civilised' and 4,791 'uncivilised' *mestiços*.[79]

On the other hand, the overrepresentation of *mestiço* children in the Benguela dispensary, an institution primarily for poor children, reflects their precarious political and socio-economic situation.[80] Whereas 'racial mixing' (*mestiçagem*) had, before the nineteenth century, often been viewed as a necessary condition of colonial rule in the tropics, negative attitudes towards miscegenation, which never were fully absent, gained urgency among Portuguese intellectuals, politicians and bureaucrats, both at home and in the colonies, in the late nineteenth century.[81] Between roughly 1880 and 1920, mounting racial prejudice and the increasing influx of competitors from the metropole contributed to the decline in power, prestige and wealth of the so-called 'creole', 'Euro-african' or 'Luso-African' elites, analytical terms used to designate those *mestiços*, 'black' *assimilados* and 'white' settlers born in the colony (*filhos do país*) who had, until then, played an eminent role in Angola's political, economic and social life.[82] In the interwar years, the growing influence of racial anthropology in the Portuguese Empire further eroded the social position of *mestiços*. Leading Portuguese anthropologists and race scientists, such as A. A. Mendes Correia and Eusébio Tamagnini, strongly opposed racial mixing in the colonies, arguing that *mestiços* were biologically inferior, or a social risk, or both.[83] Simultaneously, powerful governors and High Commissioners in Angola such as Norton de Matos and Vicente Ferreira advocated segregationist measures to protect 'racial purity' and maintain Portugal's colonial prestige, with Vicente Ferreira even proposing to 'quarter these erratic elements [*mestiços*] in duly selected and prepared places, with a different type of administration'.[84] Although detailed studies on *mestiço* children in Angola are still lacking, the evidence suggests that, as in other colonies, *mestiço* children were often not officially recognised or cared for

---

[79] Neto, 'Ideologias', 354.
[80] In 1946, *mestiço* children accounted for 18.5% of the dispensary children, while they only represented 11% of the infantile population in greater Benguela (*concelho de Benguela*) in 1940 (0–4 years) and 3.2% in 1950 (0–9 years). See Repartição de Estatística Geral da Colónia de Angola (ed.), *Censo geral da população (1940)*, vol. III, 185 and vol. IV, 55; Repartição Técnica de Estatística Geral da Província de Angola (ed.), *II Recenseamento geral da população* (1950), vol. II, 60 and vol. IV, 45.
[81] Alencastro, 'Mulattos'; Ferreira, 'Colonização étnica', 193–212.
[82] See Havik and Newitt (eds.), *Creole Societies* and Corrado, 'The Fall of a Creole Elite'.
[83] Matos, 'Aperfeiçoar a raça', 97–9; Coghe, *Population Politics (2014)*, 257–8.
[84] Ferreira, 'Alguns aspectos', 48.

by their 'white' fathers. Many grew up in poverty with their mothers, in a social limbo between two worlds.[85]

That white, *mestiço* and black infants went to the same dispensaries should not primarily, if at all, be read as an indication of a lack of racial boundaries, as some commentators suggested at the time. In a description of the dozens of mothers waiting in front of the *Gota de Leite* in Luanda to be examined by doctor Levy, one journalist exulted: 'Looking at them there together, there was one feature which made these women, who were clearly distinct by the colour of their skin, equal: they were linked to each other by the feeling of mother-hood.'[86] Yet surviving pictures of mothers and children waiting in or outside the *Gota de Leite* in Luanda in the early or mid-1930s show them grouped separately, with African mothers and children at the back of the queue.[87] Moreover, the presence of white and *mestiço* children resulted primarily from growing socio-economic problems that were, in the case of the *mestiço* children, also linked to racial exclusion.

The impact of the dispensaries on infant health is hard to measure. Statistics for the Luanda dispensary suggest a mortality rate of 5.6 per cent in the 1930s (183 out of 3,250 children admitted between 1931 and 1939).[88] This unlikely rate was very probably much lower than general mortality rates among young children in Luanda – and even lower than that of the infant dispensaries in the city of Porto in the 1930s and 1940s, which ranged between 6 and 10 per cent.[89] Defending the importance of the dispensaries at the National Colonial Congress in 1940, Damas Mora even further overstated their effect on mortality rates. He maintained that mortality rates among supervised children ranged from 1 to 3 per cent in Luanda and were lower than 1 per cent in Benguela.[90] This was, certainly for Luanda, an inaccurate interpretation of the statistics published in the *Boletim Sanitário de Angola*, just like his comparison with the 'normal' infant mortality rate of 48 per cent: this percentage merely denoted the share of children aged 0–4 in the total number of deaths in Luanda in 1938.[91] Whether these miscalculations were done on purpose to promote the importance of the dispensaries or just revealed his poor statistical skills, is unclear. Significantly, however, Damas Mora also exaggerated registration

[85] For more detail, see Coghe, *Population Politics (2014)*, 258–64. Compare with White, *Children of the French Empire*; Saada, *Empire's Children*.

[86] 'Protecção à criança', *A Província de Angola*, 26 June 1933 (quote). On this absence of racial boundaries, see also 'Iniciativa benemérita. A gota de leite para crianças pobres', *A Província de Angola*, 2 May 1931 and Sarmento, 'Dispensário'.

[87] See particularly ANTT, Agência Geral do Ultramar, Angola, Cx. 6, images 4508 and 4509 and Cx. 9, images 4862, 4863, 4867 and 4870, accessible on https://digitarq.arquivos.pt/DetailsForm.aspx?id=4650634 (last accessed 16 February 2021).

[88] *Boletim Sanitário de Angola* 1 (1937–8), 69 and 2 (1939), 52.   [89] Silva, 'Possibilidades'.

[90] Mora, 'Mortalidade infantil', 605–6, 620.

[91] Compare with *Boletim Sanitário de Angola* 1 (1937–8), 69 and 75.

numbers, stating that the three dispensaries had assisted 4,000 children in 1937, including 1,272 for Benguela, a number seven times higher than the attendance statistics in the Benguela-based journal *O Intransigente*.[92] Official data suggest that, in 1939, the three existing dispensaries assisted only 1,806 children in total (1,183 in Luanda, 186 in Benguela and 437 in Nova Lisboa), from which 693 had been admitted in that year.[93] Yet, Damas Mora conceded that even 4,000 was only a tiny fraction, less than 5 per cent of all children born each year in Angola. The utility of the dispensaries was incontestable, he added, but because of their reliance on European women, their operating range was limited to the population living around European centres.[94]

Even in these few towns, many women did not use the dispensaries regularly. In Benguela, for instance, only 89 newborns, or 8.3 per cent of all those born in 1940, were newly admitted to the dispensary that year. Here, women's reluctance reshaped the policy of the dispensary. From 1941 onwards, it no longer focused on 'preventive' services, but also offered curative treatments to ill children on a broad, systematic basis, as the other dispensaries were already doing.[95] As a result, the number of registrations soared to 833 or 77.7 per cent in 1946 and the number of 'treatments and injections' rose from 211 (1935–40) to 73,484 (1941–6). For the director of the *dispensário*, the inclusion of curative medicine had been necessary to reach more women: 'When assistance is given to backward populations, like the native one, deeply rooted in ancestral customs that contradict medical action, hygienic measures are condemned to vanish into thin air or to arouse little interest when they are not combined with curative action.'[96]

Accepting curative medicine did not necessarily make women more inclined to take advice on 'good mothercraft'. There are no detailed data for Benguela, but historians have shown for similar institutions in other colonies that African women were fundamentally eclectic in their choices. Their attitudes, as Jean Allman puts it, oscillated between the extreme poles of 'full participation' and 'complete avoidance'.[97] In Benguela, women's attitude of passive resistance and selective appropriation forced the dispensary to alter its policy. Whether the dispensary made mothers alter their hygienic beliefs and everyday practices is less certain.

---

[92] Mora, 'Mortalidade infantil', 621. Compare with the monthly statistics for 1937 in *O Intransigente*, 16 March 1937–1 March 1938, which list about 100 new admissions in 1937 and 75 children remaining from the previous year.
[93] *Boletim Sanitário de Angola* 2 (1939), 52.   [94] Mora, 'Mortalidade infantil', 621.
[95] Passos, 'Contribuição'. Compare with *Boletim Sanitário de Angola* 1 (1937–8), 70 and 2 (1939), 52.
[96] Passos, 'Contribuição', 404–5.
[97] Allman, 'Making Mothers', 31–4 (quote 31); Hugon, 'Redéfinition'.

Medical Missionaries and Maternal and Infant Healthcare

In addition to the colonial health services and philanthropic associations, Protestant missions in interwar Africa also began to invest in maternal and infant healthcare.[98] In Angola, several missions engaged with maternity work, including the American Board of Commissioners for Foreign Missions (ABCFM), which held a maternity clinic in Central Angolan Chissamba,[99] and the Baptist Missionary Society (BMS) in the Portuguese Congo, on which I will focus here. Initially, BMS medical work had concentrated on sleeping sickness, as shown in Chapter 2, but from the 1920s infant and maternal welfare was an increasingly important field of work.

This shift was reflected in the number of supervised childbirths: from 73 in 1925, the number of babies born in the maternity ward of the BMS central hospital in São Salvador rose to 200–300 annually in the 1930s.[100] From the early 1930s onwards, the two other BMS mission stations in the Congo district, in Quibocolo do Zombo and Bembe, engaged with maternity work as well. With around 250 births annually in the mid-1930s, numbers in Bembe even equalled those of the central BMS hospital in São Salvador, about 100km north.[101] Comparatively, these were substantial numbers: they largely surpassed, for example, those of the important BMS hospital of Yakusu in the Belgian Congo, where, according to Nancy Rose Hunt, far fewer than 100 births a year took place until the 1940s.[102]

The medicalisation of childbirth extended far beyond maternity confinement. Mission stations also offered pre- and post-natal consultations and mothers could bring sick children to the maternity clinic. Mission statistics suggest that, by the 1930s, these services reached a few thousand expectant mothers and infants annually, far more than those mothers who eventually chose to deliver under missionary oversight.[103] In addition, the mission

---

[98] Jennings, 'Matter of Vital Importance'. See also Vaughan, *Curing Their Ills*, 66–70 and Bush, 'Motherhood', 278–9.

[99] See Óscar Ruas, 'Relatório da visita a algumas missões protestantes e instituições de assistência indígena do Estado', 23 December 1936, 12, AHU, MU, ISAU 1665.

[100] 'Mapa do movimento de doentes durante o ano 1925', BMSA, A 124; Annual Reports of the BMS station in São Salvador to the Portuguese Government, 1926–45, BMSA, Box 12 (Africa: Angola).

[101] See A. A. Lambourne, 'Defence', 14 January 1935, 5, BMSA, A 94; Miguel António de Freitas Barros, 'Relatório anual do Encarregado do Governo da Província de Luanda (1935–1936)', 16, AHU, MU, ISAU 1727.

[102] Hunt, *Colonial Lexicon*, 255–6.

[103] Annual Reports of the BMS station in São Salvador to the Portuguese Government, 1926–45, BMSA, Box 12 (Africa: Angola). See also Saxton, 'Baby Day'; Dr. Jack Saxton, 'Report of San Salvador Hospital for 1939', BMSA, A 92 and the descriptions in Raúl de Lima, 'Relatório do Governo da Província de Luanda (1938)', 30 April 1939, 57–9, AHU, MU, DGAC 543.

hospital in São Salvador, the only BMS hospital with a permanent European doctor, gained a reputation for its obstetrical operations and other treatments for infertility, miscarriage and early infant deaths, thus also attracting women from further away.[104] Adam, a doctor sent by the BMS in Britain to evaluate the medical work of the mission field stations in Angola and the Belgian Congo, asserted that the immense popularity of the hospital stemmed from its 'powder babies': in order to reduce the number of stillbirths, expectant mothers received a course of 'grey powder'.[105] 'Grey powder', a mixture of mercury and chalk powder, was a widely used medicine against congenital syphilis in infants at the time. Presumably, BMS health workers in São Salvador followed the recommendation of their famous colleague Chesterman in the Belgian Congo in his widely used manual and extended this treatment to expectant mothers, to prevent the transmission of syphilis from mother to child, considered an important cause of miscarriage, stillbirth and neo-natal mortality.[106]

BMS maternity work also included education. Under the supervision of two European nurse-midwives, a midwife training programme was commenced at the mission hospital in São Salvador in 1924.[107] The Baptist missionaries proved far more successful in training African nurses and midwives than their secular competitors – a success that belied Damas Mora's anthropological negativism about the aptitudes of African girls. Soon, the African midwives were called on for normal deliveries, with the European personnel brought in only in difficult cases.[108] Once married, most nurses left the station, but they often went on to practise midwifery in their village.[109] Education in midwifery was not confined to future nurses; in addition to their regular education, girls enrolled at station schools were also taught the basic principles of nursing, midwifery and infant hygiene.[110] Missionaries also organised monthly 'baby days' during which the infants were weighed and examined and the mothers taught new principles in infant welfare, just as in the state dispensaries. All mothers with babies from São Salvador and its surroundings were invited to participate. All regular attendants received small yet meaningful gifts like clothes or soap, while the 'best babies' were awarded additional presents as

---

[104] See, for instance, Saxton, 'Medical Missionary's Experience' and Hancock, 'San Salvador Station Report 1940', 10 January 1941, BMSA, A 124.

[105] Adam, *Africa Revisited*, 30.

[106] See Adams, 'Ante-natal and Post-natal Syphilis' and Chesterman, *Manuel*, 236.

[107] Moorshead, *Heal the Sick*, 156.

[108] Jack Saxton, 'San Salvador Hospital: Letter to Co-workers', September 1935, BMSA, A 124; Saxton, 'Medical Missionary's Experience'.

[109] Phyllis Jessop, 'Report from Bembe for 1939', BMSA, A 92.

[110] See, for instance, 'Relatório sobre o movimento da Sociedade Missionário Baptista em São Salvador do Congo (1935), 8 February 1936, BMSA, Box 12 (Africa: Angola) and Winifred D. Cuff, 'Quibocolo Medical Report for 1939', BMSA, A 92.

further incentive.[111] Reports and pictures of these events, like the public weighing of babies on big scales, were in turn used to charm the mission's supporters at home.[112]

These educational programmes show that, like Portuguese hygienists, Protestant missionaries aimed to change local childbearing and child-rearing customs. Certainly, one can question their efficiency. The BMS sources I was able to consult are silent on how African mothers treated their infants outside mission stations. Mary Cushman, a medical missionary working for the ABCFM in Chilesso, was utterly pessimistic on the effect the courses in infant welfare had even on the *Christian* 'native' women that followed them. Mbundu women, she lamented in her memoirs, usually listened with interest, but did not change their customs, claiming that their babies were different from American ones.[113] As I have argued for the women using the state dispensary in Benguela, many (expectant) mothers in the Portuguese Congo might indeed have been choosing selectively, just taking the medical and material benefits offered by the BMS without adopting new views and habits of maternal and infant hygiene. Yet, by offering a wide range of both curative and preventive services, from treatments for infertility and neo-natal mortality to direct child-birth supervision and infant healthcare, from midwife training to infant welfare courses, Protestant medical missionaries were eventually able to reach many African women, generating a lot of welcome attention for the Protestant mission.

In various regards, maternity work was of strategic importance for the BMS in Angola. They often highlighted their successes in maternal and infant healthcare in their letters to supporters and sponsors back in Britain, not only to express pride in their work, but also to obtain more funds, as their medical work largely relied on private donations.[114] Moreover, as with sleeping sickness, the missionaries used their maternity work to legitimise the existence of the mission as a whole vis-à-vis a Portuguese administration that was not always favourable towards them but usually appreciated their efforts to improve Africans' health. Thus, at the height of a conflict with the local *chefe do posto*, who had accused the mission of illegally trading in medicines and

---

[111] Moorshead, *Way*, 83; Saxton, 'Baby Day'. On similar practices in the Belgian Congo, see Hunt, *Colonial Lexicon*, 4, 23 and 237–8. On the significance of soap, cleanliness and bodily hygiene as 'civilising' features in colonial and missionary discourse, see Burke, *Lifebuoy Men*, 17–62.

[112] See for instance Saxton, 'Baby Day'.   [113] Cushman, *Missionary Doctor*, 206–10.

[114] 'Miss Bell and Dr. Craven to the Friends who have named beds at San Salvador', 7 January 1933 and 'M. Stevens to the bed friends of San Salvador', 3 February 1934, both BMSA, A 124. For a similar argument, see Summers, 'Intimate Colonialism', 802–4, who has shown that the maternity programme of the Church Missionary Society was a huge financial and public relations success in Britain.

extorting African patients, the Rev. Arthur Lambourne defended the work of the Bembe mission with its maternal and infant welfare programme:

We conclude that before the arrival of the missionaries, the infant mortality reached 80 per cent; but now owing to the efforts made by the competent personnel of the Mission Dispensary as regards ante-natal and post-natal treatment, as well as a hygienic and effective service at the time of birth, the infant mortality is already reduced to 7 per cent amongst women [who have] delivered in the Mission.[115]

It is noteworthy that the BMS greatly expanded its maternity work in the late 1920s, at the very moment when the state had begun to set up its anti-sleeping sickness programme in the region and, therefore, had begun to monopolise the fight against this disease.[116] Maternity work had become the new niche and, like the prolonged sleeping sickness treatments mentioned in Chapter 2, offered promising opportunities to evangelise. As Nancy Rose Hunt has written on the BMS in Yakusu, 'women in childbearing crisis' were considered to be 'particularly open to conversion'.[117] For BMS missionaries, medical work not only had a value in itself; it was quintessential in spreading the gospel.[118] Referring to the hospital in São Salvador, Adam concluded: 'Here, unmistakably, the medical mission is in itself the whole Evangel [. . .] The best part of the hospital itself is the preaching hall.'[119]

This underlying rationale of Protestant missionary medicine complicated relations with the – officially Catholic – Portuguese colonial state. Certainly, BMS doctors and missionaries consistently characterised their relations with Portuguese medical officers stationed in São Salvador or Bembe as very cordial, with both parties granting mutual support and assistance if necessary.[120] Portuguese state doctors usually did the same.[121] In the early 1930s, Dr Alfredo Rezende even translated into Portuguese a widely used manual on the 'art of motherhood' written by BMS missionaries working in the Belgian Congo.[122] Yet beyond these personal and professional bonds, medical work was an object of national and religious strategic rivalry, since Portuguese missionary policy in Angola was to contain the spread of foreign Protestant influence.[123] In the interwar period, official policy towards the medical work of

---

[115] A. A. Lambourne, 'Defence' handed to the Administration office at Uige, 14 January 1935, BMSA, A 94. On this conflict, see also Grenfell, *History of the Baptist Church*, 113–4.

[116] See Chapter 3. See also Salzberg to Chesterman, 11 June 1938, BMSA, A 51.2.

[117] Hunt, *Colonial Lexicon*, 227 (quote) and 230.   [118] See, for instance, Moorshead, *Way*.

[119] Adam, *Africa Revisited*, 67.

[120] See, for instance, 'BMS Medical report São Salvador for 1918'; Winifred D. Cuff to Dr. Chesterman, 26 December 1939 and Dr. Jack Saxton, 'Report of San Salvador Hospital for 1941', all in BMSA, A 92.

[121] See, for instance, Almeida, 'Relatório Congo', 24.

[122] Millman and Millman, *Manual*. See also Adam, *Africa Revisited*, 30.

[123] See also Chapter 6.

the BMS oscillated between support and obstruction, for instance by denying foreign medical missionaries the right to practise in Angola, obliging them to take a six-month course in tropical medicine in Lisbon or accusing them of illegally trading in medicines.[124]

This rivalry also underwrote maternity work in São Salvador. Instead of integrating Protestant mission medicine into the state's health programme, as for instance the British did in Uganda and Tanganyika or to some extent the Catholic Belgians in the Congo, the Portuguese administration competed with it.[125] It was hardly coincidental that, in 1928, the colonial health services planned one of the very first state maternities precisely in São Salvador. 'The creation and use of the maternity will fill the most serious gap of the *Assistência Médica Indígena* in São Salvador, as it will then be possible to say that the assistance of the natives of the Portuguese Congo is entirely secured by Portugal', Pires dos Santos, the head of the Western Congo AMI zone, wrote.[126] Somewhat ironically, the history of this maternity would also lay bare the limits of state medicine. The construction of the maternity was completed in the beginning of the 1930s (see Figure 5.2),[127] but only became real competition for the BMS maternity, reducing the number of its confinements, in the early 1940s. This was after the Franciscan Missionaries of Mary, a Catholic female congregation that had been present in São Salvador since 1908, had taken over the maternity and set up its own infant dispensary with post-natal consultations.[128] This strategic alliance between the colonial state and the Catholic Church not only solved the problem of recruiting European lay midwives, but also convinced many Catholic African women to attend the state maternity.

The engagement of Catholic sister-midwives was enabled by significant shifts in Portuguese state-church relations and in Catholic missionary doctrine. In 1936, the Portuguese state allowed Catholic sisters to carry out nursing work in state hospitals again, after this had ended in 1911 due to the anti-clerical policy of the First Republic.[129] Also in 1936, the Vatican lifted the

[124] See Adam, *Africa Revisited*, 32 and the correspondence between Clement Chesterman, Jack Saxton and Eduardo Moreira, July–August 1939, BMSA, A 51.3.

[125] For the British, see Summers, 'Intimate Colonialism', 802–3 and Jennings, 'Matter of Vital Importance'. For the Belgian Congo, see Browne, *BMS Medical Work*, 8–9 and Hunt, *Colonial Lexicon*, 239–40, 255–6.

[126] 'Assistência Médica aos Indígenas – Sector Congo Oeste', 302.

[127] The pictures in *A Província de Angola*, 20 April 1934 and AHU, MU 975 reveal that the construction was completed by 1934 the latest.

[128] Dr. Jack Saxton, 'Reports of San Salvador Hospital for 1941 and 1944', BMSA, A 92; 'Obras novas' and José Ferreira, 'Relatório do Governo da Província de Luanda (1942)', 85–6, AHU, MU, ISAU 1667.1. See also Gabriel, *Angola*, 458–62.

[129] Ibid., 457, 466–7 and 511. On state-church relations in Angola, see Dores, *Missão da República* and Chapter 6.

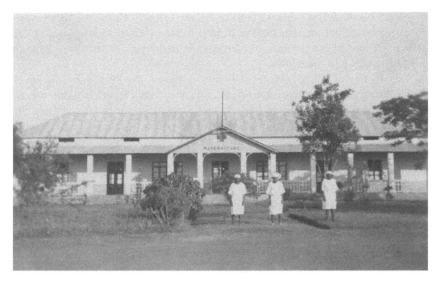

Figure 5.2 'Native maternity' of São Salvador do Congo, with African nurses/ midwives, ca. 1934.
Source: AHU, MU 975, Obras de assistência aos indígenas (1934)
Image courtesy of AHU

centuries-old ban on religious women practising as maternity nurses and mid-wives, and recommended the training of sister-midwives.[130] Not all female congregations in colonial Africa had obeyed this doctrinal prohibition, as Hunt has shown, but its official abolition contributed much to the expansion of Catholic midwifery.[131]

It has been argued that the Vatican's change in doctrine triggered a global shift, wherein the Catholic Church quickly became a leading player in maternal and child welfare services.[132] In Angola, things moved in the same direction, as the Franciscan sisters and other congregations like the Sisters of São José de Cluny began to take up maternity work and, after the Second World War, to establish their own missionary maternities.[133] By 1974, there were 12 Catholic missionary maternities in Angola.[134] In comparison with other colonies, how-ever, this process was slow and limited in scope: in 1948, Catholic missions in the Belgian Congo already directed 184 maternities.[135]

---

[130] Brásio, 'Missionação pela medicina', 466; Wall, *Into Africa*, 13–4.
[131] Hunt, *Colonial Lexicon*, 253–5.   [132] Hardiman, 'Introduction', 24.
[133] For maternity work by the Sisters of Cluny, see Conceição, 'Obra das irmãs', 16; Costa, *Cem anos*, 171.
[134] Gabriel, *Angola*, 512.   [135] Hunt, *Colonial Lexicon*, 255.

If Catholic mission medicine in general remained marginal in Angola before the 1950s, that was also because male Catholic congregations in Angola, most notably the Congregation of the Holy Spirit and from the 1930s also the Benedictines of Singeverga, were slow to professionalise their healthcare services. In part, this was due to a long, general reluctance towards undertaking missionary medicine in the Catholic Church. It was only in the mid-1920s that Pope Pius XI finally recognised its value and that associations in support of Catholic medical missionaries, which had been virtually inexistent, were established in Europe and the United States.[136] However, it was also specific to Portugal and its colonies. Whereas for instance the Belgian associations *Aide Médicale aux Missions* and *Fondation Médicale de l'Université de Louvain au Congo* (FOMULAC), both founded in the mid-1920s, had, by 1947, already sent more than 30 doctors and many nurses and midwives to Catholic mission stations in the Belgian Congo, no similar movement had emerged in the Portuguese Empire, despite high-ranking Catholic missionaries publicly lamenting their rudimentary dispensaries and the much better medical care in foreign Protestant missions.[137] Speaking at the Third International Congress of Catholic Doctors in Lisbon in 1947, the Portuguese priest Augusto Teixeira Maio blamed the country's Catholic doctors for failing to assist the missions and to alleviate the suffering of the African population in the colonies, causing an 'enormous and criminal waste of human and divine potential'.[138]

Conclusion

From the 1920s, state doctors and administrators, missionaries and lay women conceived various ways to improve infant and maternal welfare in Angola. Before 1945, however, these were implemented on a very limited scale and reached only a tiny part of the population. This stood in stark contrast to the urgency instigated by the elevated percentages of infant mortality that circulated in medical and other reports at the time. The expansion of maternal and infant welfare services was also slow compared to other colonies such as the Belgian Congo and French and British West Africa. This cannot only be explained with the eternal constraints of money and personnel; it was also the consequence of a different ideological stance towards and a slow institutionalisation of such services in metropolitan Portugal. Accordingly, schemes of maternal and infant welfare in Angola were often adopted and adapted, not from Portugal, where in the 1920s they were still exceptional or virtually non-

---

[136] Hardiman, 'Introduction', 24; Souto, 'Auxílio médico', 452–4.
[137] Compare Villela, 'Rapport' and Au, 'Medical Orders', 78–9 with Estermann, 'Conferência', 72–3 and Junqueira, *Missões católicas*, esp. 10–1, 20–4.
[138] Maio, 'Missões protestantes', 461 (quote).

existent, but across imperial boundaries from Belgian, French or British colonies in Africa. Another explanation for their limited reach lies in the particularities of the missionary field in Angola. Through their Medical Missionary Auxiliary programmes, Protestant missions like the Baptist Missionary Society were at the forefront of maternity work in Angola, but were sometimes hampered by Portugal's ambiguous policy towards Protestant missionary medicine. Catholic missions hardly invested in professional healthcare before 1945.

Yet the significance of maternal and infant welfare initiatives did not lie in numbers alone: analysis also reveals the profound tension between colonial ideology and African women's agency. Colonial schemes thrived on the idea that the key to lowering infant mortality rates was tackling African women's backwardness and ignorance of hygiene and child-rearing and that, hence, mass education through infant welfare courses in maternities or by itinerant midwives was more important than individual curative assistance. However, the successes of the Benguela dispensary after it began to offer curative treatments for sick children, and of the Protestant mission maternity in São Salvador with its obstetric operations, infertility treatments and supervised childbirths, tell a different story. Demonstrating the limits of preventive medicine, they suggest that many African women were more interested in direct medical interventions and/or material benefits than in European doctrines of motherhood – and that their demands also shaped the orientation of maternal and infant welfare programmes.

Even so, these programmes still had a narrow view of infant mortality, as they focused on hygiene, medicine and the 'art of motherhood' and ignored the broader socio-economic conditions that governed demographic regimes. Some observers, however, also considered social causes, such as poverty and undernutrition, sometimes exacerbated by colonialism itself, and hence noted that it was imperative to raise the general standard of living. In addition to blaming 'the vileness and incredible ignorance' of African women, Damas Mora attributed high infant mortality to chronic undernutrition: 'Underfed parents don't manage to conceive robust children [...]. Underfed mothers can hardly raise normal children', insisting that it was imperative to tackle both cultural and socio-economic causes.[139] At the SCIU conference in Geneva, some rapporteurs and discussants accused colonial rule itself, in particular practices of land-grabbing, labour migration and exploitation, of exacerbating infant mortality.[140] These analyses fit within a broader discourse on the social determinants of health that grew stronger towards the end of the interwar period.[141] In interwar Angola, this did not lead to much overt critique of

[139] Amaral, 'Natalidade e mortalidade', 178, 183; Mora, 'Mortalidade infantil', 605–9 (quote 608).
[140] See for instance Save the Children International Union, *Proceedings*, 36–9, 44–8 and Torday, *Mortinatalité*.
[141] Packard, 'History of Social Determinants', 44–8.

colonialism itself, but to plans for agricultural reform and education that were to enhance village food production, to villagisation schemes that were to improve general health conditions and to the promotion of family labour migration and village resettlement.[142]

---

[142] See, for some aspects, Chapters 3 and 4. For an in-depth discussion, see Coghe, 'Reordering Colonial Society'.

6   The Problem of Migration: Depopulation Anxieties, Border Politics and the Tensions of Empire

In January 1947, Captain Henrique Galvão, one of three deputies representing Angola in the National Assembly in Lisbon, submitted a secret report on Portugal's colonial rule in Africa to the Assembly's Colonial Committee.[1] The 58-page report was extremely critical of the 'native' policy Portugal had thus far pursued in its *indigenato* colonies Angola, Mozambique and Guinea, colonies wherein a legal distinction was made between 'citizens' and 'natives'. According to Galvão, the colonies were suffering heavy demographic losses from high mortality rates, notably among young children and contract labourers, and an increasing flow of African emigration into neighbouring colonies.[2] These neighbouring colonies offered better work conditions and higher wages to the labourers, imposed lower taxes and set lower prices for consumables. They also provided better medical care and attracted Angolans via well-aimed propaganda and recruiting agents.[3] All three colonies were affected, but Galvão claimed that emigration was particularly serious in Angola. He warned that 'if this exodus continued at its current pace, it would, on its own, be sufficient to depopulate Angola in about thirty years'.[4] Labour supply was already suffering and colonial rule itself would become unsustainable if the 'demographic haemorrhage' was not stemmed.[5] In addition to direct economic and political consequences, Portugal's prestige as a colonising nation was at risk: 'Either we solve this problem, in a quick and determined manner [. . .] or we will fail tragically, still in this century, and after five centuries of glory, in our mission of modern colonizers in Africa.'[6]

Galvão's alarming report was by no means the first account of African out-migration from the Portuguese colonies, yet it was the most comprehensive, the most dramatic and the most intensely discussed of its kind.[7] It was first

---

[1] Henrique Galvão, 'Exposição à Comissão de Colónias da Assembleia Nacional', 22 January 1947, AHP, Secção XXVIII, Caixa 48A, n. 10.
[2] Galvão, 'Exposição (1947)', 11–24.   [3] Ibid., 11–18.   [4] Ibid., 11.   [5] Ibid.
[6] Ibid., 1.
[7] See Wheeler, 'Forced Labour System', 387–8; Wheeler, 'Galvão Report'. Compare with the incisive but much less prominent 'Correia report' discussed in Keese, 'Why Stay?' and the many other reports mentioned in this chapter.

presented in a 'secret session' of the National Assembly's Colonial Committee and then forwarded to António de Oliveira Salazar, Portugal's dictator. It most likely then circulated within the Colonial Ministry, given that a year later, Galvão presented the new Minister with a second more detailed report on emigration and depopulation, primarily with regard to Mozambique, upon the Minister's explicit request.[8] Although the 1947 report was confidential, it also started to circulate publicly in fragments in Portugal and abroad. Aided by a 1961 English summary (written by Galvão himself), the report became one of the key references for anti-colonialists – mainly British and American – attempting to demonstrate how obsolete Portuguese colonial rule in Africa was. The full text, however, was never published.[9]

That the report gained such authoritative status was mainly due to the prestige of the author in Portugal and abroad. Galvão had for many years been one of the *Estado Novo's* foremost colonial ideologists, with first-hand colonial experience especially with regard to Angola. In 1929, long before his term as deputy for Angola (1945–9), he had briefly been *chefe de gabinete* ('head of office') of High Commissioner Filomeno da Câmara and District Governor of Huíla. From 1936 onwards, he was one of the leading inspectors of the newly established High Inspectorate of the Colonial Administration *(Inspecção Superior da Administração Colonial – ISAC)*. In this capacity, he had travelled throughout Angola and appraised many a report from the colony's administration. As a loyal supporter of Salazar's *Estado Novo*, he organised several of the colonial expositions in Portugal and its African colonies in the 1930s. However, he gradually became one of the regime's fiercest critics and finally, in the 1950s and 1960s, an overt opponent. He was incarcerated in 1952, escaped from prison in 1959 and was responsible for orchestrating two of the most spectacular acts of piracy ever carried out against the regime in 1961: the hijacking of the ship Santa Maria and a few months later of a Portuguese plane from Casablanca to Lisbon. In 1963, he pleaded for African self-determination before the Fourth Committee of the United Nations.[10]

In the 2000s, historians have (re)discovered the original 'Galvão report' from 1947 and begun to study its contents and the history of its reception.[11] However, little has been said about one of Galvão's central allegations, namely

---

[8] Henrique Galvão, 'Estudo da emigração indígena em Moçambique', 30 January 1948, AHD-MNE, MU/GM/GNP/RNP/0520/01619.

[9] For the English summary, see Galvão, *Santa Maria*, 57–71. A longer excerpt dealing with emigration can be found in English translation in Coghe and Widmer, 'Colonial Demography', 53–6.

[10] Montoito, *Henrique Galvão*; Farinha, 'Império Português' and Wheeler, 'Galvão Report'. For his work as deputy, see the autobiographical Galvão, *Por Angola*. For his work as ISAC inspector, see later in this chapter.

[11] Ball, *Colossal Lie*, 52–7; Varanda, *A Bem da Nação*, 84–5; Wheeler, 'Forced Labour System'; Wheeler, 'Galvão Report'.

that the grave shortcomings of Portugal's native policy were causing an increasing number of 'natives' from Angola, Mozambique and Guinea to take refuge in neighbouring colonies and that he had warned various colonial ministers about it, without success.

While historicising it, this chapter also takes the 'Galvão report' as a point of departure from which to explore Portuguese anxieties and policies regarding the emigration of Angolans to other colonies in the first half of the twentieth century. Based on a close reading of many barely used, mostly administrative, sources from various archives, it shows that the report was not the beginning, but rather the culmination of a long discussion: for decades, the emigration of 'native' Angolans had been a great concern within the colonial administration, first in Angola and later also in Portugal, and had triggered a whole series of policies to maintain the population within the colony's borders. Although these policies were often unsuccessful, the extensive paper trail that they left provides a fresh view on Portuguese colonial rule in Angola, showing that the issue of cross-border migration was discussed in a much broader and controversial way than Galvão suggested in 1947 and than historiography has thus far accounted for.[12] It thereby reveals that criticism of Portugal's native policy was widespread within the colonial administration in Angola before 1945, against a historiography that has attributed such criticism mainly to foreign actors or to the post-Second World War period.[13]

The migration of Africans across colonial and/or imperial borders was, of course, not unique to twentieth-century Angola. Historiography has analysed how mostly male Africans from all over the continent engaged in – often officially sanctioned, but not always voluntary – cross-border migration to 'foreign' mines and agricultural enterprises in need of manpower.[14] It has also shown the flexible use Africans made of the virtually unpatrollable intercolonial borders for other reasons: for the seasonal transhumance of cattle, for smuggling commodities or for so-called 'protest migrations' (Asiwaju) to evade taxation, forced labour, conscription and other repressive regulations. For many Africans, colonial borders offered a 'theatre of opportunities' (Nugent) and Africans' instrumentalisation of borders contributed to their longevity during and after the colonial era.[15] Compared to this literature, the

---

[12] Compare with the otherwise excellent Kreike, *Re-creating Eden*, who concentrates on South African sources and largely neglects Portuguese policies at Angola's southern border. An exception is Keese, 'Why Stay?'

[13] Compare with Wheeler, 'Galvão Report'; Keese, 'Proteger os Pretos' and Monteiro, *Portugal*.

[14] See, for instance, Crush, Jeeves and Yudelman, *South Africa's Labor Empire*; Harries, *Work, Culture and Identity*; Cordell, Gregory and Piché, *Hoe and Wage* and Lindner, 'Transnational Movements'.

[15] Asiwaju, 'Migrations as Revolt'; Musambachime, 'Protest Migrations'; Nugent, *Smugglers*; Kreike, *Re-creating Eden*.

current chapter is less concerned with the 'real' motives and actions of African migrants or the impact of migration on African communities. Centre stage is given to how Portuguese officials perceived the – allegedly massive – emigration of Angolans, that is, how they analysed the causes, numbers and consequences of this demographic loss for colonial rule, and how they devised policies to attempt to stem the tide.

First, the chapter explores debates and policies concerning 'legal' labour migration from Angola to the Portuguese colony of São Tomé and Príncipe and to foreign neighbouring colonies. These intra- and transimperial migratory movements caused great demographic and socio-economic concern to many colonial officials in Angola, and the advantages of either stopping or better monitoring them were continuously discussed. These discussions often alienated Portuguese officials in Angola from their colleagues in other parts and governing bodies of the empire. These tensions, the chapter argues, reflect the changing position and autonomy of Angola within the imperial framework. Second, the chapter deals with how Portuguese officials explained and sought to contain Angolan emigration more broadly, beyond the particular case of labour migration. From the 1920s onwards, the reduction of taxes in border regions became an important policy to reduce economic disparities with neighbouring colonies and to keep the African population within the colony. Yet many authorities also feared that Angolans emigrated because they considered other colonisers, whether they were the religious missions just across the borders or the civil authorities of neighbouring colonies, to be better equipped and more prestigious. These fears, the chapter argues, reveal profound anxieties among Portuguese officials about the country's position as a colonial power. Colonial authorities responded by reducing contact between Angolans and foreign actors as much as possible and by strengthening Catholic missionary and administrative presence in Angola's own border regions, with limited success. The conclusion returns to Galvão's report and argues that he attributed the growing problem of 'native' emigration not only to poor policies, but also to the lack of stable knowledge on the gravity of the situation among decision-makers.

Controlling Labour Migration: Angola and the Politics of Empire

Throughout the first half of the twentieth century, many observers viewed cross-border labour migration as an important cause of depopulation and an impediment to the economic development of Angola. They did not have an easy solution for the problem, however. Angola was embedded in a larger economic context and labour market in West Central and Southern Africa that stretched across colonial and imperial boundaries. While enterprises in other Portuguese and foreign colonies were eager to employ Angolan labourers to remedy local recruitment problems, Angolans themselves often viewed labour migration as an opportunity to improve their standard of living or to escape the oppression of Portuguese colonial rule. In some cases, they were also forcibly recruited. Colonial officials in Angola and in the metropole took different positions, recommending prohibiting, reducing or capitalising on transcolonial and transimperial migration. The following examples reveal the conflicts of interest between various parts of empire and Angola's changing position within the imperial framework.

Serviçais *to São Tomé and Príncipe*

The first emigration flow to be intensively discussed was the forced migration of so-called *serviçais* or indentured labourers to the cocoa plantations of São Tomé and Príncipe. As shown in Chapter 2, this labour flow, which started around 1850, elicited increasing protests from foreign governments, journalists and humanitarian groups in the late nineteenth and early twentieth centuries. They condemned it as a barely hidden form of slavery, given that *serviçais* were usually contracted against their will and not 'repatriated' after their three- or five-year contracts ended, but continuously forced into new contracts. Historians have paid much attention to this story recently, yet they have usually retold it in a rather binary fashion as a story of British and international protest versus Portuguese appeasement politics, which culminated in Cadbury's boycott of São Tomé and Príncipe cocoa in 1909 and forced Portugal to decree an official recruitment ban for Angolan *serviçais* and revise the whole recruitment system.[16] In this narrative, the resumption of recruitment in 1913, under the promise of stricter controls and the repatriation of all those labourers who volunteered for it, was accompanied by new reports about legal loopholes and illegal abuses. Together with reports about forced labour in Portugal's other African colonies, labour migration to the cocoa islands kept discussions about Portugal's labour policies and its (non-)compliance with international standards alive until the labour reforms of 1962.[17]

Focus on the international and humanitarian dimensions of labour migration to São Tomé and Príncipe has obscured the importance of long-lived 'domestic' protest in Angola against this labour drain. As shown in Chapter 1, the compiler of the 1900 census accused it of depleting the population in the Cuanza region and, in the 1900s, colonial officials and planters used local journals such as *A Defeza de Angola* and *A Voz de Angola* to object to official

---

[16] See, for instance, Duffy, *Question of Slavery*; Stone, 'Foreign Office'; Ball, 'Alma Negra'; Higgs, *Chocolate Islands*; Jerónimo, *Civilising Mission*, 38–76.

[17] Jerónimo, *Civilising Mission*, 134–93; Jerónimo and Monteiro, 'Internationalism and Empire'. For the broader anti-slavery context, see Forclaz, *Humanitarian Imperialism* and Miers, *Slavery in the Twentieth Century*.

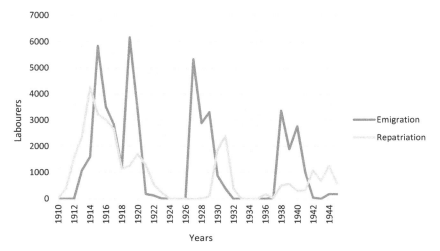

Figure 6.1 Labour migration between Angola and São Tomé e Príncipe, 1910–45.

Sources: Amadeu de Bettencourt Reys, 'Relatório da Repartição Central dos Negócios Indígenas de Angola (1942)', [1948], 306–8 and Colónia de São Tomé e Príncipe, 'Relatório do Chefe da Repartição Central dos Serviços de Administração Civil e dos Negócios Indígenas (1945)', 225–6, both AHU, MU, ISAU 1661; Duffy, *Question of Slavery*, 211 and 228–9

migration policies. They criticised not only labour migration's human toll and its potential consequences for Angola's internal stability and Portugal's colonial prestige, but also and perhaps mainly the demographic and hence economic consequences for Angola, as they feared labour shortage. Simultaneously, they accused the Colonial Ministry in Lisbon of privileging the interests of the islands' cocoa planters (and their strong lobby in Lisbon) over those of Angola.[18] Arguably, these protests, along with the international scandal, contributed to the recruitment ban of 1909. But, most importantly, they laid bare the intra-imperial tensions over Angolan labour migration that would shape Portuguese policies over the next decades. More than international humanitarian and legal arguments, I argue, economic and demographic rationales and political decisions in Angola, in combination with the fluctuating power relations between Angola, São Tomé and Príncipe and the metropole, determined the rhythm and volume of this labour migration.

As Figure 6.1 shows, the recruitment of Angolan *serviçais*, after the first pause in 1909, came to a halt three more times between 1918 and 1945. In the

---

[18] See concisely Duffy, *Question of Slavery*, 176–9 and 207–8.

1920s, their number fell spectacularly from 6,169 in 1919 to a mere 12 in 1923 and zero in 1924–6. This steep decline coincided with the establishment of the system of High Commissioners in Angola (and Mozambique) that secured the colonies greater autonomy from the metropole.[19] Unlike his colleague in Mozambique Brito Camacho, who in 1921 (temporarily) ended Mozambique's role as backup for the unstable labour supply from Angola, Norton de Matos did not officially prohibit labour migration to the cocoa islands.[20] Yet he used his large executive powers to enforce stricter recruitment controls. Like other recruitment operations for private enterprises, this was to occur on a strictly voluntary basis.[21] Knowing that '"forced labour" [was] the only way to get workers to São Tomé', given the 'natural aversion of the black people of Angola against leaving their homeland and going to distant and mysterious islands, from where it was said that one never returned', Norton de Matos had thus deliberately created an impasse.[22]

The unofficial recruitment pause coincided with mounting anxieties of labour shortage in Angola.[23] Supporting Norton de Matos's plans to boost Angola's agricultural and industrial production,[24] many European planters and traders opposed 'native' labour migration to São Tomé and Príncipe on the grounds that Angola needed all existing manpower for its own development. When, in 1925–6, the resumption of recruitment was discussed, the *Associação dos Agricultores de Angola* (Association of Angolan Farmers) vigorously campaigned against it in the local press, particularly in the Luanda newspaper *O Comércio de Angola*. They argued that it would only increase the private gains of the cocoa planters and ruin Angola's imminent economic take-off.[25] Angola, a planter from Benguela proclaimed, 'is a great empire in formation; its colonisation has thus far only been outlined. Emptying it from its main element for such achievement is more than a contradiction – it is a treason against our country'.[26] Some also argued that Mozambique was a better labour reservoir, since it allowed tens of thousands annually to work in the South African mines.[27]

These protests, however, were in vain. Although São Tomé and Príncipe were no longer world-leading exporters of cocoa, the islands' planters were still ambitious and influential. Under their pressure and that of the Colonial

---

[19] On this system, see Introduction and Chapter 3.

[20] Mozambique had sent ca. 40,000 labourers to São Tomé and Príncipe between 1908 and 1921. See Nascimento, 'Recrutamento'.

[21] See 'Decreto 73', 17 December 1921, in Secretaria de Colonização e Negócios Indígenas (Província de Angola), *Legislação provincial (1921)*, 21–3 and Matos, *Província de Angola*, 246–7. For the general goal of 'free labour', see ibid., 126–32.

[22] Quotes from Matos, *Memórias e trabalhos*, vol. III, 232–3.   [23] See also Chapter 4.

[24] On his and other interwar plans, see Castelo, *Passagens para África*, 61–106.

[25] *O Comércio de Angola*, 13 April 1926, 1.   [26] *O Comércio de Angola*, 4 September 1926, 4.

[27] *O Comércio de Angola*, 15 May 1926. See also below.

Ministry, which feared that labour shortage would further ruin the former 'jewel of the Portuguese empire', Acting Governor-General Artur de Sales Henriques concluded a new 'modus vivendi' between Angola and São Tomé and Príncipe in April 1926, which obliged Angola to provide up to 5,000 male adult labourers annually for 10 years.[28] Even if Angola had managed to impose new rules, such as minimum wages, the reduction of the contracts to three years and the compulsory repatriation of all labourers at the end of their contracts, the *modus vivendi* and a similar one concluded with Mozambique a few months earlier clearly demonstrate the importance the Colonial Ministry attached to the still lucrative cocoa plantations. Their labour demands were deemed more important for the empire than those of enterprises in Angola and Mozambique – and possible international protest. In its view, the colonies were not autonomous but had to provide mutual support as each was only 'one part of an indestructible national unity'.[29]

The antagonism between colony and metropole was not absolute. The next High Commissioner António Vicente de Ferreira (1926–8) defended the *modus vivendi*, arguing that the planters' protests were exaggerated and that there was no labour shortage.[30] Referring to a new labour survey conducted at the end of 1926, he maintained that Angola's labour reservoirs were easily large enough to feed its economy: from the ca. 588,000 able-bodied men aged 18–45, only two-thirds were reportedly needed for European enterprises or 'native' agriculture. The manpower problem, he concluded, was not one of scarcity but of 'distribution and rational use'.[31]

The *modus vivendi* of 1926 did not end the opposition of many settlers and colonial officials in Angola to the intra-imperial labour drain, on the contrary. In the early 1930s, the cocoa estates on São Tomé and Príncipe themselves halted recruitment to cope with falling international demand due to the world economic crisis. When they wanted to resume recruitment in 1932–3, they met strong opposition again from within Angola.[32] They were not only accused of having violated the terms of the 1926 agreement, by halving the workers' salaries and not repatriating many of them at the end of their contracts, but some entrepreneurs and officials also advanced (again) Angola's own labour needs. Yet discussions between the administrations of São Tomé and Príncipe, Angola and Mozambique and within the Colonial Ministry reveal that the power relations between colony and metropole had shifted under the *Estado Novo*. In his report for the *Conselho Superior das Colónias* (High Council of

[28] Ministério das Colónias, 'Diploma Legislativo Colonial 108', 19 June 1926, *DG Série I* (1926), 626–31.
[29] Ibid., 626 (quote).   [30] See *A Província de Angola*, 21 July 1926.
[31] Ferreira, *Situação de Angola*, 49–53 (quote 49).
[32] For this paragraph, see Conselho Superior das Colónias, 'Parecer 702', 9 December 1935, AHU, CSC, Livro 5 (1934–6) and the correspondence in AHU, MU, GM 2833 and GM 2878.

the Colonies), the Colonial Ministry's most important consultative institution, Francisco Caeiro wrote that 'excessive decentralisation' in the 1910s and 1920s and 'exaggerated hopes to immediately use all colonial hands in the local economy' had given Angola and Mozambique considerable leverage in previous negotiations. Now the time was ripe to impose Portugal's 'real national interest'.[33] Guided by 'the spiritual and political idea of the unity of the Empire', a key idea of the *Estado Novo's* imperial nationalism, the High Council sided with the cocoa estates and recommended restarting recruitment and even loosening regulations.[34] The Minister of Colonies followed these recommendations and in 1936 decreed the resumption of recruitment in Angola.[35]

Even then, intra-imperial tensions over the distribution of the empire's workforce did not disappear. When Angola's economy burgeoned in the late 1930s and early 1940s, the labour scarcity argument regained force.[36] New detailed calculations suggested that barely 10,000 out of 590,000 able-bodied men were not immediately needed to support the colony's economy.[37] Angola, Governor-General Álvaro de Freitas Morna concluded, was not in a position to deliver thousands of *serviçais* yearly without jeopardising its own economy: 'with regard to the labour force, the two problems – that of Angola and that of São Tomé – are antagonistic'.[38] While his prerogatives as Governor-General did not allow him to alter the *status quo*, he instructed provincial governors to rigorously control recruitment operations and severely punish any use of force.[39] Dwindling recruitment figures under his government (1942–3) suggest that few Angolans were willing to go to São Tomé and Príncipe voluntarily and that, hence, many of those 9,000 recruited from 1937–41 had probably still been recruited by force – a situation that was violently criticised by Henrique Galvão in 1937–8 and just as violently denied by many leading Portuguese officials and agencies.[40] Many of them may have been work or tax defaulters, as both the Governor-General and the Colonial Minister condoned their recruitment in 1938.[41] Falling recruitment numbers also indicate that, within the imperial framework, the central government in Angola had some room for manoeuvre, probably aided by the growing importance of Angolan export products and increasingly critical reports about labour conditions on São

[33] Conselho Superior das Colónias, 'Parecer 702', 26–7 (quotes).
[34] Ibid., 13 (quote). On the *Estado Novo*'s imperial nationalism, see Polanah, 'Imperial Mystique'.
[35] Ministério das Colónias, 'Decreto 27.063', 2 October 1936, *DG Série I* (1936), 1159–60.
[36] Clarence-Smith, 'Impact'; Newitt, 'Portuguese African Colonies'.
[37] Morna, *Angola*, 214–8.   [38] Ibid., 239–48 (quote 244).   [39] Ibid., 246–8.
[40] Galvão to Vieira Machado, 'Carta Confidencial', 22 December 1937 and Henrique Galvão, 'Relatório sobre o recrutamento em Angola de mão de obra para S. Tomé', 6 January 1938, ANTT, AOS/CO/UL-8E, pasta 2. For the denials, see further in this chapter and footnote 179.
[41] Lopes Mateus to Vieira Machado, 6 January 1938 and Viera Machado to Lopes Mateus, 10 January 1938, AOS/CO/UL-8E, pasta 2.

Tomé and Príncipe during the Second World War.[42] After 1945, labour migration from Angola did not end, but Angolans were increasingly replaced with Cape Verdian workers fleeing the devastating famines in the archipelago, Mozambican 'undesirables' and autochthonous *forros* ('freedpeople'), as Morna had proposed.[43]

The Perils of Transimperial Labour Migration

The cocoa planters on São Tomé and Príncipe were not the only external employers eager to recruit Angolan labour. Mining and railway corporations in Angola's adjacent colonies also coveted Angolan labourers to remedy local labour shortages. From the 1910s to 1940s, official and less official recruitment attempts from enterprises in the Belgian Congo, Northern Rhodesia (now Zambia), South West Africa (now Namibia) and even South Africa generated protracted discussions about whether and on what terms to officially allow cross-border labour migration. While these discussions took place against the same backdrop of intra-Angolan labour shortage and depopulation anxieties, the constellation was fundamentally different from the São Tomé and Príncipe case. There was no intra-imperial solidarity at stake here and virtually no-one within the Portuguese empire wanted Angola to become a major reservoir for transimperial labour migration. Yet observers generally knew that it was impossible to simply close off the colony and that, if duly paid, taxed and repatriated, labour migrants could constitute an important source of revenue in Angola's underdeveloped border regions. As Mariano Machado, a high representative of the Benguela Railway, put it in 1919: 'In principle, I am, like everybody, against the emigration of the natives of our Overseas Provinces, but given the material impossibility to prevent such emigration from happening clandestinely, the only solution is to adequately regulate it, thus securing the greatest benefit for the Colony and the natives.'[44]

The example of Angolan labour migration to the Belgian Congo illustrates this dilemma very well. After a first failed attempt in 1910, Robert Williams & Co. eventually managed in 1917 to obtain an official concession from the colonial government in Luanda to recruit Angolan labourers for the Union Minière du Haut-Katanga (UMHK) in the Belgian Congo, of which Williams had been one of the co-founders in 1906.[45] The concession seemed advantageous for all sides: for the quickly expanding UMHK, it offered a (partial)

---

[42] Clarence-Smith, 'Impact'; Keese, *Living with Ambiguity*, 166.

[43] Keese, 'Forced Labour'. Compare with Morna, *Angola*, 244–5.

[44] Mariano Machado to Afonso Costa, 15 October 1919, AHD-MNE, 3. Piso, A. 12, M. 168.

[45] See Perrings, 'Good Lawyers'. On Robert Williams, also concessionaire of the Benguela railway connecting the Katanga mines with the port of Lobito, see Katzenellenbogen, *Railways*.

solution to the acute recruitment crisis it was facing; for Portuguese officials in northeastern Angola, the taxation of returning workers promised a new important source of income after the collapse of rubber prices; and many Angolan workers hoped to earn more cash, needed to pay the 'native tax', than they would at home.[46] Over the next two years, Robert Williams & Co. recruited almost 3,000 Angolans for the copper mines in Katanga, but in 1919, the Portuguese did not renew the concession. According to Charles Perrings, the reason was not so much the violence and lies of labour recruiters, but the fact that the recruiting agency insisted on engaging women as well, thus jeopardising the return of the male workers at the end of their contracts. Moreover, the establishment in 1917 of the Angolan Diamond Company (Diamang) in northeastern Angola, the region closest to Katanga, was fuelling domestic labour demand. However, even after the official expiration of the concession, Williams & Co. still managed to recruit some 600 Angolan workers.[47]

The end of the official concession foreshadowed Angola's official labour migration policy, and its contradictions, in the 1920s. For the sake of domestic development, High Commissioner Norton de Matos formally prohibited all emigration of Angolan 'natives' to territories other than São Tomé and Príncipe in 1921. In practice, he allowed exceptions for the construction of railways near the Angolan borders, as this would serve Angola's interests, but maintained the ban on recruitment for the Katanga mines on the basis that this type of labour migration tended to become permanent.[48] This official policy continued throughout the 1920s, even though it was difficult to control. Like other borders in interwar Africa, Angola's borders were by definition porous and a 'theatre of opportunities' as the Portuguese colonial state was unable to patrol them effectively.[49] When, for instance, in 1921–2, Norton de Matos refused to allow the Belgian Colonel Paulis to recruit Angolan labourers for the Matadi-Léopoldville railway, Paulis reportedly gave up his negotiation attempts because Angolan labourers had begun to cross the border to enter his service anyway.[50] Whether or not labour migrants were enlisted by corrupt Portuguese traders and officials or 'seduced' by foreign labour recruiters illegally operating in Angola, as common Portuguese accusations went, the

---

[46] See also 'Recrutamento dos trabalhadores d'Angola para a Katanga', 10 September 1918, enclosed in Machado to Costa, 15 October 1919, AHD-MNE, 3. Piso, A. 12, M. 168.

[47] Perrings, 'Good Lawyers', 244–5. On Diamang, see Cleveland, *Diamonds in the Rough.*

[48] See 'Decreto 73', 17 December 1921, in Secretaria de Colonização e Negócios Indígenas (Província de Angola), *Legislação provincial (1921)*, 21–3; Matos, *Província de Angola*, 246–7. For Norton's different appraisal of railway and mine labour, see also Governor of Belgian Congo Rutten to High Commissioner Norton de Matos, Boma, 9 July 1923 and Norton de Matos to Rutten, 2 September 1923, MAEAA, AE 3238, Folder 1359.

[49] See the literature in footnote 15.

[50] See AHU, MU, AGC 2441, Processo 27 and AR, I 254 (Union Minière), dossier 338.

agency and mobility of Angola's border populations constantly undermined official restrictions.[51]

The colonial administration was aware of this problem. When reports of clandestine labour migration to neighbouring colonies grew increasingly frequent in the late 1920s, some officials (again) asked whether it would not be better to agree labour conventions with the surrounding colonies, modelled on those Mozambique had negotiated with its neighbours. In 1930, Carlos Roma Machado, a high-ranking colonial engineer who had helped to demarcate Angola's southern border with South West Africa in the 1910s and 1920s, put the issue on the agenda of the Third National Colonial Congress in Lisbon.[52] Indeed, starting in the late nineteenth century, the Portuguese government had concluded a series of conventions with the Chamber of Mines in Transvaal and, from 1913 onwards, with Southern Rhodesia to regulate, control and tax the 'inevitable' labour migration of Mozambicans to the flourishing mines and agricultural enterprises across the border. These conventions created the largest colonial labour migration system in southern Africa. They allowed the Witwatersrand Native Labour Association (WNLA) and the Rhodesian Native Labour Bureau (RNLB) to recruit tens of thousands of Mozambican labourers under well-established conditions every year: the workers were to be repatriated at the end of their contracts and therefore would receive part of their salary only after returning to Mozambique, and Portuguese 'curators' or 'protectors of natives' were to monitor the whole system. This included protecting Mozambican workers from abuse, but also ensuring the profitability of the system for the Portuguese state by enforcing individual labour contracts and extracting various fees from the workers. In practice, these arrangements were not impervious. Many Mozambicans circumvented official recruitment schemes and hence the taxes and restrictions these entailed, triggering increasing concerns about clandestine migration among colonial officials in the 1930s and 1940s. Yet the conventions managed to legalise at least part of the migration flow and generated important tax revenues.[53]

The Portuguese government would not emulate this policy for Angola, however. Initially, the world economic crisis of the early 1930s turned labour emigration into a less pressing issue, as mines in South West Africa, Northern Rhodesia and the Belgian Congo curtailed production and strongly reduced or even halted recruitment. The number of Angolans employed in the mines of

---

[51] For such accusations, see, for instance, 'Recrutamento dos trabalhadores d'Angola para a Katanga (1918)' and Machado [de Faria e Maia], 'Trabalho dos indígenas'.

[52] Machado [de Faria e Maia], 'Trabalho dos indígenas', esp. 1–6, 12–3, 20 and 24–6.

[53] See especially Harries, *Work, Culture and Identity*; Katzenellenbogen, *South Africa*; Newitt, *History of Mozambique*, 482–516; Tornimbeni, 'State'.

South West Africa, for example, dropped systematically from a monthly average of 2,204 in 1929 to a mere 37 in 1934.[54] And when the labour migration issue resurfaced together with the economic recovery in the second half of the 1930s, the Colonial Ministry's main advisory bodies strongly advocated a closed border policy for Angola. Going against more pragmatic voices from within the colony, they underlined the different position Angola had in the imperial framework compared to Mozambique.

This is obvious from the responses given to the *Sociedade de Recrutamento*. In 1937, this formerly unknown 'Recruiting Society' petitioned the colonial government in Angola to conclude a *modus vivendi* with all neighbouring colonies and Transvaal.[55] The Recruiting Society demanded the same extensive recruitment provisions as those granted to the WNLA for Mozambique and, in return, offered the Angolan government part of the expected profits. It underscored the advantages of such a solution, claiming that the clandestine emigration of tens of thousands of 'natives' from Angola's poor and underdeveloped border territories in the south and the east could not be stopped, and that the government had thus far not benefited from this exodus. The society's request divided the government in Luanda. While the Civil Administration Department (*Direcção dos Serviços de Administração Civil*) opposed the proposal, arguing that the colony greatly needed labour itself and that it was better to prevent emigration by developing the border zones, Governor-General António Lopes Mateus (1935–9) was extremely sceptical about the chances of border development and considered a *modus vivendi* the lesser of the two evils. Francisco Serra Frazão, the interim Director of the Native Affairs Department and one of the more ardent defenders of 'native' rights, agreed: 'On this topic I must say that there is the urgent need to conclude a treaty with the neighbouring colonies. [...] I know that there is no abundance of people in this colony [...] but, if they go there, even without us knowing, why don't we make sure, then, that, if they go, they go in concordance with the law.'[56]

The government in Angola, however, did not have the authority to conclude such an international agreement and the question was deferred to the Colonial Ministry. In Lisbon, the proposal was first rejected by the *Junta Central de Trabalho e Emigração* (Central Labour and Emigration Board), a distinguished

---

[54] Compare Union of South Africa, *Report for 1930*, 96 with Union of South Africa, *Report for 1934*, 108. For Katanga and Northern Rhodesia, see Perrings, *Black Mineworkers*, 99–109 and Macola, *Kingdom of Kazembe*, 217–8.

[55] For the following, see in great detail Conselho do Império Colonial, 'Parecer 18 da nova 3a secção (Regulamentação da emigração)', 19 December 1942, AHU, MU, CIC, Livro dos pareceres de 1942.

[56] Francisco dos Santos Serra Frazão, 'Relatório da Curadoria Geral dos Indígenas (1939–40)', 25 June 1941, 43, AHU, MU, ISAU 1725.

consulting body in imperial labour issues, in 1939.[57] Three years later the *Conselho do Império Colonial* (Council of the Colonial Empire, the successor of the *Conselho Superior das Colónias*) did the same.[58] For both advisory boards, a *modus vivendi* that allowed individuals or societies to recruit Angolan labourers for non-Portuguese colonies was out of the question. It would only denationalise the Angolan workers and further increase the emigration figures at the very moment when Angola needed its entire labour force to supply its own burgeoning economy and the cocoa islands. The five members of the *Conselho do Império Colonial* who examined this question (Lopo Vaz de Sampayo e Mello, Marcello Caetano, Vicente Ferreira, Álvaro de Fontoura and António Leite de Magalhães), all leading figures of Portuguese colonial thinking in the 1930s and 1940s, were unanimous that the Mozambican model was not to be applied to Angola. The tax income to be gained from such a *modus vivendi*, they stated, would not compensate for the loss in manpower and economic production the colony would suffer: 'The abundance of money was never synonymous with wealth. The economic conditions of the colony of origin do not get any better with the gold brought back by repatriated workers; and in the meantime local agriculture and industry, the only secure and stable source of wealth, must do without the indispensable workers.'[59] The council's solution to the emigration problem was to prohibit it wholesale. To keep the population in the colony, it recommended improving the economic and material conditions along the border or, if this proved insufficient, to consider the large-scale resettlement of border populations to other regions.

As in the 1920s, this prohibition was not a viable solution, as the example of the South African mines reveals. In the face of Portugal's official position, even the powerful WNLA did not reach an agreement to recruit Angolan labourers, despite the support of the South African government.[60] When, however, the WNLA in 1939 resumed its recruitment of 'tropical Africans' – that is, Africans living north of the 22° parallel – official Portuguese policy could not prevent the company from building recruiting stations on the south-eastern border of Angola nor from hiring 'clandestine' emigrants.[61] Accordingly, Angolan workers appeared in the official employment statistics of the South African Chamber of Mines in 1940. In the 1940s, they numbered around 7,500 annually.[62]

---

[57] Junta Central de Trabalho e Emigração, 'Parecer 42', 12 April 1939, AHU, MU 729 and the corresponding debate in 'Acta da Sessão 83' (23 November 1938) and '85' (12 April 1939), AHU, MU, DGAPC 996, Proc. 20.
[58] Conselho do Império Colonial, 'Parecer 18'.   [59] Ibid., 5.
[60] Wilson, *Labour*, 69. For this support, see Foreign Office Research Department, 'Portuguese Possessions in West Africa', 6 May 1944, 9, TNA, FO 371/60249.
[61] Crush, Jeeves and Yudelman, *South Africa's Labor Empire*, 35, 45–7 and 108; Gemmil, 'Growing Reservoir'.
[62] Crush, Jeeves and Yudelman, *South Africa's Labor Empire*, 234–5.

Avoiding 'Clandestine' Migration: Border Politics and the Problem of Prestige

Discussions about Angolan migration were not restricted to the (often temporary) labour migration of male adults. In the interwar years, the 'clandestine' migration of individuals, families, clans or entire villages for all kinds of reasons became a broadly and critically debated issue within the colonial administration. In their search for the causes of this flight, local administrators, provincial governors and imperial inspectors oscillated between self-criticism and self-victimisation. On the one hand, many of their reports identified grave shortcomings of Portuguese native policy as important push factors that drove Angolans across the border. Although, as Alexander Keese has argued, many of these reports probably still underrated the role of Portuguese forced labour practices in Angolan emigration, virtually all of them emphasised the nefarious effects of excessive taxation and economic, administrative and religious underdevelopment in Angola's border regions.[63] On the other, many reports also accused foreign government officials and missionaries of unfair strategies to drain Angola's 'native' population. Angola, these reports suggest, was attacked from all sides; it was a colony under siege. Portuguese officials not only lamented the causes of population flight: an analysis of their reports shows that they also advanced a whole series of practical – and at times radical – solutions to stem the tide, many of which copied practices from across the border. These, however, were not (or only insufficiently) implemented, due to diverging rationales and conflicting interests between the different echelons of the colonial administration and the limited control over foreign actors.

Tax Competition and Migration

Interwar administrative reports frequently blamed the difference in taxation between Angola and its neighbouring colonies as one of the main causes of 'native' emigration. Many Portuguese administrators and district governors claimed that border populations in the Belgian Congo, Northern Rhodesia or South West Africa were not subject to 'native tax' payments, or to rates that were much lower than on the Angolan side.[64] Several saw this as a deliberate policy. According, for instance, to José Ribeiro da Cruz, former administrator

---

[63] Keese, 'Why Stay?'
[64] See, for instance, Casimiro Marques, 'Relatório anual da Circunscrição Civil de Camaxilo, 1926–1927', 10 August 1927, ANA, Cx. 907; Augusto Casimiro, 'Relatório do Governo do Distrito do Congo, 1923–1926', 11 December 1928, 5, AHU, MU, AGC 47A and Bento Roma, 'Relatório da Intendência do Cubango', 10 July 1929, 24–8, AHU, MU, GM 599.

of Camaxilo on Angola's northeastern border (1932–8) and Director of the Native Affairs Department in 1941–2, 'native' taxation in the Belgian Congo was very low in border areas and increased the further one went toward the interior.[65] Others accused their colonial neighbours of temporarily exempting Angolans from tax payments when they crossed over to settle. Tax exemption, they asserted, was part of a broader policy of economic incentives with which Angola's neighbours actively sought to attract Angolans to their territories and which also included higher salaries, land to settle and fields to cultivate.[66]

Such complaints, while symptomatic of a broader Portuguese discourse of Angola as a colony 'under foreign attack', are in part supported by evidence from Angola's colonial neighbours. Belgian administrators at the Congo-Angola border, for instance, frequently reported that tax differences indeed constituted a major reason that Angolans chose to resettle in the Belgian Congo.[67] Given further evidence for other borders, it is probable that, between 1918 and 1945, taxes were mostly lower on the other sides of the border and contributed to Angolan emigration, especially in times of crisis.[68] However, it remains unclear whether Angola's neighbours deliberately planned a tax competition strategy, as some Portuguese officials asserted. Studies of taxation in colonial Africa have mostly used a national or imperial analytical framework and more research into inter-imperial tax competition and transimperial adaptation processes is needed, in general as well as for Angola's neighbours.[69]

Caution is also needed because Portuguese accusations of systematic tax competition often rested on a partial misreading of the tax policies in the adjacent colonies. In South West Africa, for example, the absence of direct taxation at the northern border was probably less a deliberate policy of attraction than the consequence of self-perceived weakness. For many years, the South African administration in Windhoek believed that it was not strong enough to implement taxation in its outlying northern territories without risking armed revolts.[70] In contrast to the Portuguese, who had brutally

---

[65] José Ribeiro da Cruz, 'Relatório do chefe dos serviços, interino, da Repartição Central dos Negócios Indígenas (1941)', [1942], 54, AHU, MU, ISAU 1725.

[66] See, for instance, Direcção dos Serviços e Negócios Indígenas, 'Organização social indígena. Seu estado actual – usos e costumes', 1930, 7, AHU, MU, AGC 2336; Sociedade Pro-Angola, 'Memorial', [ca. 1934], 4, AHU, MU, GM 2813 and Norberto Correia's 1929 report on southern Angola, analysed and quoted in Keese, 'Taxation', 127–9 and Keese, 'Why Stay?'.

[67] See, for instance, 'Rapports annuels AIMO du Territoire de Kahemba (Prov. de Léopoldville)', 1935, 33; 1936, 19 and 1946, 7–8, MAEAA, RA/AIMO 102 and 'Rapport annuel AIMO du Territoire de Malonga (Prov. d' Elisabethville)', 1932, 46, MAEAA, RA/AIMO 137.

[68] Keese, 'Taxation', 128, 130; Santos, 'Peasant Tax', 66–7; Kreike, Re-creating Eden, 68.

[69] See Gardner, Taxing Colonial Africa; Frankema and van Waijenburg, 'Metropolitan Blueprints' and, for Portuguese Africa, Havik, 'Colonial Administration'; Havik, Keese and Santos (eds.), Administration and Taxation. For a transimperial perspective, see De Roo, 'Customs'.

[70] Hayes, 'Famine of the Dams', 123.

conquered southern Angola, the South Africans – and before 1915 the Germans – governed their part of Ovamboland and the Okavango Region further east through indirect rule. It was only in the 1930s that Windhoek effectively introduced taxation in these regions.[71] In the Belgian Congo, then, the 'native' tax was not just a 'symbol of sovereignty', as Serra Frazão wrongly assumed. As in Angola, it was an essential source of revenue for the colony and a means with which to coerce the Congolese population into wage labour.[72]

Portuguese complaints about foreign tax schemes might also have distracted attention from the fact that tax levels in Angola were so high that they constituted already in and of themselves an important incentive to leave the colony. Many Angolans, particularly those living far from the colony's main economic centres, had difficulty paying their tax. When this, from the 1920s onwards, could no longer be paid in grain or cattle, but only cash (or cash crops), it was not uncommon, as Kreike has shown for southern Angola, that people were forced to sell their livestock, on the spot and at very low prices, to meet their tax requirements.[73] Wage labourers were not necessarily better off than peasants or pastoralists. Theoretically, minimum wages were bound to the tax level: the Native Labour Code (*Código do Trabalho Indígena*) of 1928 stipulated that, depending on the kind of labour, monthly wages were to amount to 25 to 40 per cent of annual tax liabilities. However, many private employers, at times even the prosperous mining company Diamang, circumvented this and paid less.[74] To escape the heavy tax burden and the punishment for tax defaulters, which usually consisted in several months of forced labour on public roads or – against legal stipulations – private estates, many men fled into areas of lesser administrative control within Angola or (temporarily) left the colony, alone or with their families.[75]

Moreover, tax collection was often a violent process in which *chefes de posto* and their *cipaios* (African policemen) resorted to unlawful extractions and arbitrary exactions: it was not uncommon that village or family members

---

[71] Ibid., 141; Kreike, *Re-creating Eden*, 67–8; Fisch, *Südafrikanische Militärverwaltung*, 209. Alexander Keese's argument that taxation in northern Namibia existed is backed with sources from 1937 and hence does not contradict this. See Keese, 'Taxation', 128.

[72] Compare Serra Frazão, 'Reabilitação dos negros. Estudo crítico sobre diversos aspectos de Angola', 1942, 237, AHU, T 215 with Seibert, 'More Continuity', 384 and 'Rapport Annuel du Service des Affaires Indigènes et de la Main-d'Oeuvre (1935)', 51, MAEAA, RA/AIMO 2.

[73] Kreike, *Re-creating Eden*, 62–5; Keese, 'Taxation', 117–20.

[74] Ministério das Colónias, 'Decreto 16.199', 6 December 1928, DG Série I (1928), 2243–84, art. 197. For infractions see, for instance, Raimundo Serrão, 'Relatório do Governador da Huíla, Março–Abril 1934', 30 April 1934, 19, AHU, MU, DGCO-RAST 377 and Nunes de Oliveira, 'Relatório da inspecção à Colónia de Angola (1944)', 4 February 1945, 204–8, AHU, MU_ISAU_A2.01.002/012.00067.

[75] Keese, 'Taxation', 122–31. See also Ross, *Report*, 24; Frazão, 'Reabilitação', 236–7. On the illegal employment of tax defaulters on settler estates, see also Keese, 'Why Stay?', 86–7.

were taken as hostages until taxes were paid.[76] The central administration in Luanda did not officially endorse such practices and often instituted disciplinary processes, but for a long time failed to eradicate such abuses.[77] Even when punished, administrators were rarely removed from the colonial service, but transferred to other places.[78] Still in 1937, the Director of the Native Affairs Department found it necessary to warn that 'the administrator who, to collect taxes, captures wives, forces people to sell livestock at poor prices and makes the natives sell the very products they need for their diet, is a bad official. He has indeed collected the taxes, but he has also destroyed the native economy and caused hunger in the village.'[79]

Yet the recurrent warnings about tax emigration did not leave Portuguese taxation policies in Angola unaffected. To end population flight, many Portuguese officials advocated reducing tax levels in border areas and/or adapting them in light of those in adjacent colonies.[80] Angola did not need the consent of the metropole for this: it enjoyed complete autonomy in the nature, level and distribution of 'native' taxation. At least until the end of the Second World War, it was the central government in Luanda that established the tax rates in the colony and decided on reductions or exemptions for certain groups or areas.[81] The regulations of 1931, for instance, stipulated that the Governor-General was to fix the tax rates on an annual basis, in collaboration with the Native Affairs Department and after hearing the district governors, who in turn were supposed to listen to the proposals of the local administrators, especially those in border regions.[82] The declared aim of this indented consultation system was to keep tax rates compatible with the incomes of the African population, which varied considerably over time and space.

---

[76] Kreike, *Re-creating Eden*, 62–5; Keese, 'Taxation', 123–5. For Portuguese Africa more broadly, see Havik, 'Ilhas Desertas' and Havik, Keese and Santos (eds.), *Administration and Taxation*.

[77] By way of example, see the disciplinary process against the administrator of Bailundo in 1935–6, AHU, MU, GM 2805. See also Havik, 'Ilhas Desertas', 187–8.

[78] See Henrique Galvão, 'Relatório da Inspecção Superior aos Serviços Administrativos de Angola, vol. I', 66 and 78 and the annexed 'Cadastro disciplinar', 10 August 1938, ANTT, AOS/CO/UL-8E, pasta 1.

[79] Manuel Pereira Figueira, 'Relatório do Curador Geral dos Indígenas da Colónia de Angola (1936)', 30 June 1937, 9, AHU, MU, ISAU 2243.

[80] In addition to footnote 64, see also Augusto Mario Borges de Sousa, 'Relatório do governador interino da província de Malanje (Abril–Dezembro 1940)', 30 June 1941, 5–6, AHU, MU, ISAU 1667 and Manuel da Cruz Alvura, 'Relatório do Governador da Província de Malange (1944)', 31 May 1945, 188–9, AHU, MU, ISAU 1663.

[81] See the legislation in Governo Geral de Angola, *Regulamento do recenseamento (1920)*, art. 5–9; Colónia de Angola, *Regulamento do recenseamento (1931)*; Ministério das Colónias, 'Decreto-lei 23.228 que promulga a Carta Orgânica do Império Colonial Português', 15 November 1933, *DG Série I* (1933), 1891–1915, art. 170. See also Oliveira, 'Relatório Inspecção (1944)', 214.

[82] Colónia de Angola, *Regulamento do recenseamento (1931)*, art. 4.

Certainly, the system was, in practice, less flexible than some administrators wanted. Taxes were not always reduced to compensate for poor harvests or other adverse economic conditions.[83] Readjustments were the outcome of complex processes of negotiation between the often-diverging interests of the local population, their administrators and the upper echelons of the colonial administration.[84] African taxpayers played an active role in this process. In border areas, they frequently sought to capitalise on Portuguese concerns over inter-colonial tax differences to reduce taxes. In the northeastern *circunscrição* of Chitato, for instance, the inhabitants of Canzari in 1942 threatened their *chefe de posto* with resettling in the Belgian Congo, where taxes were considerably lower, if the government did not undo a recent tax increase. Sensitive to the issue, both the provincial governor and the Native Affairs Director supported their request.[85] As this example demonstrates, the success of their demands not only depended on the goodwill of the local administrator, but on the latter's ability to convince his superiors that reductions were appropriate and practical. Administrator José Ribeiro da Cruz, for example, reported that he repeatedly failed in his attempts to do so in the mid-1930s.[86] Often, as Henrique Galvão reported for the border region with Namibia, larger groups also used their bargaining power to negotiate tax reduction or even temporary exemption as a precondition to resettling in Angola.[87]

Overall, readjustments were frequent and led to a great variation in tax rates in Angola, with border regions in particular benefiting from the lowest rates. In 1929–30, for example, the 'native' inhabitants of the border *circunscrições* of Baixo Cunene, Alto Zambeze and Dilolo and the border intendancy (*intendência da fronteira*) of Cubango, all of which were situated along the southern and eastern borders, paid only 20 or 25 ags., whereas the standard rate in the colony, which had been applied in all central districts but also along the richer northwestern and southwestern border, was 80 ags.[88] At least in Baixo Cunene, rates had been lowered explicitly to reattract 'natives' who had resettled across the border.[89] Over the next 15 years, many border regions continued to benefit from advantageous 'native tax' rates, and in some areas, tax was even temporarily suppressed, as Map 6.1 suggests.

These examples demonstrate that the colonial administration in Angola did engage, at least to some extent, with a flexible tax policy as a way to influence migratory flows. Nevertheless, except for the temporary suppression of

[83] Keese, 'Taxation', 119–20.
[84] For a detailed example, see Amadeu de Bettencourt Reys, 'Relatório da Repartição Central dos Negócios Indígenas (1943)', 1948, 186–200, AHU, MU, ISAU 1661.
[85] Amadeu de Bettencourt Reys, 'Relatório da Repartição Central dos Negócios Indígenas (1942)', 1948, 180–2, AHU, MU, ISAU 1661.
[86] Cruz, 'Relatório (1941)', 54–5.   [87] Galvão, *Huíla*, 138 and 258.
[88] Galvão, *Informação económica*, 22–3.   [89] Galvão, *Huíla*, 137–8.

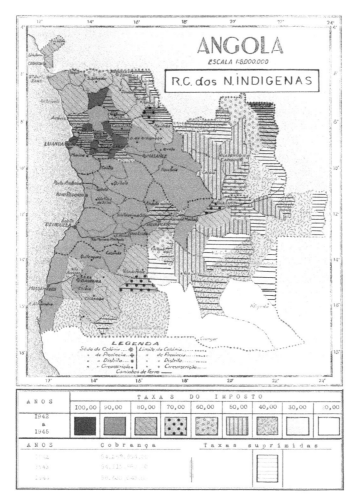

Map 6.1 Levels of 'native tax' in Angola, 1942–5.[90]
Source: 'Mão de obra: elementos estatísticos', [1945], AHU, MU, ISAU 1661 (Colours and patterns have been changed to make the map legible in black-and-white)
Image courtesy of AHU

taxation in some areas, the tax burden in Angola's border regions probably remained higher than in most, if not all, surrounding colonies, thus foiling the

[90] Tax rates varied between 1942 and 1945. The values on the map are close to those in 1944 and probably those of 1945. It is unclear, however, when and for how long the 'native tax' was suppressed in some areas. Compare with the 'Mapas da Cobrança' for 1944 in 'Mão de obra: elementos estatisticos', [1945], AHU, MU, ISAU 1661.

ultimate aspiration of tax equality.[91] The colonial administration did not engage with further reductions for two reasons, each of which reveals tension between colony and metropole.

First, Angola's finances had grown increasingly dependent upon 'native tax' income. When the 'hut tax' (*imposto de cubata*), as a first form of direct taxation, was introduced in 1907, the Colonial Ministry highlighted three sources of legitimacy. It was presented as financial compensation for expenses incurred in policing and developing the territory; as a political symbol for the recognition of Portuguese sovereignty by Angolans; and as an instrument of civilisation that would create regular working habits among the 'native' population and induce many of them to undertake waged labour for Europeans.[92] Over time, however, the growing financial importance of the 'native tax' overtook political and civilisational arguments.[93] Given the reluctance of Portugal to invest in its empire, the 'native tax', which became an individual 'head tax' in 1920, was increasingly seen as indispensable to the rapid development of the colony.[94] It was a significant and growing share of the colony's budget, averaging around 25 per cent in the 1920s and some years more than 30 per cent. This was the result of a rising number of taxpayers, due to greater administrative coverage and tighter fiscal control, and successive increases in tax between 1923 and 1929.[95]

Between 1930 and 1945, the share of the 'native tax' in the colony's total revenue gradually decreased to 13.6 per cent (1945), including a reduction of its nominal value between 1930 and 1936, as the world economic crisis and falling prices for agricultural produce left many Angolans unable to pay their taxes.[96] It continued, however, to be an essential source of income for the colony as the emerging *Estado Novo* imposed new financial constraints on Angola. Having eliminated Portugal's budget deficit in 1928–9, Minister of Finance António de Oliveira Salazar, in 1930 also briefly Minister of Colonies, began to apply the same model of financial austerity to the colonies.[97] His aim was not only to make the empire as a whole self-sufficient, as others had tried before, but to achieve balanced budgets in every single colony. To control the implementation of this policy, he placed the budgets of the colonies under the

---

[91] See footnote 68.

[92] Secretário de Estado dos Negocios da Marinha e Ultramar, 'Decreto criando na província de Angola um imposto sobre habitações denominadas "cubatas"', 13 September 1906, *COLP* (1906), 583–4. See also Couceiro, *Angola*, 229–31.

[93] See, for instance, the complaints in Galvão, *Huíla*, 137 and Frazão, 'Reabilitação', 237.

[94] Matos, *Província de Angola*, 183–5.

[95] See *Anuário Estatístico de Angola* (1933), 209, 212–3; Havik, 'Colonial Administration', 186–93; Santos, 'Peasant Tax', 59–69.

[96] *Anuário Estatístico de Angola* (1939), 464, 472–3; (1940–3), 555–6, 566; (1944–7), 467–8.

[97] For Salazar's budget reforms in Portugal, see Meneses, *Salazar*, 46–52.

strict control of the Colonial Ministry.[98] Large cuts in government spending were the most visible aspect of this policy, as discussed with regard to health expenditure in Chapter 3,[99] but it also placed constant pressure on income. The priority given to balancing the budget in times of economic crisis and falling revenues led to even greater pressure on African taxpayers and, as may be assumed, to less willingness on the part of the administration to endlessly reduce tax rates, even if the heavy tax burden was causing severe hardship in African communities and driving tax migration in border regions.[100]

Second, further tax reductions in border areas were hampered by fears of sovereignty loss. The vicissitudes of a project that aimed to end tax migration to the Belgian Congo through the conclusion of a bilateral treaty illustrates this very well. In the late 1930s, the central administration in Luanda proposed the establishment of a common tax zone on either side of the border that would reach inland as far as 100–150 km. In that zone, it would only be possible to change tax rates via mutual consent of both parties. Although Governor-General Lopes Mateus backed this radical project, it was probably never submitted to any of the surrounding colonies, as both the Council of the Colonial Empire in Lisbon and the Minister of Colonies voted against it. They gave two reasons for so doing: first, the treaty would infringe too much upon Portugal's sovereignty, as it would need the consent of its neighbours to modify taxes; and second, it would trigger emigration from the regions beyond the common zone, where tax rates would be much higher.[101]

The spectre of growing internal tax migration was a compelling argument and had already been raised by several high-ranking officials in Angola in previous years.[102] The former argument about sovereignty, however, is still more illuminating, as it illustrates the increasingly nationalist ideology that underpinned Portugal's colonial policy. In fact, the idea of establishing a common 'native tax' zone was reminiscent of the common customs tariff zone that had existed between Angola, the Congo Free State, and French Congo from 1892 to 1911, in order to end tax competition and curtail cross-border smuggling of export goods.[103] Such a loss of national sovereignty was no longer acceptable in the 1930s, when, as shown in Chapter 3, it became

[98] Havik, 'Tributos e impostos', 33–4
[99] See also Galvão and Selvagem, *Império ultramarino – Angola*, 268.
[100] Havik, 'Colonial Administration', 181–2 and Santos, 'Peasant Tax', 64–7. See also the complaints in 'Imposto indígena', *A Província de Angola*, 14 April 1931.
[101] See Conselho do Império Colonial, 'Parecer 37', 28 March 1938, AHU, MU, CIC, Livro dos pareceres 2a Secção 1938 and the correspondence in AHU, MU, CIC, Cx. 3, Processos Consulta 2ª Secção, 1936–41, Processo 41.
[102] See, for instance, Galvão, *Huíla*, 139; Conselho de Governadores de Angola, 'Relatório e propostas da reunião extraordinária (7–11 May 1935)', 9–10 and 'Proposta 17 (8 May 1935)', AHU, MU, ISAU 1730.
[103] De Roo, 'Customs'.

increasingly taboo to openly adapt the colony's policy to that of its neighbours. The following reaction of the Governor of Malange is illustrative of this mindset. While his administrators advocated orienting or basing their policies on various aspects of Belgian native policy, including tax levels, the governor stubbornly refused to allow that 'our administration subordinates its norms and its goals to the conditions of native life in the Belgian Congo'. Angola's policy had to be guided by its own resources and its own way of colonisation, not its neighbours.[104]

The Threat of Foreign Missionaries

In the late 1920s and 1930s, Portuguese officials identified the existence of mission posts across Angola's borders as another main cause of 'native' emigration. The missions were accused of attracting Angolans by providing better education and medical assistance or actively recruiting Angolan workers for mines abroad.[105] This 'missionary threat' appears in reports from all over the colony, but the situation in the southeastern province of Bié appears to have been particularly acute. In several of his mid-1930s annual reports, Provincial Governor António de Almeida included a very suggestive map in which Bié appeared to be surrounded and assaulted by a multitude of foreign missions, Catholic and Protestant alike (Map 6.2).[106] Like his colleague from the southwestern Huíla Province, Almeida was convinced that at least some of these mission posts had been deliberately established to draw the Angolan population across the border, not without success. He maintained that they not only recruited male adults for the mines, but also children for their mission schools.[107] In a similar vein, southern border expert Carlos Roma Machado suggested that missionaries from Namibia crossed the border to convince the Cuamato and Kwanyama people in southern Angola to have their daughters educated in their mission posts. Many, he added, never returned home, but were sent south to work as maids.[108]

Many missionaries of the Congregation of the Holy Spirit, the most important (and until the 1930s only male) Catholic order in Angola, agreed with this

---

[104] Alvura, 'Relatório Malange (1944)', 189–90.

[105] See, for instance, Bento Roma, 'Relatório Cubango (1929)', 36; António de Almeida, 'Relatório do Governador da Província de Bié (1935–1936)', 31 December 1936, 77, AHU, MU, ISAU 1727; António Lopes Mateus, 'Relatório do Governador Geral de Angola, primeiro trimestre de 1935', Abril 1935, 15–16, AHU, L 5725.

[106] Beyond Map 6.2 from 1938, see also Almeida's reports for 1934–5, 85, AHU, MU, GM 2894 and 1935–6, 69, AHU, MU, ISAU 1727.

[107] Compare with Eurico Eduardo Rodrigues Nogueira, 'Relatório do Governo da Província da Huíla (1940)', June 1942, 100, AHU, MU, ISAU 1667.2.

[108] See his articles in the daily journal O Século in 1929–30, reprinted in Machado [de Faria e Maia], Na fronteira sul, 139–41 and 145–8.

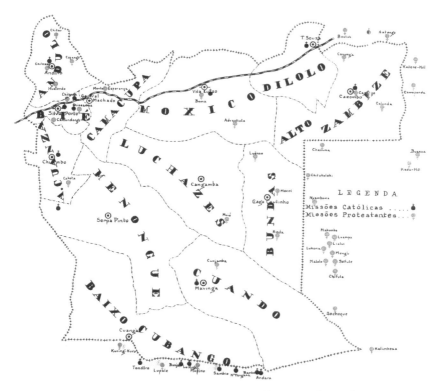

Map 6.2 Foreign mission stations encroaching upon the southeastern
province of Bié, 1938.
Source: António de Almeida, 'Relatório do governador da província do Bié (1938)', 31
December 1938, 72, AHU, MU, DGAC 543
Image courtesy of AHU

interpretation. According to Louis Keiling, the Alsatian superior of the vast
Cubango Mission Province (*Préfecture Apostolique*) in southern Angola, the
Protestant border missions in Northern Rhodesia only served one purpose, as
he wrote to his superior-general in Paris in 1929: 'I have found out that all
these Protestant mission posts have not done a great deal with regard to
evangelisation; they serve another purpose, the clandestine emigration to the
English Barotseland.'[109] Not all Spiritans, as the *Pères du Saint-Esprit* or
Holy Ghost Fathers were also called, used such strong words, but they
generally confirmed that border missions caused many to emigrate, especially

---

[109] Keiling to Superior-General, 12 January 1929, AGCSSp, 3L1.17a3.

young people.[110] On earlier occasions, Keiling himself had already deplored the fact that many Kwanyama boys were attracted by these missions; these same boys would later come back to seek girls to marry, thus precipitating the gradual displacement of all the young people across the border.[111] When the Spiritans finally opened a mission post in Cuamato (west of Kwanyama territory) in 1940, its superior José Maria Felgueiras estimated that half of the population had already crossed the border 'because of religious motives'.[112]

As I have argued more extensively elsewhere, the fear that foreign missions were 'stealing' and 'denationalising' Angolan natives was not entirely new. The border debate partly mirrored how Portuguese officials feared the impact of foreign Protestant missions within Angola itself since the latter's arrival in the late nineteenth century. For Portuguese officials, the main problem was not their Protestantism, even if that conflicted with Portuguese Catholic identity, but their non-Portuguese origin. They believed that the growing number of Protestant missionaries, mainly from Great Britain, the United States, Canada and Switzerland, would not adhere to the Portuguese imperial project. Instead of turning Angolan 'natives' Portuguese, they would either deliberately or unconsciously 'denationalise' them, for instance by spreading other languages and customs. This was, some of them emphasised, already obvious in the way how many Protestantised 'natives' self-identified as American or British. Such fears were also nurtured by Portuguese feelings of inferiority vis-à-vis the Protestant missions, which they believed to be more numerous, richer and better equipped than their Catholic competitors, and hence more attractive 'in the eyes of the natives'. Moreover, stories circulated in Angola and Portugal that Protestant missionaries deliberately ridiculed Portugal as a small and powerless country compared to the United States or Great Britain. Because of its French origins and its majority non-Portuguese missionaries in Angola, the Congregation of the Holy Spirit had sometimes also faced accusations of denationalisation and pressure to engage more Portuguese. Distrust was much less strong, however, and after the coup of 1926, the colonial state increasingly built on them to limit Protestant missionary influence, by engaging them in a spatial strategy of containment throughout Angola.[113]

Convinced of the attraction of religious missions for Angolans, many colonial officials proposed that the missionary policy (or what they considered as such) of neighbouring colonies be replicated: that the Portuguese would also establish mission stations near the border. A chain of 'purely national' Catholic

---

[110] See, for instance, Mittelberger to Superior-General, 15 August 1932, AGCSSp, 3L1.17a3.
[111] Keiling to Superior-General, 27 September 1927, AGCSSp, 3L1.17a2.
[112] Quoted in Nogueira, 'Relatório Huíla (1940)', 101–2.
[113] For a fuller presentation of this argument, see Coghe, *Population Politics (2014)*, 405–14.

missions, as an administrator from the northeastern Lunda district put it, should form a defensive 'barrier' against the 'pernicious influence' of the foreign missions and thus keep the population within the colony.[114] From the mid-1920s, local administrators, district governors and, at times, even the Governor-General or the Minister of Colonies, pressured the Spiritans to establish mission posts in sensitive border areas, notably in the south and east.[115] They later did the same with the Benedictines of Singeverga, a Portuguese order that had taken charge of the southeastern district of Moxico in 1933, thus becoming the second male Catholic order in Angola.[116] In return, colonial state officials offered ample material support, notably housing facilities in former administrative posts, state farms (*granjas*) or 'lay missions'.

This overt support for Catholic missions constituted a break with the anticlerical policy of the First Republic. Especially during the first years, the Republic's new political elite had promulgated a series of laws and decrees aimed at minimising the role of the Catholic Church in the Portuguese state. Most notably, in 1910, it forbade all religious orders in Portugal and, in 1911, declared the separation of State and Church, thus turning religion into a private affair. Having sparked strong opposition from the clergy and a large portion of the Portuguese population, this laicisation policy was somewhat attenuated after 1918.[117] Certainly, the impact of republican anti-clericalism was less directly felt in the colonies: despite some local conflicts, especially in the first years, Catholic missionary congregations (except Jesuits) were not expelled. Many, like the Spiritans in Angola, even continued to receive funding from the colonial state.[118] But the Republic invested much, both politically and financially, in a non-religious alternative, the so-called *missões laicas* ('lay missions'). Between 1917 and 1926, a few dozen lay missions were established in Angola and Mozambique, with the aim to 'civilise' and nationalise the 'native' population through technical, moral and hygienic education and the Portuguese language.[119] With the demise of the Republic in 1926, the lay missions were abolished, partly on the grounds that badly prepared lay missionaries had proven ineffective in winning over the 'native' minds.

[114] António Gonçalves, 'Relatório Anual da Circunscrição de Fronteira do Chitato (1927–8)', 30 September 1928, ANA, Cx. 907. See also Galvão, *Huíla*, 163 and Machado, *No sul de Angola*, 399–402.

[115] See, for instance, Keiling to Superior-General, 27 September 1927, 15 December 1927 and 25 May 1928, AGCSSp, 3L1.17a2 and Mittelberger, 15 August 1932 and Keiling to Superior-General, 2 July 1931, AGCSSp, 3L1.17a3. See also later in this chapter.

[116] Almeida, 'Relatório Bié (1935–36)', 70–1. On the Benedictines, see Gabriel, *Angola*, 443–4, 564–6.

[117] See, for instance, Neto, 'Questão religiosa'; Moura, *Guerra religiosa*.

[118] Dores, 'Séparation'. See also Correia, *Civilizando Angola e Congo*, 73–4, 88–93.

[119] See Madeira, 'Popular Education'; Janeiro, 'Primera República'; Dores, *Missão da República*, 174–82.

Simultaneously, the Catholic missions were officially reinstated as key allies of the colonial state. In the new statute for the Catholic missions in the Portuguese colonies, Colonial Minister João Belo portrayed them as the colonial state's 'civilising' and nationalising agents *par excellence* and promised them more financial support.[120] Yet, despite the rapprochement between State and Church during the early *Estado Novo*, only one new Catholic mission post was opened at an important border location before the late 1930s, in Omupanda (1926).[121]

One important reason was that they did not have sufficient personnel to staff new mission posts, as mission superiors Keiling (in Cubango) and Bonnefoux (in southwestern Cunene) continually told the colonial administration.[122] The correspondence between the Spiritans in southern Angola and the Mother House in Paris is replete with such complaints and corresponding requests for more missionaries.[123] These reinforcements were supposed to come from the Portuguese branch of the order, but they did not. The pro-religious policy of the *Estado Novo* did not resolve the chronic lack of vocations that Portugal had experienced since the late nineteenth century, further reinforced by the anti-clerical policy of the First Republic.[124] It was, therefore, with regret that the superior of the Omupanda mission acknowledged in 1932 that the lack of personnel impeded the expansion of his station. 'The Father Oblates of Mary [Immaculate], our neighbours in the south,' he stated, 'wonder why we don't multiply our missions. In our place, they say, they would already have split up Omupanda in three or four new missions along the border, with good hopes to make them all prosperous.'[125] Ten years later, the Governor of Huíla was still hoping for such a development.[126]

Yet another reason was that missionaries and state officials agreed that religious competition was a major cause of cross-border migration, but did not agree on whether and how to stop it. Keiling, for example, was particularly reluctant to give in to government demands for the establishment of new posts in what he considered to be remote and sparsely populated areas such as the Baixo Cubango, a *circunscrição* on Angola's southeastern border, simply for the sake of emigration control. To the intendant of Cubango, he justified his refusal with the lack of personnel, but highlighted another reason to his

---

[120]   Ibid., 182–93.
[121]   See Keiling to Superior-General, 27 September 1927, 15 December 1927 and 26 July 1928, AGCSSp, 3L1.17a2.
[122]   See, for instance, Galvão, *Huíla*, 163; Bento Roma, 'Relatório Cubango (1929)', 36–7; Manuel Pereira Figueira, 'Relatório do Curador Geral dos Indígenas da Colónia de Angola (1938)', 30–2, AHU, MU, ISAU 2243.
[123]   See, for instance, Keiling to Superior-General, 6 May 1933, reprinted in Brásio (ed.), *Spiritana – Angola, Vol. 5*, 607–11.
[124]   Péclard, 'Eu sou americano', 367.
[125]   Mittelberger to Superior-General, 15 August 1932, AGCSSp, 3L1.17a3.
[126]   Nogueira, 'Relatório Huíla (1940)', 99.

superior-general in Paris: 'That region is a desert,' he pointed out, 'there are not even 2,000 souls in it; it is at the end of the world without communication with our other missions. I think that when it comes to establishing a mission, we must above all ascertain that there is a population, that there are souls to save, and not only consider political purposes.'[127] Overall, the Holy Ghost Fathers were sympathetic to Portuguese requests for missionary expansion into new areas, but unwilling to fully subordinate themselves to the Portuguese *raison d'état* by backing administrative occupation indiscriminately.

The missionaries' reluctance to settle in border regions reveals the different 'logics of occupation' for State and Church. The administrative occupation in Angola obeyed (in theory) the imperative of comprehensive territorial control, which pushed the colonial state to distribute administrative personnel evenly over the territory.[128] The Congregation of the Holy Spirit, however, preferred to apply its scarce human and material resources to the most promising and most strategic locations, where there was fertile land, hygienic living conditions and a large population well-disposed towards mission work, preferably within reasonable distance of other mission posts.[129] Significantly, the congregation found enough missionaries to open a host of new branches that met these requirements in Angola's interior: in the late 1920s and 1930s, the number of both Spiritan mission stations and missionaries almost doubled, to 50 and 124 respectively.[130] Furthermore, missionaries and colonial officials took different stances on the Catholic border missions in the surrounding colonies. Whereas colonial officials regarded their influence as no less pernicious than that of Protestant missions, since both were draining the population from Angola, the Spiritans did not see them as a threat, but rather as collaborators. One of the arguments Keiling advanced against the foundation of a mission post in the Baixo Cubango, besides the lack of population, was precisely the presence of two German Catholic mission stations nearby, to which he had given jurisdiction of that area.[131]

Despite – or perhaps because of – these fundamental conflicts of interest, the colonial state continued to promote Catholic missionary expansion in Angola's border regions. Under the relentless pressure and explicit recommendation of Minister of Colonies Francisco Vieira Machado (1936–44), three further

---

[127] Compare Bento Roma, 'Relatório Cubango (1929)', 37 with Keiling to Superior-General, 1 May 1929, AGCSSp, 3L1.17a3.

[128] See Matos, *Província de Angola*, 81–6.

[129] See, for instance, Bonnefoux to Superior-General, 19 October 1927, AGCSSp, 3L1.14a8; 'Missão nova na região do Cubango' and Pinho, 'Rapport du visiteur des missions d'Angola et Congo (Octobre 1931–Mars 1932)', AGCSSp, 3L1.18.2bis.

[130] Brásio (ed.), *Spiritana – Angola, Vol. 5* lists many of them. For numbers, compare Melo, *Angola*, 42–3 with 'Panorama missionaire de l'Angola [1940]', in Brásio (ed.), *Spiritana – Angola, Vol. 5*, 747–57 and *Missões de Angola e Congo* 20 (1940), 14 and 315.

[131] Keiling to Superior-General, 1 May 1929, AGCSSp, 3L1.17a3.

Catholic mission stations were opened along Angola's southern and south-eastern border: one in far-eastern Cuando (1939), along the border with Northern Rhodesia, by the Benedictines of Singeverga; and two by the Holy Ghost Fathers, in Cuamato (1940), west of Omupanda, and at the border post of Cuangar (1940), in the Baixo-Cubango area.[132] It was Vieira Machado's explicit aspiration to use missionaries as the vanguard of Portuguese colonisation in these areas, to counterbalance the Protestant missions over the border and prevent the Angolan population from migrating. To overcome the missionaries' resistance, Vieira Machado promised additional subsidies for each of the three foundations.[133] Missionary logic, however, often prevailed. After two years, the Spiritans concluded that the mission station in Cuangar was not viable, in part because of the lack of population, and moved the station to Capico, more than 200 km to the north and much further away from the border, a decision strongly criticised by imperial inspector Nunes de Oliveira.[134] Vieira Machado continued to encourage Church representatives, including the Bishop of Silva Porto during his visit to Angola in 1942, to establish more mission posts in southeastern Angola, but to no avail.[135]

The Administrative Occupation of Border Areas

Portuguese fears that foreign Protestant missions, either in Angola or across the border, were superior to their 'own' Catholic allies in terms of numbers, resources and prestige, and used their superiority to subtract and 'denationalise' Angola's 'native' population, was part and parcel of a broader discourse about colonial prestige. In very similar ways, Portuguese officials frequently complained about the deficiencies of their *administrative* presence in border areas and its nefarious effects on African emigration. Border stations were too often left unstaffed and the administrators sent there were often inexperienced, unmotivated and/or living in poor conditions. As border areas enabled direct comparison between adjacent colonial systems, many observers feared that Portuguese border posts represented the colonial state in a disadvantageous manner. While they were concerned with the effects of this 'poor representation' on Portugal's international prestige as a colonial power, the following examples show that many of them also worried that, because of the

---

[132] António Ildefonso dos Santos Silva, 'Relatório da Diocese de Silva Porto (1942)', 27 February 1943, 10, AHU, MU, DGEns 2344; Brásio (ed.), *Spiritana – Angola, Vol. 5*, 672–3, 676–7; Junqueira, 'Pelo sul de Angola', 74–5.

[133] Brásio (ed.), *Spiritana – Angola, Vol. 5*, 676–7.

[134] Costa, *Cem anos*, 312–5; Oliveira, 'Relatório inspecção (1944)', 232.

[135] See Vieira Machado, 'Despacho sobre o relatório da diocese de Silva Porto (1942)', 20 October 1943, AHU, MU, DGEns 2344.

perspicacity of the 'natives', the situation greatly contributed to cross-border population flight.

The Neutral Zone between Angola and South West Africa (1915–28) was probably the area in which the most direct contact and comparisons occurred.[136] Following a long and unresolved dispute with Germany over the location of the inter-colonial border and South Africa's takeover of South West Africa, this strip of territory, roughly 450km long and 11km wide, was put under the joint administration of a Portuguese and South African 'Resident' in 1915, pending its definitive delimitation. The Neutral Zone rapidly became a thorn in the flesh of the Portuguese administration. On the one hand, officials like Carlos Roma Machado, the engineer who directed the Portuguese border delimitation missions of 1916, 1920 and 1926–8, claimed that Portugal had been dispossessed of its 'historical' and 'incontestable' rights over the entire zone.[137] On the other, they lamented that many Angolan 'natives' had taken refuge there to avoid labour and tax obligations and that the South African government did not take any action to prevent this and perhaps even encouraged it.[138] They also deplored the fact that the South African government did not ratify the agreement reached between Portuguese and South African military officials in 1917, according to which resettlement was only to be allowed with the mutual consent of both colonial powers.[139] As the Neutral Zone caused 'great embarrassment', the Portuguese administration wanted to abolish it as quickly as possible.[140] This could not be done, however, before a joint commission had delineated the exact course of the border and the Portuguese suspected the South Africans of slowing down the process. Despite Portuguese pressure, the issue remained unresolved until the Cape Agreement of 1926 and the definitive border demarcation between 1926–8.

Between 1915 and 1928, Portuguese officials expressed great concern at the effects of the Neutral Zone on Portugal's prestige and African migration. The confidential report that Ernesto Machado, the chief of the Portuguese General Staff in Angola, wrote to the Governor-General about his mission to South Angola in 1925 is particularly illuminating in this regard.[141] Due to Portugal's

---

[136] On the history of the Neutral Zone from a South African perspective, see Vigne, 'Moveable Frontier'. For a Portuguese view, see Machado [de Faria e Maia], *Na fronteira sul.*

[137] See his newspaper article in *Diário de Notícias*, 12 October 1921, reprinted in ibid., 55–62.

[138] See, for instance, Dias, 'Fronteira' and Machado [de Faria e Maia], *Na fronteira sul*, 111–2. See also Kreike, *Re-creating Eden*, 67 and 74.

[139] See Eckl, *Herrschaft*, 294–308 and Fisch, *Südafrikanische Militärverwaltung*, 77–9.

[140] See, for instance, High Commissioner Norton de Matos to Minister of Colonies, 10 February 1921 and 28 March 1922, AHU, MU, DGAPC 590, Proc. 265D.

[141] For the following, see Ernesto Machado, 'Relatório da minha missão especial no sul de Angola em Janeiro–Fevereiro de 1925' and particularly the annex 'A Zona neutra e a residência de Namakunde' [1925], AHU, MU, DGAPC 590, Proc. 265E.

misguided native policy, Machado complained, the Neutral Zone functioned as a 'hideout for those who do not want to pay taxes, for those who want to evade labour recruitment, for idlers, criminals and vagabonds'.[142] As such, it profoundly undermined Portuguese authority. Yet, reassessing the reports from various Portuguese Residents, he maintained that the Neutral Zone also damaged Portugal's prestige because Residents lacked the means to appropriately represent Portugal. Whereas the South African Resident possessed many horses and carriages, the Portuguese Resident was forced to travel on an old and unhealthy horse. In addition, Machado complained, the South African Resident killed 80 to 100 oxen per year and distributed the meat among his employees and locals, whereas his Portuguese counterpart was not allowed to kill oxen at all. Consequently, the Portuguese Residents attempted to avoid direct comparison. On public holidays, for example, when the South Africans used to slaughter several oxen, the Portuguese Resident would leave the Neutral Zone, pretending to visit family or friends. In Machado's opinion, the discrepancy between Portuguese and South African means of representation was not only humiliating and embarrassing vis-à-vis the South Africans, but it also discredited the Portuguese in the eyes of the 'natives'. These surely would notice the difference between the 'poor' Portuguese 'who did not eat meat' and the grandeur of their South African colleagues.[143] Machado urged the Governor-General to settle the border dispute and eradicate the Neutral Zone as quickly as possible and, meanwhile, to increase the official 'representation budget' (*fundo de representação*).

The Neutral Zone was abolished in 1928, but this did not eradicate the problem. Similar accounts of unequal material conditions between Portuguese administrators and their neighbours continued at other points along the border. Though usually told with the purpose of triggering better funding for administrators' field work, there is little reason to doubt the veracity of these stories, so diverse were the authors and so well-known the financial problems of Angola's territorial administration during the crisis-ridden 1930s. Almost invariably, these somewhat anecdotical stories were imbued with strong sentiments of shame. In 1942, for example, Native Affairs Director José Ribeiro da Cruz related how, in 1933, when he administered the *circunscrição* of Camaxilo in northeastern Angola, he went to an appointment with the administrator of Kahemba in the Belgian Congo at the border between both colonies. While he had been obliged to ask well in advance for a temporary shelter of grass to be constructed for him, the Belgian administrator simply arrived with a tent and a foldout desk, which he erected in no time whatsoever. Almost 10 years later, Ribeiro da Cruz emphasised that he had experienced this blatant

---

[142] Machado, 'A Zona neutra', 1.   [143] Ibid., 2–3 (quote 2).

difference in equipment and comfort, displayed in front of the local populations, as so humiliating that he never attended such meetings again, even though it would have been useful to talk to the Belgian authorities. Like his colleagues in the Neutral Zone, Ribeiro da Cruz considered eschewing direct confrontations and comparisons as the best way to preserve Portugal's prestige.[144]

Perhaps the most incisive and comprehensive analysis of the deficiencies of Portuguese border occupation can be found in the reports that imperial inspector Henrique Galvão and his colleague in Angola, administrative inspector Óscar Ruas, wrote after inspecting the colonial administration in Angola in 1937–8.[145] During this inspection, the first of its kind in the Portuguese colonies after the creation of the ISAC in 1936, Galvão and Ruas toured the Cuando-Cubango region at Angola's southeastern border extensively – a region about which Galvão had already written during his short term as Governor of Huíla in 1929.[146] They claimed that part of the region had not been visited by any white person for decades and that it was much more populous than generally assumed. However, the people living there were only the remainder of a much larger population, the majority of which had crossed the border, where foreign civil servants and missionaries provided medical assistance and agricultural aid and where Angolans could sell their products and buy consumer goods. Moreover, on the border with Namibia, Galvão and Ruas found one of the few administrative posts (Mucusso) unoccupied; one (Luiana) governed by a *chefe de posto* who had gone almost mad from prolonged isolation; and another (Dirico) occupied by an administrator living in 'a ruin of adobe which makes one envy the houses of many natives from the Alto Zambeze'. Moreover, he did not have any sure means of transportation, had not been able to pay the native policemen for months and depended upon the aid of German missionaries and the South African authorities on the other side of the Cubango river for everything.[147]

Galvão and Ruas depicted the situation of this isolated colonial administrator in his 'lands at the end of the world' in a way that differed fundamentally from the usual colonial narratives.[148] Portuguese propaganda of the 1930s

---

[144] Cruz, 'Relatório (1941)', 16–18.
[145] Óscar Freire de Vasconcelos Ruas, 'Relatório da inspecção administrativa de Angola', 30 December 1937, AHU, MU, ISAU 1665 and, with some overlaps, Henrique Galvão, 'Relatório da Inspecção Superior aos Serviços Administrativos de Angola, vol. I', 10 August 1938, ANTT, AOS/CO/UL-8E, pasta 1.
[146] Galvão, *Huíla*, 240–56. For the following, see particularly the diary of this journey in Ruas, 'Relatório inspecção administrativa (1937)', 70–96, also copied into Galvão, 'Relatório Angola (1938)', 86–108.
[147] See also Ruas, 'Relatório inspecção administrativa (1937)', 53–6; Galvão, 'Relatório Angola (1938)', 85–6 (quote 86).
[148] Quote from Galvão, *Huíla*, 242.

frequently presented the dangers and deprivations at the fringes of the empire as heroic sacrifices, preludes to great achievements.[149] The inspectors thus described their journey through no man's land, plagued by fatigue, danger and deprivation, according to the long heroic tradition of colonial explorers – and the travel narrative Galvão published a few years later also lauded the abnegation of Portugal's unknown heroes in this region.[150] In their inspection reports, however, Galvão and Ruas did not transform the obvious vulnerabilities at Angola's borders into a story of heroism: of how local officials managed to deal with problems in a way that recalled Portugal's imperial greatness. Rather, the *chefes de posto* were portrayed as symbols of Portugal's imperial decay. Instead of being exalted as the 'nation's forgotten heroes', they were pitied as poor fellows trying to survive in a hostile environment.[151] As Ruas put it, the *chefe de posto* of Dirico 'divides his time between two concerns: the [European] food that never arrives and the lion that comes around almost every day'.[152] Moreover, their miserable living conditions were felt to cause the greatest dishonour to Portugal. Galvão and Ruas described these scattered posts as being 'more detrimental than useful, as they only serve to exhibit deficiencies that diminish our prestige'.[153] They feared that this brought ridicule down on Portugal in the eyes of both its foreign competitors and the 'native' population, who supposedly saw this weakness as a further reason to leave the colony.[154]

Beyond material shortcomings, observers frequently invoked another problem of border representation as cause of emigration, as they commented that border district posts were often vacant or held by the least capable civil servants, who had often been sent there as a disciplinary measure.[155] Galvão and Ruas used as an extreme example the secretary of the Cuando *circunscrição*, who had allegedly exacted the cruellest acts of violence (including crucifixions) upon the population in N'Riquinha close to the border with Northern Rhodesia. Before his actions were exposed and halted in 1936, many locals had already taken refuge across the border.[156] The problem of vacancies was not restricted to the border areas, but a consequence of both an administrative system that promoted short terms and frequent rotations, and hence

---

[149] See Roque, 'Razor's Edge'.   [150] Galvão, *Outras terras*, vol. II, 35–93.

[151] Roque, 'Razor's Edge', 117 (quote).

[152] Ruas, 'Relatório inspecção administrativa (1937)', 94.

[153] Galvão, 'Relatório Angola (1938)', 85 (quote).   [154] Ibid., 71.

[155] See, for instance, Bento Roma, 'Relatório Cubango (1929)', 28; A. Soromenho, 'Relatório do Governador de Distrito da Lunda (1931)', 211, AHU, MU, GM 601.

[156] See Ruas, 'Relatório inspecção administrativa (1937)', 51; Galvão, 'Relatório Angola (1938), 63–4 and 78.

much movement and administrative fuzz, and an acute shortage in civil
servants due to poor wages and adverse career possibilities in the 1930s.[157]
Yet, the problem was particularly pressing in border *circunscrições*, especially
in the east, far from the rich and densely populated coastal and central highland
areas. This situation was further aggravated by high living costs, reduced
comfort levels and the psychological burden of isolation. Moreover, during
the expenditure cuts of the early 1930s, the colonial government had abolished
the 'isolation bonus' (*bonus de isolamento*) for administrative staff in remote
areas, thus losing an important incentive and corrective.[158]

In the face of these adverse circumstances, it proved very difficult to get
'good' *chefes de posto*, administrators and secretaries to go to remote border
areas. This is obvious from the efforts made by Governor-General António
Lopes Mateus (1935–9). From the beginning of his term, Lopes Mateus
expressed great concern about the situation. He admitted that it had been
wrong to tolerate vacancies or to systematically send the 'least protected'
and least capable administrators to the most distant and isolated areas, given
the accrued responsibility they had there. However, when he tried to remedy
the situation, he met with covert resistance on the part of the men that had been
designated to go. They arrived late or not at all, invented all kinds of excuses
(notably diseases), and, if they arrived, many quickly left for the closest
town.[159] The problems encountered in the administrative occupation of
Angola's border regions are thus illustrative of the 'internal intermediarity'
of colonial rule.[160] In part, however, they also resulted from a lack of urgency
in the Colonial Ministry: despite the incessant recommendations of Governor-
General Lopes Mateus and ISAC inspectors, it was only in 1945 that the new
Minister of Colonies, Marcello Caetano (1944–7), having personally visited
the colony, re-established the isolation bonus.[161]

---

[157] On these frequent rotations, see Messiant, *Angola colonial*, 92; Havik, 'Administration', 216.

[158] See Galvão, 'Relatório Angola (1938)', 63–4; Ministério das Colónias, 'Decreto 23.940',
31 May 1934, *DG Série I* (1934), 702.

[159] António Lopes Mateus, 'Relatório do Governador Geral de Angola, primeiro trimestre de
1935', April 1935, 7, AHU, L 5725; Conselho de Governadores de Angola, 'Relatório e
propostas da reunião extraordinária (7–11 May 1935)', 14, AHU, MU, ISAU 1730; António
Lopes Mateus, 'Relatório da Colónia de Angola (1936)', 14 August 1937, 14–7, AHU, MU,
ISAC 546.

[160] On this concept, see Introduction.

[161] Ministro das Colónias, Telegrama 162 Esp., 29 October 1945, ANTT, AOS/CO/UL-1D, pasta
16. For the recommendations, see the references in footnote 159 as well as Henrique Galvão,
'Parecer', 27 August 1936, AHU, MU, ISAU 62; Galvão, 'Relatório Angola 1938', 63–6;
Ruas, 'Relatório inspecção administrativa (1937)', 57–8; Oliveira, 'Relatório inspecção
(1944)', 230.

Conclusion: A Problem of Ignorance?

Analysing the causes of Angolan emigration, Portuguese observers usually oscillated between two conclusions. While they blamed inadequate Portuguese policies and practices, they also exteriorised culpability by ascribing emigration to the 'unfair' (or simply astute) policies of neighbouring colonies. This view fitted with the widespread rhetoric of a colony 'under attack': illegal labour recruiters, foreign colonial governments and proselytising missionaries were all supposedly seducing, abducting and denationalising Angola's 'natives'.

Henrique Galvão, as pointed out in this chapter's introduction, largely shared this analysis.[162] Yet he also analysed the problem of 'native' emigration on a meta-level as the consequence of the unresolved intermediarity of Portuguese colonial rule. Galvão claimed that the highest echelons of the administration, in Luanda as well as in Lisbon, had ignored the gravity of the situation. Already in his 1938 report, he had denounced an 'incredible ignorance' at all levels of what was really going on in the colony: 'Luanda does not know Angola, [the provincial capital] Silva Porto does not know [the province of] Bié – and a great deal of the [local] administrations do not know the very *circunscrição* they govern.'[163] This negligence was particularly troubling at the lowest administrative level of the *chefes de posto*, the 'real informer[s] and author[s] of the reports' that were eventually written by their superiors. According to Galvão, they were not always competent or diligent, often lacked the transportation to appropriately monitor their territory, and were not controlled efficiently by their superiors. Consequently, the reports the *chefes de posto* wrote were often fictitious: 'Faced with urgent demands for information, the requirements of the population surveys and the difficulties they struggle with, they do not refrain from sending the report ... but they refrain from seeing what should only be reported if duly seen and counted.'[164]

Galvão's critique was reflected in the epistemic worries of provincial governors concerning the volume and nature of Angolan emigration. Many of their annual reports from the late 1930s and early 1940s reveal how they struggled to make sense of the sparse and often contradictory intelligence on African migration received from their subordinates. The Governor of the southeastern province of Bié, António de Almeida, for example, noticed that the official population numbers in some of the *circunscrições* along the border with the Belgian Congo and Northern Rhodesia had fallen significantly between 1936 and 1938, but that local reports denied the existence of mass emigration. In the absence of other possible causes for the population decrease, Almeida

---

[162] Galvão, 'Exposição (1947)', 15–8.   [163] Galvão, 'Relatório Angola (1938)', 4 (quotes).
[164] Ibid., 4–5.

concluded that inaccurate counting was most likely, but nevertheless announced that he would personally inspect his province to better understand the statistics.[165] His colleague in the Malange province complained in 1945 that he did not receive enough information to assess and quantify the importance of various migration flows that had apparently been occurring simultaneously in recent years: temporary male labour migration to and permanent family resettlement in the Belgian Congo on the one hand, and the return of numerous families to escape military recruitment in the Belgian Congo on the other.[166] The detailed population numbers he gave for the eastern part of his province, with various border *circunscrições*, show yearly variations but no decline, and even growth for the period 1938–46.[167]

In his 1947 report, Galvão also openly expressed mistrust of the population numbers and movements advanced by the border administrations. 'We are dealing', he stated 'with a phenomenon whose salience can be seen by direct observation, by in situ study, by analysis of facts at different times and locations – but which at no time, other than in rare places, has been precisely documented.'[168] According to Galvão, the only solution to this epistemic problem had been to personally inspect the border regions. His conclusion that Angola, Mozambique and Guinea had together lost about 1 million people in the last 10 years was not only based on a critical analysis of the official numbers, but reportedly also on information gathered directly from African emigrants and chiefs, Portuguese curators and settlers, foreign recruiters and residents, and direct inspection of frontier territories.[169]

For Galvão, the key issue was his failure to convince the Colonial Minister of the gravity of the situation, and hence to solve the problem of intermediarity between the administration in Angola and the Colonial Ministry in Lisbon. In fact, the ISAC for which Galvão worked had been founded precisely to bridge the intelligence gap between colony and metropole: through *in loco* inspections and the critical analysis of administrative reports, the inspectors were to inform the Colonial Ministry directly about the most important problems of colonial rule.[170] Nevertheless, Galvão complained in 1947 that his repeated warnings about growing 'native' emigration had been ignored for more than 10 years.[171] Indeed, after returning from his inspection journey through

---

[165] António de Almeida, 'Relatório do governo da província de Bié (1938)', 31 December 1938, Vol. II, 425–6, AHU, MU, ISAU 1663.1.

[166] Alvura, 'Relatório Malange (1944)', 187–8.

[167] Manuel da Cruz Alvura, 'Relatório do governador da província de Malange (1945–46)', 175–7, AHU, MU, ISAU 1705.

[168] Galvão, 'Exposição (1947)', 13.   [169] Ibid., 14.

[170] Ministério das Colónias, 'Decreto 26.180 (Reforma do Ministério das Colónias)', *DG Série I* (1936), 9–36, art. 27–32.

[171] Galvão, 'Exposição (1947)', 3–4.

Angola in 1937, he had alerted the Minister of Colonies Vieira Machado (1936–44) and even Salazar himself about the 'massive flight' that was taking place along Angola's borders.[172] And, in various *pareceres* (reviews) of reports from administrative entities in Angola that addressed the issue, Galvão had again urged the Minister of Colonies to investigate the question.[173] Yet he was (knowingly?) mistaken when he asserted that the Colonial Minister had remained inactive. Upon receiving Galvão's first warning in December 1937, Vieira Machado promptly requested the Governor-General of Angola to send him more information on the subject 'with greatest urgency', adding that 'until now, [he had] no knowledge about the fact that the natives in Angola [were] emigrating en masse'.[174] Moreover, his *pareceres* in the early 1940s led to various inquiries by senior colonial officials.[175] And when he re-addressed some basic problems of native policy, including the depopulation of the border areas, to Vieira Machado's successor Marcello Caetano in 1944, Caetano instructed Galvão to personally study these issues on his next visit to the African colonies, which led to a new report.[176] Arguably, by warning the Minister and triggering further inquiries, the ISAC had largely fulfilled its function as 'watchdog of the empire'.[177]

The problem of intermediarity between colony and metropole was not due to *lack* of intelligence, but to the diminished credibility of that intelligence. In its first decade, ISAC inspectors clearly had limited authority. Critical reports were often successfully challenged by the administrations in the colony that the ISAC was supposed to control or by other agencies that advised the Minister of Colonies. In his report to Caetano, Galvão himself complained that, back in 1938, Vieira Machado had preferred to believe the optimistic reports of the Bank of Angola rather than the pessimistic ones of his inspector.[178] Even more importantly, Galvão's previous reports on illegal recruiting methods and labour conditions regarding São Tomé and Príncipe in 1938 had backfired, when they were violently refuted by the colonial administration in São Tomé and the *Junta Central de Trabalho e Emigração*, an

---

[172] Galvão to Vieira Machado, 'Carta confidencial', 22 December 1937 and Henrique Galvão, 'Relatório sobre o recrutamento em Angola de mão de obra para S. Tomé', 6 January 1938, 4, 12, ANTT, AOS/CO/UL-8E, pasta 2.

[173] See footnote 175.

[174] Chefe de Gabinete do Ministro das Colónias to Governador Geral de Angola, 23 December 1937, ANTT, AOS/CO/UL-8E, pasta 2.

[175] For Galvão's *pareceres* from 25 July 1941 and 27 March 1944 and the ensuing inquiries, see Amadeu de Menezes, 'Emigração de indígenas de Angola', 18 Febr. 1943, AHU, MU, ISAU 2243 and 'Processo 21', AHU, MU, DGAPC 556.

[176] Henrique Galvão, 'Parecer 15', 18 September 1944 (with Caetano's handwritten recommendations), AHU, MU, ISAU 1725. For the report, see Galvão to Caetano, 'Carta-relatório n. 2', (15 March 1945), ANTT, AMC, Cx. 8.

[177] Quote from Garner, *Watchdogs of Empire*.

[178] Galvão to Caetano, 'Carta-relatório n. 2', [15 March 1945], 45, ANTT, AMC, Cx. 8.

advisory board created in 1914 to control the labour flow to the cocoa islands.[179] As a consequence, Vieira Machado had questioned Galvão's credibility and even implicitly asked Salazar for permission to remove Galvão from office: 'With everything that I have sent to his Excellency, I believe that it is not unfair to conclude that either Senhor Inspector Galvão's information show a thoughtlessness incompatible with the minimum requirements of reflection for a highranking official or that he consciously ill-informed your Excellency and his Minister.'[180] Eventually, Galvão was not fired, but Vieira Machado stopped trusting him and did not use him for further inspections in Angola.

In conclusion, one cannot say that the Colonial Ministry completely neglected the problem of 'native' emigration in Angola. Yet Galvão was probably right when he assumed that it had underestimated its gravity and not taken decisive action. One reason certainly was the paucity and instability of colonial knowledge about migration movements: not only was it difficult to gather precise intelligence, but this intelligence often seemed unexplainable and contradictory, or was contested by other actors during its long journey up the command chain to the Colonial Ministry. Moreover, the problem was also hard to solve. If one considers the main causes of Angolan emigration advanced by colonial officials at the time, stopping it would have necessitated stronger economic development as well as a thorough reform of many aspects of Portugal's 'native' policy and administrative practices in Angola. And while the administration in Angola at times used its prerogatives to engage with such reforms, by lowering taxes or promoting new Catholic missions in border regions, the Colonial Ministry was often unwilling to support these or other reforms, giving priority to financial austerity, the interests of São Tomé and Príncipe and exalted nationalist visions of Angola's exclusive Portugueseness and Portugal's imperial sovereignty.

---

[179] See footnote 40 and the documents from January to March 1938 in ANTT, AOS/CO/UL-8E, pasta 2, subpasta 4.
[180] Vieira Machado to Salazar, 5 May 1938, ANTT, AOS/CO/UL-8E, pasta 2, subpasta 4.

Conclusion

From the late nineteenth until the mid-twentieth century, colonial actors conceived and tried to implement a wide array of interventions aiming to improve the 'quantity and quality' of the 'native' population in Angola. These population politics were inextricably linked to the pervasive idea of a demographic crisis: virtually all colonial actors assumed that the 'native' population was declining or at best stagnating, and suffering from ill-health. The emergence of these depopulation anxieties was intimately connected with a major epidemic of sleeping sickness in the 1890s and the changing political, economic and ideological imperatives of colonial rule in what had been a Portuguese colony for many centuries. These new imperatives emphasised the importance of a healthy and growing 'native' population for the success and legitimacy of modern colonial rule, and the importance of Angola for the future of the Portuguese nation. The ideal of a growing and healthy population was firmly linked to the changing labour demands of the colonial economy: depopulation scares usually intensified in phases of economic expansion, as in the 1890s, 1920s, or during and directly after the Second World War, when they dovetailed with fears of labour scarcity. Depopulation anxieties persisted until the late 1940s, but over the decades, primary explanations gradually shifted from excessive mortality caused by epidemic and endemic diseases to low birth rates, high infant mortality and rampant emigration.

This depopulation discourse was driven by reports of disease-stricken empty villages, deserted border districts and 'incompetent' African mothers. It also built on statistical data: over and again, new population counts and estimates reignited demographic worries as they seemed to confirm population decline and very low population densities (i.e. underpopulation) in Angola. Certainly, some contemporaries knew or at least suspected that these data, which after the First World War were being produced by a growing number of actors including medical doctors, were still largely inaccurate and often contradictory. However, this did not prevent them from instrumentalising the flawed statistics at their disposal. Accordingly, one important field of intervention for this book has been to push the analysis of colonial demography beyond the production side of the story and to explore how population numbers, percentages and indices subsequently circulated and were interpreted, debated and used. While some eminent colonial doctors wielded population numbers and indices to demonstrate the positive impact of colonial health campaigns, colonial administrators and governors struggled to come to terms with the sometimes contradictory and inexplicable variations in population size registered in border districts. And while doctors in the 1930s employed inflated infant mortality figures to promote interventions, critics such as Henrique Galvão used similar figures to lay bare the regime's inaptness and inhumanity.

Population politics in Angola targeted all three principal determinants of population change: mortality, fertility and migration. Excessive mortality was initially the prime concern. From the late nineteenth century, Portuguese doctors and scientists avidly participated in the international 'scientific scramble for sleeping sickness', the deadly disease that was wreaking havoc in much of sub-Saharan Africa, including northern Angola and Príncipe. While they managed to eradicate the disease from Príncipe in 1914, campaigns in Angola were more fragmentary and less successful before the coordinated campaigns of the late 1920s that integrated anti-sleeping sickness measures into a more comprehensive 'native healthcare' scheme. The AMI scheme also targeted other epidemic and endemic diseases, and high infant mortality. Simultaneously, it aimed to shift the focus from curative to preventive medicine, which implied changing habits of hygiene and child-rearing and improving the social determinants of health, for instance through education or the establishment of model villages. Low fertility also became a concern in the interwar years, as some observers pointed to the nefarious influence of polygamy, single male labour migration and STDs on the birth rates. However, such concerns did not trigger generalised fertility scares in Angola, partly because evidence of low birth rates and high STD incidence in eastern Angola was deemed less important than the high fertility rates found in studies in many other parts of the colony. Migration became a major focus after the First World War, when the colonial administration began to devise policies to prevent Angolans from migrating to neighbouring colonies. While official cross-border labour migration was greatly restricted and repeatedly prohibited, other policies drew on positive incentives: in border regions, the administration lowered taxes, encouraged the establishment of Catholic missions and tried to improve its representation seen as crucial for Portuguese prestige among 'natives'.

Population policies in Angola were neither homogeneous nor uncontested, varying greatly across regions and population groups. Both the anti-sleeping sickness measures and the broader AMI programme focused on the north-west, where sleeping sickness was ravaging one of the colony's key economic areas. Before 1945, state medicine was less present and intrusive in the rest of the colony, with the exception of the main towns, where European doctors and biomedical infrastructures (including infant dispensaries) were concentrated.

In the densely populated (yet reputedly healthier) highlands of central Angola, as well as in the less populous eastern and southern border regions, it was mainly Protestant missionaries who provided medical assistance to 'native' Angolans. This unequal distribution of state medicine testifies to the priority that, partly because of international pressure, was given to tackling sleeping sickness, but also to the failure to extend the AMI programme to the rest of the colony in the 1930s. After the health services had experienced a remarkable increase in funding and personnel in the 1920s, the world economic crisis, political opposition and the austerity policy of the early *Estado Novo* limited health budgets and staff, and clipped the wings of the AMI programme. Simultaneously, training programmes and job opportunities for inexpensive African medical auxiliaries remained rather modest: while some African nurses were successfully trained, state-sponsored midwifery training schemes failed and the idea of educating African doctors was completely abandoned.

Above all, the implementation of Portuguese population policies hinged on the beliefs, attitudes and (re)actions of the colonial subjects at whom they were directed. Population policies were usually designed without asking the opinion or consent of 'native' Angolans, yet in their role as chiefs, villagers, labourers, migrants, tax-payers, patients, mothers, nurses and midwives, they were not passive recipients of Portuguese intervention. Rather than open revolts, eschewing population counts and medical interventions was a common form of resistance by Angolan villagers. African nurses not only mediated the spread of Western biomedicine, but also carved out spaces of agency for themselves and protested against racial discrimination. African women, then, were not as receptive to Western doctrines of motherhood and infant welfare as state doctors and Protestant missionaries had hoped. Many preferred curative interventions over lessons in mothercraft. While they actively sought the medicalised infertility treatments and supervised childbirths that some missionary stations offered for themselves, their demand for biomedical treatments for their ill children also induced state dispensaries in cities like Benguela to abandon their focus on preventive, hygienic measures. Thus, African women actively shaped the orientation of maternal and infant welfare programmes in Angola.

The comparative and transimperial perspectives adopted in this book show that neither depopulation fears nor most of the policies to foster population growth and health were unique to Angola. Anxieties over the 'quantity and quality' of the population existed in many African colonies and European metropoles at the time and often mutually reinforced each other. Population policies in Angola were not only premised on intellectual, political and socio-economic conditions and developments within the Portuguese Empire. To a considerable extent, they resulted from the intra- and transimperial circulation of views, knowledge and practices, and hence broader shifts in European colonialism in Africa. Senior colonial officials, from leading doctors, (district) governors and Native Affairs directors in Angola to experts in tropical medicine and elder colonialists in the metropole, were embedded in intra- and transimperial networks that facilitated the exchange of views, ideas and practices between colonies and empires. Understandings of and strategies against sleeping sickness, for instance, transcended national frameworks through international conferences, journals and personal exchanges. Similarly, the AMI scheme, methodological innovations in colonial demography, or urban infant dispensaries analysed in this book were all interventions in African lives that travelled across colonial and imperial borders. Moreover, Portuguese actors were not only on the receiving end of such transimperial flows. Doctors like Ayres Kopke, Annibal Correia Mendes and Bernardo Bruto da Costa actively contributed to the scientific 'scramble for sleeping sickness', by formulating new aetiological theories, undertaking drug research or conceiving and implementing innovative eradication measures. Others, like António Damas Mora, conceived new 'best practices' in healthcare and novel ways to foster inter-imperial exchange.

However, this book has also shown that transimperial and other cross-border circulations were not simply a given, but governed by power relations as well as mutual and self-perceptions that often prevented or obscured the 'flow' of knowledge and practices. Sometimes, 'foreign' knowledge and practices were neglected or dismissed. African understandings of and remedies for sleeping sickness, for instance, were widely disregarded by European doctors for not fitting biomedical standards. Portuguese experiences with this disease did not find much resonance on the international stage either, partly because the Portuguese failed to bring them to the attention of international audiences in an appropriate way, as experts in the early 1920s criticised, but also because contemporaries did not think that they could be valuable, given Portugal's growing reputation for backwardness in the late nineteenth and twentieth centuries, an exclusionary practice that many historians of colonial medicine in Africa seem to have reiterated. Sometimes, however, effective transfers of knowledge and practices were simply not accounted for. In its analysis of the interwar reforms in African healthcare, this book has shown that national pride and international rivalry caused European colonialists to repeatedly conceal such transfers and even emphasise the 'exceptional ingenuity' and 'superiority' of their methods and practices. Whether inter-imperial comparisons and borrowings occurred and whether this was hidden or openly acknowledged depended on shifting nationalist tendencies, but above all on how colonial nations perceived their position and that of their competitors on the ladder of prestige. When undertaking transimperial history, historians should hence not only focus on networks of exchange and collaboration, but also on the inter-imperial competition and other exclusionary practices that underwrote colonial politics of comparison and often prevented or obscured such exchange and collaboration.

While other historians have already drawn attention to the negative and stereotyped images of Portuguese colonialists and colonialism among their European competitors, this book has shown to what extent Portuguese colonialists themselves nurtured deep-seated anxieties about the position and prestige of their country as a colonial power. This not only led to nationalist exaltations and exaggerations of Portuguese medical discoveries and innovations on the international stage, but also influenced Portuguese policies toward, and local interactions with, the Angolan population. While they contributed, for instance, to the establishment of the AMI programme or the mass atoxylisation campaigns in the late 1920s, they also affected Portuguese dealings with Angolans living in border areas or near foreign (Protestant) missions in unexpected ways. Many a Portuguese official feared that Angolans might recognise the 'inferior' material conditions of the Portuguese and their Catholic missionary allies compared to those of their 'foreign' neighbours. Haunted by the loss of prestige the Portuguese nation might suffer 'in the eyes of the natives', they sought strategies to avoid direct comparison, by reducing their own contact and exchange with other colonial powers and keeping Angolans away from their 'denationalising' competitors.

Overall, this book makes an argument against a current in both Portuguese and international historiography that emphasises the exceptionalism of twentieth-century Portuguese colonialism. If we look through a comparative and transimperial lens at pre-1945 population politics, Portuguese colonialism in Angola does not look 'exceptional' but at most a local variation of European colonialism in Africa (just as population politics in French Congo or British Uganda would be). Ideologies, discourses and practices concerning the demography and health of Angola's 'native' population were very similar to those in neighbouring colonies and often resulted from transimperial exchanges, particularly with French and Belgian colonies in Central Africa. Differences of course existed, and many of them have been duly identified in this book, but they were gradual and not fundamental. Moreover, as for instance the comparative analysis of sleeping sickness approaches has shown, differences were often more pronounced between Angola and other Portuguese colonies than between Angola and its neighbours, due to diverging environmental, economic, political and financial conditions between the Portuguese colonies, their different positions within the empire and the often region-specific transimperial networks in which local Portuguese experts were embedded.

Portuguese population policies in Angola can hardly be considered backward on the level of implementation either. The colonial state invested as much as others, if not more, in measuring the African population. Censuses started very early and were conducted or coordinated almost annually by the Native

Affairs Department since 1913; AMI doctors not only conducted fertility inquiries as elsewhere in colonial Africa, but also established medical registries similar to those in French and Belgian Central Africa; and the scientific census of 1940 was among the earliest in sub-Saharan Africa. Shifts towards rural African healthcare and growing investments in medical infrastructure and staff in the 1920s matched developments in much of French and Belgian Africa, although this development stagnated in the 1930s. There is also little to suggest that anti-sleeping sickness campaigns in Angola were much less (or more) successful than in the rest of West Central Africa. Certainly, some medical interventions failed or took more time than planned like the midwifery training programmes and the state maternity clinics, but such 'innovations' were slow to take root in many other colonies as well. A more salient particularity was the dearth of medical research (infrastructure) and the almost non-existent involvement of Portugal's School, later Institute of Tropical Medicine in Angola before 1945. Significantly, research from Angola was, in the 1920s, mainly published in two medical journals in Angola itself, a rather uncommon procedure in colonial Africa, but before and after that, publications on medicine in Angola were rather rare. However, in the light of the historiography on colonial medicine and the colonial state in Africa before 1945, none of this is sufficient to qualify Portuguese population policies in Angola as exceptional, or to invoke some exceptional Portuguese colonial incompetence.

Epilogue: Demography and Population Politics, 1945–75

In the historiography on post-Second World War demographic developments, it has often been argued that fears of de- and underpopulation regarding Africa subsided and gave way to a new discourse that problematised rapid population growth and imminent overpopulation instead. Karl Ittmann and Monica van Beusekom, for instance, have identified such changes in the population discourse among colonial experts in French West Africa and parts of British Africa, most notably Kenya and Nigeria.[1] This discursive reversal was not only due to local changes, nor was it nurtured by *colonial* experts alone. After the Second World War, the demographic development of Africa was increasingly viewed through the lens of a *global* discourse that considered unbridled population growth in the so-called 'Third World' an ecological and political risk for the planet and one of the main reasons for persistent underdevelopment, poverty and global inequality. Excessive population growth was a constitutive feature of this new 'Third World'.[2]

The global overpopulation discourse had its intellectual origins in the interwar period, as Alison Bashford has shown, but gained momentum in the wake of the Second World War due to three concurrent developments. While strong population growth was observed in more and more world regions beyond the initial 'danger zones' of South and East Asia, demographic transition theory became the leading paradigm in population studies, predicting further population growth in the 'Third World'. Moreover, the fear of global overpopulation and the search for solutions reflected strategic concerns in the Western world about its position vis-à-vis the decolonising 'Third World' in the Cold War. This explains why the discourse was pushed by a small but powerful epistemic community of 'population experts', many of whom were employed or

---

[1] van Beusekom, 'From Underpopulation to Overpopulation'; Ittmann, 'Where Nature Dominates Man'; Dörnemann, *Plan Your Family*.

[2] The term 'Third World' was coined by the French demographer and Director of the *Institut National d'Études Démographiques* in Paris, Alfred Sauvy, in the early 1950s, see Kalter, *Discovery*, 42–6.

supported by US-based research organisations and foundations, such as the Office of Population Research, the Ford Foundation and the Population Council.[3]

Demographic transition theory was first advanced in 1929 by Warren Thompson, but reformulated and publicised by American population scientists Frank Notestein and Kingsley Davis in the mid-1940s. It posited that all societies would eventually move from a pre-modern equilibrium of high fertility and high mortality to one of low fertility and low mortality as industrialisation and modernisation progressed. In the transitional phase, however, societies would experience strong population growth, since mortality rates would fall much quicker than birth rates; high birth rates would persist before populations adapted their reproductive behaviour to the new conditions of modernity.[4] Under the influence of modernisation theory, adepts of the demographic transition theory also asserted that fertility reduction and modernisation mutually reinforced each other: not only would modernisation lead to lower fertility rates, but lower fertility rates would conversely induce modernisation. They would, as Ansley Coale and Edgar Hoover argued in their influential study on India, increase the GDP, not only per capita but in total. These were strong arguments in favour of 'family planning' programmes. Reducing birth rates was now 'conceptualised as a shortcut on the path to modernisation'.[5]

Demographic transition and modernisation theories greatly contributed to incorporating Africa in the global overpopulation discourse. Around 1950, demographic data for most parts of Africa were still of poor quality, yet more and more observers, among them the compilers of the first authoritative United Nations Demographic Yearbook, believed that the continent's total population was increasing rapidly, due to falling mortality rates and persistently high fertility. This conclusion was not only based on new data, but followed the predictions of the demographic transition model.[6] Historical demographers nowadays largely corroborate this chronology. Struggling with the same deficient data, they tend to agree that population growth in Africa might already have taken off in the interwar years as colonial powers greatly reduced 'crisis mortality' caused by famines and epidemics, before accelerating and becoming very evident after 1945. As for the causes, they point either to falling overall

---

[3] Bashford, *Global Population*; Connelly, 'To Inherit the Earth'; Connelly, *Fatal Misconception*; Frey, 'Experten'; Frey, 'Neo-Malthusianism'.
[4] Hodgson, 'Demography'; Szreter, 'Idea of Demographic Transition'.
[5] Dörnemann and Huhle, 'Population Problems', 143–5 and 155–6 (quote 144).
[6] Badenhorst, 'Population Distribution', 24; Statistical Office of the United Nations (ed.), *Demographic Yearbook for 1949–50*, 11.

mortality, due to improvements in basic healthcare, or to fertility rates that were even increasing, or both.[7]

Several historians, however, have suggested that this reversal did not occur everywhere at the same time, and that in some African colonies such as (French) Gabon, the Belgian Congo and some parts of (British) Uganda, fears of de- and underpopulation persisted until decolonisation or even beyond.[8] The case of Angola also complicates the overpopulation narrative for the late colonial period, but on other grounds. On the one hand, it shows that there were strongly diverging views on the direction demographic development was taking in the 1930s and 1940s, thus revealing not only the lack of uncontested data, but also competing narratives about the impact of medical interventions and the 'success' of Portuguese population politics. On the other, when more and more experts accepted the existence of population growth, this did not provoke fear of imminent overpopulation among Portuguese colonialists.

In Angola, the depopulation thesis began to be challenged in the 1930s and, in the 1940s, claims of population decline and population growth increasingly overlapped and competed. As Chapter 4 showed, senior colonial officials in Angola such as Alberto de Lemos and António Damas Mora claimed already in the early 1930s that the 'native' population had begun to grow again thanks to colonial health programmes. However, there were also more cautious voices, such as former High Commissioner Norton de Matos, who by 1940 was not yet convinced of this demographic reversal, or people like imperial inspector and deputy Henrique Galvão, who warned still in the late 1940s that the colony was rapidly depopulating. Galvão not only pointed to rampant emigration, as discussed in Chapter 6, but also the colony's failure to invest sufficiently in basic healthcare and maternity and child welfare in order to lower mortality rates and reverse the alleged fertility decline.[9] Galvão thereby dismissed official population statistics as erroneous, biased by the fear of colonial officials to tell the truth.[10]

Galvão's critique of the quality of demographic data was not entirely unfounded. With the censuses of 1940 in Angola and Mozambique, the Portuguese were among the first to organise colony-wide 'scientific' censuses in sub-Saharan Africa that were much more detailed and complete than the usual administrative enumerations.[11] Yet, not even Alberto de Lemos, the head

---

[7] For a critical discussion, see Doyle, 'Demography and Disease', 41–5.

[8] See, for instance, Cinnamon, 'Counting and Recounting'; Sanderson, 'Congo belge'; Hunt, 'Colonial Medical Anthropology'; Hunt, 'Rewriting the Soul' and Doyle, *Crisis and Decline*.

[9] Henrique Galvão, 'Exposição à Comissão de Colónias da Assembleia Nacional', 22 January 1947, 18–24, AHP, Secção XXVIII, Caixa 48A, n. 10.

[10] Ibid., 9–10.

[11] For this idea of Portugal's primacy in modern colonial censuses, see Cordell, Ittmann and Maddox, 'Counting Subjects', 7–8; Durand, 'Adequacy'; Lorimer, 'Introduction', 4–5. On the censuses themselves, see Heisel, 'Indigenous Populations' and Heisel, 'Demography'.

of the Statistical Office in charge of the Angolan census operations, believed that the results were entirely accurate. He criticised that, with five months, the 'statistical moment' had been much too long, allowing for all kinds of omissions or repetitions; that some sparsely populated areas had not been incorporated; and that local census agents had possibly over- or underestimated population numbers.[12] Due to these methodological problems, which were typical of many demographic endeavours in colonial Africa and partly repeated in the censuses of 1950, 1960 and 1970, the total number of inhabitants and their geographical distribution was necessarily inexact.[13] Moreover, the colonial censuses suffered from the same sex and age distortions that had affected previous administrative enumerations. These resulted from both African misreporting strategies and European misjudgements: while Angolans deliberately underreported (young) adult men in order to avoid tax, labour duties and military conscription, enumerators often overreported (young) adult women, since they tended to overestimate the age of married women with children.[14]

However, even if the census data could not offer watertight evidence as to whether and at what rate the population was growing, more and more observers in the late 1940s and 1950s interpreted them as important proof of growth. The 1940 census had revealed a considerably larger 'native' – or, in official census language, 'non-civilised' – population than previously assumed, totalling 3.67 million. Moreover, early colonial demographers like Alexandre Sarmento interpreted a series of indices calculated from the census data, such as the large proportion of children under 15 (40.3 per cent), the low sex ratio of 89.6 (men per 100 women) signalling a majority of women and an estimated birth rate of 35.8 per thousand, as proof of a growing population.[15] From now on, demographers at the National Institute of Statistics (*Instituto Nacional de Estatística*) in Lisbon, which had supervised the census operations, also endorsed the idea of population growth. To estimate the evolution of the Angolan population in the 1940s for the first United Nations Demographic Yearbook of 1948, they applied the very optimistic annual growth rate of 2.7 per cent that had been observed in Mozambique between 1930 and 1940.[16] This implicitly challenged Galvão's outcry that Angola was depopulating at an ever-increasing pace. Certainly, the 1950 census, published in the mid-1950s, eventually indicated a much lower total growth rate of 'only' 1.0 per cent per

[12] Lemos, 'Introdução ao primeiro censo', 60, 64–6.
[13] See, for instance, Lemos, 'Censo da população de 1950', 8–11.
[14] Durand, 'Adequacy', 183, 185 and 188; Morgado, 'Da razão dos sexos'; Heisel, 'Demography', 446–7. See also van de Walle, 'Characteristics', 45–50. Compare also with Chapter 4.
[15] Sarmento, 'População indígena de Angola', 636 and 644–8. Similarly Santos, *Perspectivas económicas*, 33–4. See also Chapter 4.
[16] Morgado, 'Estimativas'. See also Statistical Office of the United Nations (ed.), *Demographic Yearbook for 1948*, 75.

year (and a total 'native' population of 4.03 million) but this nevertheless corroborated the idea that sustained population growth was taking place.[17] According to the 1950 census, even the 'Bushmen' in southern Angola, long considered a 'dying race', were growing in numbers.[18]

Unlike what happened in parts of West and East Africa, however, this and further evidence of population growth that became available in the 1950s and 1960s did not spark fears of imminent overpopulation in Angola. At a time when population growth in Africa and the 'Third World' was increasingly problematised and equated with underdevelopment, why did Portuguese colonialists appear unworried?

First, population growth in the 1940s and 1950s was probably less pronounced in Angola than in many other parts of Africa. Demographic studies published in the 1960s suggest that natural population increase only amounted to 0.7 per cent per year in the 1940s and between 1.0 per cent and 1.5 per cent in the 1950s, against 2 per cent and more in many parts of West, East and Southern Africa.[19] To some extent, Angola's limited growth fitted a larger (West) Central African pattern. Certainly, Angola was not part of the so-called 'Central African infertility belt', a zone stretching from Gabon through northern Congo and what is now South Sudan to Uganda where birth rates remained particularly low until at least the end of the 1960s, due to STDs, malnutrition and labour migration.[20] Uncoincidentally, concern over declining or stagnating populations in this region remained high until decolonisation or beyond, as various historians have noted.[21] Average birth rates for Angola in the 1940s and 1950s were calculated at 45 per thousand (equal to a total fertility rate of 5.8 children per woman in the 1940s) or more than 50 per thousand, figures way above the threshold of low fertility.[22] But Angola did show the persistently high mortality rates typical of Central Africa as a whole. Whereas mortality rates in East, North and Southern Africa declined markedly in the 1940s and 1950s, Central Africa was, in the mid-1950s, considered the 'only major region of the world where the existence of a systematic decline of mortality has not yet been established'.[23] With regard to Angola, Don Heisel and Ansley Coale from the Office of Population Research at Princeton

---

[17] Lemos, 'Censo da população de 1950', 15–6; Sarmento, 'Subsídios', 510.

[18] Coghe, 'Reassessing Portuguese Exceptionalism', 197–8.

[19] Heisel, 'Demography', 458; Coale and Lorimer, 'Summary', 157–61; Singer, 'Demographic Factors', 248, 260; Rela, 'Angola', Issue 29 (1970), 54–5. Compare also with Badenhorst, 'Population Distribution', 32–3.

[20] Doyle, 'Demography and Disease', 41–5. See also Romaniuk, 'Infertility'; Caldwell and Caldwell, 'Demographic Evidence' and Hunt, 'Colonial Medical Anthropology'.

[21] See footnote 8.

[22] Heisel, 'Indigenous Populations', 189; Heisel, 'Demography', 458; Carvalho, *Population noire*, 75.

[23] United Nations Population Division, 'Framework', 289.

University calculated mortality rates at 38 per thousand.[24] For Heisel, Angola's pattern of limited growth with high fertility and high mortality was still typical of pre- or early-demographic transition societies. Writing in 1966, he warned that rapidly falling mortality could lead to explosive population growth, but that this was unlikely to happen soon because of the destabilising effects of the colonial war that had begun in 1961.[25]

Second, even if Angola's overall population density had increased to 3.3 inhabitants/km² in 1950 and would further increase to 3.9 in 1960, it was still very low even by African standards.[26] In 1960, the United Nations estimated the world's average population density at 22 inhabitants/km² and sub-Saharan Africa's at 8. Only in some Sahelian and other (West) Central and Southern African countries were population densities in Africa lower than in Angola. Angola also had by far the lowest density of all Portuguese colonies in Africa.[27] Moreover, many regions within Angola were still considered under-populated in light of the labour demands from the colonial economy. The Congo region in Northern Angola illustrates this very well. In the late 1950s, Nuno Alves Morgado, a leading colonial demographer at the Centre for Demographic Studies in Lisbon, concluded in various studies (based on medical registries) that the population of the Congo district was growing very swiftly, due to natural increase and the return of migrants from the Belgian Congo. This 'demographic explosion' did not excite any fear of overpopulation, however, since its burgeoning economy, as Morgado stressed, was still dependent upon the constant influx of temporary migrant labourers from South and Central Angola.[28] Morgado wrote this before the colonial war, which began with a revolt in northwestern Angola in 1961, caused presumably 200,000–300,000 people, mainly Bakongo, to take refuge in the former Belgian, now independent Republic of Congo, and before the ensuing labour shortage obviated any possible discussion of overpopulation in the region.[29]

As in the interwar period, when labour force surveys heightened fears of de- and underpopulation, the way in which Morgado and other observers evaluated demographic change was based on socio-economic criteria and ideas of optimum density.[30] More than absolute population figures, it was the perceived relationship between these figures and socio-economic and environmental

---

[24] Heisel, 'Indigenous Populations', 189; Coale and Lorimer, 'Summary', 158.
[25] Heisel, 'Indigenous Populations', 192–5.
[26] Sarmento, 'Subsídios', 511–2; Morgado, 'Povoamento em África', 107. Compare to Coale and Lorimer, 'Summary', 154–5.
[27] Statistical Office of the United Nations (ed.), *Demographic Yearbook for 1961*, 101–5 and 120.
[28] Morgado, *Aspectos*, 62 (quote); Morgado, 'Crescimento'.
[29] Pélissier, 'Conséquences démographiques', 47–64. See also Bender, *Angola under the Portuguese*, 158.
[30] See Chapter 4.

conditions that underwrote population discourses. This was also true for other parts of the continent. Van Beusekom, for instance, has argued that the discursive shift from under- to overpopulation in French West Africa around 1945 was not so much caused by new population data acknowledging population increase – which were only produced a decade or so later – but by increasingly pessimistic interpretations of the agricultural potential of Sahelian soils and of French abilities to 'modernise' agriculture in order to sustain growing populations.[31] In a similar vein, emerging fears of overpopulation in East Africa were largely related to concerns about soil erosion and the limited 'carrying capacity' of the land.[32]

Portuguese observers were not similarly pessimistic for Angola. Unlike the French in West Africa and the British in East and Southern Africa, soil degradation, resource depletion and the scarcity of arable land were not (yet) central issues for most Portuguese colonialists. Instead, they stressed the enormous potential of Angola in ways reminiscent of the late nineteenth century. Evaluating Angola's demography in the light of its economy, A. C. Valdez Thomas dos Santos maintained in 1949 that 'only in very limited areas one can observe a light surplus population pressure on the land, so that the possibilities of demographic development, even within the present economic type, are still great', before concluding that 'one can claim without fear for error that, quantitatively, the population is below the economic possibilities of the soil and subsoil, however meagre they may appear'.[33] In Angola, strong population growth was still seen as a prerequisite for economic development – and not as a hindrance to it, as proponents of demographic transition theory and birth control were claiming.[34] Still 20 years later, José Rela concluded in his study on the relation between population and economic growth in Angola that annual rates of population growth between 1.5 to 2 per cent were 'absolutely necessary for the economic development and industrialisation of these regions'.[35]

Third and finally, population growth was also welcomed for political reasons. The idea of an under-populated colony with plenty of 'empty space' was already present in 'white colonisation' plans in the interwar years[36] and gained even more purchase in colonial discourse after 1945 as it 'legitimised' the increasing influx of white Portuguese settlers. This nexus pervaded the work of social scientists and demographers working in Portugal's foremost colonial research institutes, the *Centro de Estudos Políticos e Sociais* of the

[31] van Beusekom, 'From Underpopulation to Overpopulation'.
[32] Ittmann, 'Where Nature Dominates Man'. See also Hodgson, 'Taking Stock'.
[33] Santos, *Perspectivas económicas*, 47 and 50.   [34] Packard, *History of Global Health*, 184.
[35] Rela, 'Angola', Issue 29 (1970), 55.
[36] See for instance Ferreira, 'Alguns aspectos', 39–42 and the overview of 'white colonisation' plans in Castelo, *Passagens para África*, 65–80.

Junta de Investigações do Ultramar and the *Instituto Superior de Ciências Sociais e Política Ultramarina* (ISCSPU), the Portuguese 'Colonial School'.[37] Óscar Soares Barata, for instance, who lectured in demography at the ISCSPU, argued that, even after the considerable population growth of the 1940s and 1950s, Angola still had one of the lowest population densities in Africa in the early 1960s and hence offered 'space for much larger human masses than those that could be expected to result from the simple natural growth from those who were already there'. Population growth being a precondition for progress and development, colonial policies should foster both the increase of the 'native' population and the immigration of Portuguese settlers, he concluded.[38] Similarly, demographer Morgado saw great potential for 'demographic absorption' in Angola. This allowed him 'not only to view the rapid increase of the autochthonous population with optimism, but also to consider the accelerating influx of European migrants as perfectly viable'.[39]

By the early 1960s, this process was already well underway. In the decades after the Second World War, Portuguese migration to the colonies, mainly Angola and Mozambique, reached unprecedented heights. The official number of white settlers in Angola almost quadrupled from 44,083 in 1940 to 172,529 in 1960 and almost doubled to approximately 324,000 in 1973. The latter increase during the 1960s and early 1970s occurred 'against the tide', at a moment when 'the wind of change' (Macmillan) had already bestowed independence upon many African states and when national liberation movements in Angola were already fighting the colonial state.[40]

Many settlers were attracted by the post-war economic boom in Angola and the prospect of greater freedom and social mobility compared to the oppressive dictatorial rule in the metropole. Yet the Portuguese state also played an active part in Angola's belated shift towards becoming a settler colony in the 1950s and 1960s. In an attempt to reroute largely clandestine Portuguese emigration from destinations in Brazil and Western Europe (particularly France) to its colonies, it promoted a series of white and racially-mixed settlement schemes, established settlement boards for coordination and eased restrictions on emigration to the colonies previously intended to limit the influx of poor and unskilled workers.[41] With the constitutional reform of 1951, the colonies were

---

[37] On these institutes, see Castelo, 'Investigação científica', 399–401.
[38] Barata, 'Aspectos', 125–6 and 131–2 (quote 132).
[39] Morgado, 'Povoamento em África', 108 (quotes).
[40] Castelo, *Passagens para África*, 215–28. See also, for Mozambique, Penvenne, 'Settling against the Tide' (first quote). For the decolonisation process in Africa, see Allman, 'Between the Present and History'.
[41] Castelo, *Passagens para África*, 107–61; Castelo, 'Reproducing Portuguese Villages'. On Portuguese emigration to other destinations, see the excellent overview in Pereira, 'Dictature salazariste'.

tied even more closely to the metropole, now officially termed 'Provinces' of a Greater Portugal. In the reconfigured ideology of the *Estado Novo*, the migration of Portuguese nationals to the colonies now served several purposes: to redistribute the metropole's surplus population in under-populated parts of the empire, thus reducing demographic pressure in mainland Portugal; to accelerate the development of these 'Provinces'; and to make them culturally more Portuguese (or 'lusotropical', as the new state ideology in favour of racial and cultural miscegenation went) and hence inalienable vis-à-vis the international community.[42]

In conclusion, demographic discourse in colonial Angola did not switch from one fear to another. From the late 1940s until the eve of decolonisation, leading colonial experts and officials welcomed the purported, yet still modest, growth in Angola's 'native' population for inducing economic development in an under-populated colony. Politically, a positive view of population growth in general and the capacity for demographic absorption in Angola allowed the regime to legitimise and support increasing numbers of Portuguese settlers. Thus, the case of Angola contributes to further nuancing the timing and geographical scope of the 'global overpopulation' discourse after the Second World War.

Partly because of the continued positive stance towards population growth, there was no sea-change in population politics after 1945 either. Although further in-depth research is needed in some domains, medical and other demographic interventions largely continued along the same lines as in the formative interwar years: they were geared towards curbing mortality and keeping fertility high, shaped by inter-imperial competition and collaboration, and international discussions about the legitimacy of Portuguese colonial rule.

In the late 1940s, the medical services thus set up a new campaign of mass chemoprophylaxis in Angola, hoping to finally eradicate sleeping sickness. This campaign bore strong resemblances to the interwar atoxylisation campaign analysed in Chapter 3, as it also relied on the screening of the whole population in HAT-endemic areas and the compulsory treatment of healthy individuals with 'preventive' drugs. The main differences consisted in the use of a new drug, pentamidine, which was also the drug of choice in similar campaigns in French, Belgian and some British colonies, and in the fact that this pentamidinisation campaign effectively almost eradicated the disease in Angola in the 1950s and 1960s, before it flared up again in the 1990s during the civil war.[43] The predominance in colonial Angola of preventative campaigns with potentially harmful drugs over ecological and spatial approaches,

---

[42] Morgado, 'Povoamento em África', 102. On lusotropicalism, see Castelo, *Modo português*; Anderson, Roque and Santos (eds.), *Luso-Tropicalism*. See also Introduction.

[43] Coghe, 'Sleeping Sickness Control', 79–89. See also Lachenal, *Médicament*.

which were only explored in a few areas, was partly due to path dependency, but also the epidemiological features of the *gambiense* form of HAT. Since the 1990s, mass screening and drug treatment has been the preferred method of the national government, the WHO and international NGOs in Angola as well.[44] In these post-colonial campaigns, however, only the infected were and are treated. The indiscriminate *preventive* use of unsafe drugs between the mid-1920s and mid-1970s was typical of how *colonial* population politics privileged population health over individual health.

From the 1950s onwards, Angola's medical services also established programmes against other endemic diseases such as malaria, leprosy, tuberculosis and venereal diseases. These were based on similar logics as the interwar AMI programme, but covered larger areas, were better funded and mostly organised in collaboration with the Institute of Tropical Medicine (IMT) in Lisbon, whose experts conducted prospective studies and coordinated field work through regular research missions and the permanent Mission for the Prospection of Endemic Diseases in Angola founded in 1950. This new role for the IMT, which had not played any role of significance in interwar Angola, coincided with its general revival after 1945. With significant increases in staff and funding, the IMT now regularly organised national and international conferences, international exchanges and research missions to all Portuguese colonies, many documented in its new journal, the *Anais do Instituto de Medicina Tropical*. In 1955, the establishment of an Institute of Medical Research in Luanda further enhanced research and training in tropical medicine in Angola.[45] Simultaneously, the colonial state also extended its efforts to improve basic healthcare, maternal and infant welfare as well as social determinants of health, such as nutrition and housing, issues that had been placed on the agenda in the interwar years.[46] However, this was the task of the regular health services, which, despite the important reforms undertaken in 1945, remained underfunded and overburdened.[47]

As in the interwar years, Angola's health programmes were not detached from those of its colonial neighbours. As Philip Havik has concluded, their general orientation and modus operandi, their expanding budgets and staff and the increasing role of metropolitan-based experts in them matched broader shifts in European colonial healthcare.[48] 'Despite being ruled by an authoritarian and corporatist regime', Havik emphasises, 'Portugal and its colonies were not impervious to international trends and debates in public health'.[49] After

---

[44] Stanghellini and Josenando, 'Situation of Sleeping Sickness'; Simarro et al., 'Human African Trypanosomiasis Control'; Aksoy et al., 'Human African Trypanosomiasis'.
[45] Havik, 'IHMT', 87–9; Havik, 'Public Health and Disease Control', 151 and 156–9.
[46] See, for instance, Nunes, 'Alimentação' and Shapiro, *Medicine*, 365–7.
[47] Havik, 'Public Health and Disease Control', 151, 156–7 and 162.   [48] Ibid., 160–73.
[49] Ibid., 171 (quote).

1945, inter-imperial exchange in health matters continued along the same lines and with some of the same tensions as in the interwar years, but it was much more strongly institutionalised. Portuguese medical experts participated in working group meetings, conferences, training programmes and disease control projects organised by (overlapping and competing) international and inter-colonial organisations of regional co-operation in Africa. These were most notably AFRO, the African Regional Bureau of the WHO created in 1951 and operating from Brazzaville since 1952, and the Commission for Technical Co-operation in Africa South of the Sahara (CCTA). Founded in 1950 to promote information exchange and mutual collaboration between its member states (Great Britain, France, Belgium, Portugal, South Africa and Southern Rhodesia) on a range of technical and social issues, the CCTA hosted regular meetings and conferences on public health issues such as nutrition and medical co-operation, and coordinated a Permanent Inter-African Bureau for Tsetse Fly and (human and animal) Trypanosomiasis (BPITT).[50] Beyond these arenas of exchange and collaboration, inter-imperial competition and international pressure were, as in the interwar years, key to Portuguese alignment. The expansion of French, British and Belgian colonial development and welfare schemes after 1945, the challenges posed by global decolonisation and, from the 1960s, the increasing pressure on Portugal from the international community and nationalist independence movements were strong incentives for Portugal to step up its health investments and emulate best practices in an attempt to defend the legitimacy of its colonial rule.

To an even greater extent than in the 1920s, Portugal's colonial health policies were also discussed on the international stage, as they got caught up in the logics of international anti-colonialism. From the late 1950s, heated debates on the merits and shortcomings of health provisions in the Portuguese colonies took place within international organisations such as the UN General Assembly and the WHO. Yet official reports by these institutions contradicted each other. In 1962, the UN Special Committee on Territories under Portuguese Administration presented a report to the General Assembly that praised the work of the IMT missions to study and combat endemic diseases, but strongly criticised the quality of basic healthcare, high infant mortality rates and malnutrition in Portugal's African colonies. WHO experts who visited the Portuguese colonies in the same year, by contrast, wrote a much more positive report.[51] While a growing number of delegates from mainly communist or newly independent countries used critical reports to denounce medical shortcomings and, for instance, appalling infant mortality rates as a

---

[50] On WHO and AFRO, and its relationship with CCTA, see Cueto, Brown and Fee, *World Health Organization*, 77–85, 92–5 and Havik, 'Regional Cooperation', 130–9.
[51] On these reports, see Shapiro, *Medicine*, 313–25.

proxy to delegitimise Portugal's colonial rule itself, Portuguese health officials and government members countered with carefully selected (and unverifiable) statistics and friendly opinions substantiating the country's continuous efforts at fulfilling its 'civilising mission'.[52]

The Portuguese colonial state did not abandon its pronatalist stance either. Unlike the United States in Puerto Rico or a host of newly (or less newly) independent states across the 'Third World' such as India, Sri Lanka, Colombia and Kenya, the Portuguese did not turn to the 'family planning' programmes of US-based organisations like the Population Council and the Ford Foundation.[53] It was not until well after independence that Angola introduced the first (largely ineffective) programme of birth control in the mid-1980s.[54] Together with other factors, the absence of such programmes contributed to continuously high fertility rates, which probably rose further between the late 1950s and the mid-1980s (like in some other sub-Saharan African countries), and to a very slow fertility decline since the 1990s, giving Angola one of the highest fertility rates in the world until today.[55] To some extent, one can argue, this is also a legacy of Portuguese population politics.

---

[52] See the extensive discussion in Ibid., 301–87.

[53] Connelly, *Fatal Misconception* and Dörnemann and Huhle, 'Population Problems'. For Colombia and Kenya, see specifically Huhle, *Bevölkerung* and Dörnemann, *Plan Your Family*.

[54] Agadjanian and Prata, 'Trends', 8

[55] Ibid., 6, 17; Nieto-Andrade et al., 'Women's Limited Choice', 75. See also https://data .worldbank.org/indicator/SP.DYN.TFRT.IN?most_recent_value_desc=true (last accessed 26 February 2021).

Bibliography

Primary Sources

Archival Sources

AEG	Archives d'État de Genève, Geneva
AGCSSp	Archives Générales de la Congrégation du Saint-Esprit, Chevilly-Larue
AHD-MNE	Arquivo Histórico-Diplomático do Ministério dos Negócios Estrangeiros, Lisbon
AHP	Arquivo Histórico Parlamentar, Lisbon
ANA	Arquivo Nacional de Angola, Luanda
ANTT	Arquivo Nacional da Torre do Tombo, Lisbon
AHU	Arquivo Histórico Ultramarino, Lisbon
AR	Algemeen Rijksarchief, Brussels
BArch	Bundesarchiv Berlin-Lichterfelde, Berlin
BMSA	Baptist Missionary Society Archives, Angus Library, Regent's Park College, Oxford
IHMT	Biblioteca do Instituto de Higiene e Medicina Tropical, Lisbon
LON	League of Nations Archives, Geneva
MAEAA	Ministère des Affaires Étrangères – Archives Africaines, Brussels
STABI	Handschriftenabteilung Staatsbibliothek zu Berlin
TNA	The National Archives, London

Periodicals

Angolan Newspapers (and the years consulted)

A Defeza de Angola (1906–7)
A Lucta de Angola (1932–7)
A Província de Angola (1923–41)
A Voz de Angola (1908–11)
Jornal do Comércio (1920–2)
Mossamedes (1933–6)
O Comércio de Angola (1925–9)
O Intransigente (1936–7)

Portugal. Órgão do nacionalismo português em Angola (1930)
Voz do Planalto (1933–5)

Law Repositories

BOA   Boletim Oficial de Angola
DG   Diário do Governo
COLP   Collecção Official da Legislação Portuguesa

Other Official Publications

Annuário Estatístico da Província de Angola (1897–1901)
Anuário Estatístico de Angola (1933–50)
Boletim Sanitário de Angola (1937–61)

Other Printed Primary Sources

'Acta da sessão, 09.11.1901', *Jornal da Sociedade das Sciências Médicas de Lisboa* 66 (1901), 405–10.
'Assistência Médica aos Indígenas – relatório do chefe da zona do Congo', *Boletim da Assistência Médica aos Indígenas e da Luta contra a Moléstia do Sono* 3.3 (1929), 295–301.
'Assistência Médica aos Indígenas – sector Congo Oeste [Summary of the Report of Dr. Pires dos Santos for the second half of 1928]', *Boletim da Assistência Médica aos Indígenas e da Luta contra a Moléstia do Sono* 3.3 (1929), 302–6.
'Condition matérielle des indigènes: discussion', in Exposition Universelle Internationale de 1900 (ed.), *Congrès International de Sociologie Coloniale tenu a Paris du 6 au 11 août 1900*, 2 vols. (Paris: Arthur Rousseau, 1901), 275–324.
'Conferência sanitária luso-belga', *Boletim da Assistência Médica aos Indígenas e da Luta contra a Moléstia do Sono* 2.12 (1928), 375–85.
Doença do somno: como evitar a infecção, com uma descriçao da glossina palpalis e illustrações d'esta e de outras moscas picantes para uso dos viajantes e residentes na Africa tropical (Lisbon: Imprensa Nacional, 1910).
'General Act of the Conference of Berlin concerning the Congo, signed at Berlin, February 26, 1885', *The American Journal of International Law* 3 (1909), 7–25.
'Maneira prática de destruir as glossinas palpalis (moscas de Gabão)', *Archivos de Hygiene e Pathologia Exoticas* 1.2 (1906), 291–2.
'Medical Work at San Salvador', *The Herald. The United Monthly Magazine of the Baptist Missionary Society, Zenana Mission and Medical Auxiliary* 28 (1914), 125–6.
'Medical Work: Report of the Medical Mission Auxiliary, 1919–1920', *The Missionary Herald of the Baptist Missionary Society, New Series*, 8 (1920), 83–6.
'Missão nova na região do Cubango', *Missões de Angola e Congo* 10.1 (1930), 7.
'Missão volante da Lunda', *Boletim da Assistência Médica aos Indígenas e da Luta contra a Moléstia do Sono* 3.3 (1929), 310–1.

'Obituary Mercier Gamble, M.D.', *The British Medical Journal* (1939), 700.

'Obras novas numa missão antiquíssima', *Anais das Franciscanas Missionárias de Maria* (1939), 181–5.

'O caso dos enfermeiros nativos: uma injustiça prestes a acabar', *Angola. Revista de Doutrina e Estudo* 14.99–104 (1945), 2–5.

'Os enfermeiros nativos e europeus perante a questão dos vencimentos', *Angola. Revista de Doutrina e Estudo* 4.1 (1936), 11.

'Os médicos da Escola da Índia', *Boletim da Assistência Médica aos Indígenas e da Luta contra a Moléstia do Sono* 3.4–6 (1929), 429–32.

Proceedings of the First International Conference on the Sleeping Sickness (London, 1907), British Parliamentary Papers, Session 1908 [Cd 3778].

'Review of "A. Correia Mendes et al., La maladie du sommeil à l'Île du Prince"', *Sleeping Sickness Bureau Bulletin* 2 (1910), 1–7.

Abbatucci, S., 'Une révolution thérapeutique dans le traitement de la maladie du sommeil', *Annales de Médecine et de Pharmacie Coloniales* 24 (1926), 83–7.

Adams, John, 'Ante-natal and Post-natal Syphilis', *Public Health* 36 (1922–23), 271.

Adam, T. B., *Africa Revisited: A Medical Deputation to the Baptist Missionary Society's Congo Field* (London, 1931).

Aguiar, José Maria d', 'La maladie du sommeil et la tsé-tsé à Novo Redondo', in Sociedade de Geografia de Lisboa (ed.), *XV Congrès International de Médecine (Lisbonne, 19–26 Avril 1906)* (Lisbon: Adolpho de Mendonça, 1906), Vol. 3, 294–300.

Albuquerque, Armando Cardoso de, 'O combate à doença do sono em Angola: métodos utilizados e resultados obtidos', *Boletim Sanitário de Angola* 11 (1953–1957), 159–214.

Almeida, Carlos de, 'Relatório do chefe da Missão do Congo referente ao triénio 1923–1924; 1924–1925; 1925–1926', *Revista Médica de Angola* 5 (1927), 22–79.

Almeida, Eurico de, *Laboratório da Zona Sanitária do Cuanza* (Luanda: Tip. Minerva, 1930).

Alto Comissariado da República em Angola and Direcção dos Serviços de Saúde e Higiene (eds.), *Diploma Legislativo do Alto Comissariado n.° 463 de 9 de Dezembro de 1926 e diversos diplomas referentes á doença do sono publicados desde 1911 a 1924* (Luanda: Imprensa Nacional, 1927).

Amaral, Antero Antunes do, *Relatório da missão médica de reconhecimento nosográfico de Catete, 1930–1931* (Lisbon: Agência Geral das Colónias, 1935).

'Natalidade e mortalidade indígenas', *Boletim Sanitário de Angola* 2 (1939), 171–85.

Athayde, Luiz de Mello e, 'O perigo do despovoamento de Angola', *Boletim da Sociedade de Geografia de Lisboa* 36.7–9 (1918), 227–43.

Azevedo, Antonio d', *Algumas palavras sobre a doença do somno: dissertação inaugural* (Lisbon, 1891).

Azevedo, João Fraga de, 'The Anglo-Portuguese Contribution to Tropical Medicine', *Anais do Instituto de Medicina Tropical* 8.1 (1951), 689–721.

Cinquenta anos de actividade do Instituto de Medicina Tropical (1902–1952) (Lisbon, 1952).

Azevedo, João Fraga de and Faria, João Pedro de, *Quatre siècles au service de la santé humaine* (Lisbon: Agência Geral do Ultramar, 1970).

Badenhorst, L. T., 'Population Distribution and Growth in Africa', *Population Studies* 5.1 (1951), 23–34.

Bagshawe, A. G., 'Review of "Bruto da Costa et al – Sleeping Sickness. A Record of Four Years' War"', *Tropical Diseases Bulletin* 7 (1916), 340–4.

Barata, Óscar Soares, 'Aspectos das condições demográficas de Angola', in Instituto Superior de Ciências Sociais e Política Ultramarina (ed.), *Angola: Curso de Extensão Universitária, 1963–64* (Lisbon: ISCSPU, 1964), 115–32.

Barradas, João Fernandes, 'Relatório da Missão à Quissama (15 December 1908)', in Governo Geral da Província de Angola, Repartição do Gabinete (ed.), *Relatórios* (Luanda: Imprensa Nacional, 1910), 3–40.

Barreto, Sant'Ana, *Sobre a doença do sono na colónia da Guiné* (Bolama: Imprensa Nacional da Guiné, 1928).

Barros, Armando A. de, 'Gonorreias nos quiocos do Moxico', *Anais do Instituto de Higiene e Medicina Tropical* 10.3,1 (1953), 793–806.

Barroso, António José Sousa de, 'Relatório da viagem ao Bembe (1884)', in Mário António Fernandes de Oliveira (ed.), *Angolana II (1883–1887): Documentação sobre Angola* (Luanda: IICA, 1971), 439–73.

Bastos, Augusto, 'Monographia de Catumbella', *Boletim da Sociedade de Geografia de Lisboa* 28–30 (1910–12), passim.

Bauvallet, M., 'Résultats d'une enquête démographique dans le Bas-Dahomey', *Bulletin de la Société de Pathologie Exotique* 24 (1931), 604–8.

Bettencourt, Annibal, 'Doença do somno: conferência feita no Real Instituto Bacteriológico Câmara Pestana, em 7 de Agosto de 1902', *Revista Portuguesa de Medicina e Cirurgia Práticas* 6.139–144 (1902), 193–240, 241–72, 286–303, 323–8, 344–52 and 374–82.

'A doença do somno', *A Medicina Contemporânea* 21 (1903), 93–5.

Bettencourt, Annibal, Kopke, Ayres, Rezende, Gomes de and Mendes, Annibal Correia, *La Maladie du sommeil: rapport présenté au Ministère de la Marine et des Colonies par la Mission envoyée en Afrique Occidentale Portugaise* (Lisbon: Imprimerie de Libanio da Silva, 1903).

'On the Etiology of Sleeping Sickness', *British Medical Journal* 2207 (1903), 908–10.

Blanchard, Maurice, 'La formation des auxiliaires médicaux dans les colonies françaises: l'école de médecine de l'AOF à Dakar', *Bulletin de l'Office International d'Hygiène Publique* 27.8 (1935), 1575–92.

Bolzman, Lara, 'The Advent of Child Rights on the International Scene and the Role of the Save the Children International Union, 1920–1945', *Refugee Survey Quarterly* 27.4 (2008), 27–37.

Bombarda, Miguel, 'Doença do sono em Angola', *A Medicina Contemporânea* 18 (1900), 413–4.

'Doença de somno', *A Medicina Contemporânea* 18 (1900), 421–2.

'Criação de uma Escola de Medicina Colonial', *Jornal da Sociedade das Sciências Médicas de Lisboa* 66 (1901), 329–37.

Braga, A. Rodrigues, 'L'Afrique orientale portugaise et la maladie du sommeil', *Archivos de Hygiene e Pathologia Exoticas* 2 (1909), 192–4.

Brandão, Paes, 'Diário da marcha do chefe do Conselho do Libollo a região da Quibala', *Portugal em África* 11 (1904), 76–9, 138–40, 223–7, 287–91, 349–55, 406–12.

Brásio, António, 'A missionação pela medicina', *Acção Médica* 12.45–8 (1948), 462–7.

(ed.), *Spiritana Monumenta Historica – Series Africana I, Angola, Vol. 5 (1904–1967)* (Pittsburgh/Leuven: Duquesne University Press/Nauwelaerts, 1971).

Brito, Eduino, 'Aspectos demográficos dos Balantas e Brames do Território de Bula', *Boletim Cultural da Guiné Portuguesa* 8.31 (1953), 417–70.

Broden, Alphonse and Rodhain, Jerôme, 'L'Atoxyl dans le traitement de la trypanose humaine', *Annales de la Société Belge de Médecine Tropicale* 1 (1921), 179–226.

Browne, Stanley George, *B.M.S. Medical Work in Congo* (London: Baptist Missionary Society, [195–]).

Brown-Séquard, Charles-Édouard, 'Des effets produits chez l'homme par des injections sous-cutanées d'un liquide retiré des testicules frais de cobaye et de chien', *Comptes Rendus des Séances de la Société de Biologie* 41 (1889), 415–22.

Bruce, David et al., 'Discussion on Trypanosomiasis', *The British Medical Journal* 2277 (1904), 367–79.

Brumpt, Émile and Joyeux, Charles, *Un Voyage médical dans l'Afrique du Sud* (Paris: Libraires de l'Académie de Médecine, 1923).

Cadbury, William, *Labour in Portuguese West Africa*, 2nd edn. (London: Routledge, 1910).

Camoesas, João, 'Sobre a organização da Assistência Médica Indígena', *Boletim da Assistência Médica aos Indígenas e da Luta contra a Moléstia do Sono* 3.2 (1929), 140–55.

Carvalho, Carlos A. da Costa, *La population noire de l'Angola* (Lisbon: Centro de Estudos Demográficos, INE, 1979).

Carvalho, Paulo de, Kajibanga, Víctor and Heimer, Franz-Wilhelm, 'Angola', in Damtew Teferra and Philip G. Altbach (eds.), *African Higher Education: An International Reference Handbook* (Bloomington: Indiana University Press, 2003), 162–75.

Casement, Consul, *Report on the Trade and Commerce of Angola for the Years 1897 and 1898* (London: HMSO, 1899).

Castellani, Aldo, 'Etiology of Sleeping Sickness', *The British Medical Journal* 2202 (1903), 617–8.

'Trypanosoma in Sleeping Sickness', *The British Medical Journal* 2212 (1903), 1218.

Castro, Ferreira de, 'Cura(?) da doença do somno pelo atoxyl', *A Medicina Moderna* 14 (1907), 123–5.

Castro, J. F. Sampaio e, 'Da preparação e aperfeiçoamento do pessoal técnico auxiliar dos serviços de saúde de Angola', *Anais do Instituto de Medicina Tropical* 10.4,1 (1953), 2871–9.

Cazanove, 'Essai de démographie des colonies françaises', *Bulletin de l'Office International d'Hygiène Publique* 22.8 (1930), supplément.

Chesneau, Pierre, 'Natalité et mortalité infantile en Nord-Annam', *Annales de Médecine et de Pharmacie Coloniales* 35 (1937), 688–743.

Chesterman, Clement, *Manuel du dispensaire africain* (London: Christian Literature Society, 1932).

Clapier, P., 'Enquête démographique et état actuel de la trypanosomiase au pays Bangala (Afrique Equatoriale Française)', *Bulletin de la Société de Pathologie Exotique* 13 (1920), 830–47.

Coale, Ansley J. and Lorimer, Frank, 'Summary of Estimates of Fertility and Mortality', in William Brass (ed.), *The Demography of Tropical Africa* (Princeton: Princeton University Press, 1968), 151–67.

Collaço, Luiz Fernandes, 'Relatório do Serviço de Saúde em Dondo', in *Estatistica Medica dos Hospitaes das Provincias Ultramarinas (1877)* (Lisbon: Imprensa Nacional, 1883), 83–101.

Colónia de Angola, *Regulamento do recenseamento e cobrança do imposto indígena, aprovado por Diploma Legislativo 237 (26 de Maio de 1931)* (Luanda: Imprensa Nacional, 1931–2).

Conceição, Lourenço Mendes da, 'A obra das Irmãs de San-José de Cluny em Angola', *Angola. Revista de Doutrina e Estudo* 4.17 (1937), 9–17.

Cook, Albert, 'Sleeping Sickness in Uganda', *Journal of Tropical Medicine* 5 (1902), 49–50.

Corre, Armand, 'Contribution a l'étude de la maladie du sommeil (hypnose)', *Gazette Médicale de Paris* 5.46 (1876), 545–7, 563.

'Recherches sur la maladie du sommeil', *Archives de Médecine Navale* 27 (1877), 292–356.

Correia, Alberto Carlos Germano da Silva, 'A doença do sono em Angola', *Revista Médica de Angola* 4.4 (1923), 157–76.

'A variola em Angola', *Revista Médica de Angola* 4.3 (1923), 232–4; 423–60.

'O clima, a nosografia e o saneamento de Loanda', *Revista Médica de Angola* 4.2 (1923), 377–482.

'Os processos práticos de hospitalização dos indígenas e a sua assistência médica em Angola', *Revista Médica de Angola* 4.2 (1923), 179–200.

'Os Luso-descendentes de Angola: contribuição para o seu estudo antropológico', in *III Congresso Colonial Nacional de 8 a 15 de Maio de 1930: Actas das Sessões e Teses* (Lisbon: Tip. Carmona, 1934), [1–57].

Correia, Joaquim Alves, *Civilizando Angola e Congo: os missionários do Espírito Santo no padroado espiritual português* (Braga: Tipografia Sousa Cruz, 1922).

Costa, Alfredo Gomes da, 'Relatório anual do chefe da zona sanitária do Cuanza Norte (1927)', *Revista Médica de Angola* 6 (1928), 21–98.

'Assistência Médica ao Indígena e combate à doença do sono', in Fernando Mouta (ed.), *Generalidades sobre Angola* (Luanda: Imprensa Nacional, 1935), 59–64.

Costa, Bernardo Francisco Bruto da, 'Estudos estatísticos sobre a mortalidade geral e sobre a doença do sono na Ilha do Príncipe desde 1908 até Julho de 1911', *Archivos de Hygiene e Pathologia Exoticas* 4 (1913), 63–76.

Sleeping Sickness in the Island of Príncipe (London: Baillière, Tindall & Cox, 1913).

Vinte e três anos ao serviço do país no combate às doenças em África (Lisbon: Livraria Portugalia, 1939).

Costa, Bernardo Francisco Bruto da, Sant'Anna, José Firmino, Santos, A. Correia dos and Alvares, M. G. Araújo de, *Sleeping Sickness: A Record of Four Years' War against it in Principe, Portuguese West Africa* (London: Baillière, Tindall & Cox, 1916).

Costa, Eduardo Augusto Ferreira da, *Estudo sobre a administração civil das nossas possessões africanas: memoria apresentada ao Congresso Colonial Nacional (1901)* (Lisbon: Imprensa Nacional, 1903).

Costa, Francisco Felisberto Dias, *Relatorio do Ministro e Secretario d'Estado dos Negocios da Marinha e Ultramar* (Lisbon: Imprensa Nacional, 1898).

Costa, Pedro Joaquim Peregrino da, 'Médicos da Escola de Goa no Quadro de Saúde das Colónias (1853 a 1942)', *Boletim do Instituto Vasco da Gama* 57 (1943), 1–62 and 58 (1943), 1–88.

Costa-Sacadura, Sebastião Cabral da, *Despopulação em Portugal* (Lisbon: Imprensa Africana, 1923).

As maternidades e a família (Lisbon: Imprensa Lucas, 1939).

Couceiro, Paiva, *Angola: dois anos de governo, Junho de 1907–Julho de 1909: história e comentários*, 2nd edn. (Lisbon: Edições Gama, 1948).

Curto, António Duarte Ramada, 'Relatório do Chefe do Serviço de Saúde de Angola', in Ministerio dos Negocios da Marinha e Ultramar (ed.), *Estatistica Medica dos Hospitaes das Provincias Ultramarinas (1887)* (Lisbon: Imprensa Nacional, 1890), 319–48.

Cushman, Mary Floyd, *Missionary Doctor: The Story of Twenty Years in Africa* (New York: Harper & Brothers, 1944).

Daniels, C. -W, 'Cases of Trypanosomiasis in England, mainly at the London School of Tropical Medicine', *Journal of the London School of Tropical Medicine 1* (1911–1912), 67–80.

Dias, Gastão Sousa, 'A fronteira do sul de Angola', *Boletim da Agência Geral das Colónias* 4.31 (1928), 15–25.

Diniz, José de Oliveira Ferreira, *Negócios Indígenas: relatório do ano 1913* (Luanda: Imprensa Nacional de Angola, 1914).

Negocios Indígenas: relatório do ano 1916 (Lisbon: Tipografia do Anuário Comercial, 1917).

Populações indígenas de Angola (Coimbra: Imprensa da Universidade, 1918).

A missão civilisadora do estado em Angola (Lisbon: Centro Tipografico Colonial, 1926).

'Contribuïção para o estudo da demografia indígena de Angola', *Boletim da Agência Geral das Colónias* 6.58 (1930), 32–53.

Distrito do Mochico, 'Relatório dos serviços de saúde (1927)', *Boletim da Assistência Médica aos Indígenas e da Luta contra a Moléstia do Sono* 2.12 (1928), 339–42.

Durand, John D., 'Adequacy of Existing Census Statistics for Basic Demographic Research', *Population Studies* 4.2 (1950), 179–99.

Estermann, Carlos, 'Conferência na Sociedade de Geografia no dia 19 de Janeiro de 1935', *Missões de Angola e Congo* 15 (1935), 38–40, 72–4 and 104–7.

Exposition Universelle Internationale de 1900, *Congrès International de Sociologie Coloniale: procès-verbaux sommaires* (Paris: Imprimerie Nationale, 1900).

Faria, José Alberto de, *Administração sanitária* (Lisbon: Imprensa Nacional, 1934).

Ferreira, António Vicente, *A situação de Angola* (Luanda: Imprensa Nacional, 1927).

'Alguns aspectos da política indígena de Angola [1934]', in António Vicente Ferreira (ed.), *Estudos ultramarinos, Vol. III* (Lisbon: Agência Geral das Colónias, 1954), 35–50.

'Colonização étnica da África Portuguesa [1944]', in António Vicente Ferreira (ed.), *Estudos ultramarinos, Vol. IV* (Lisbon: Agência Geral das Colónias, 1955), 149–264.

Ferreira, J. Bettencourt, 'A doença do somno', *Jornal da Sociedade das Sciências Médicas de Lisboa* 65 (1901), 301–15.

Galvão, Henrique, *Huíla: relatório de governo* (Famalicão: Tipografia Minerva, 1929).

Informação económica sôbre Angola (Lisbon, 1933).

Outras terras, outras gentes: viagens na África Portuguesa: 25.000 km em Angola, 2 vols. (Lisbon: Livraria Popular de Francisco Franco, 1941–2).

Por Angola: quatro anos de actividade parlamentar (Lisbon: Edição do Autor, 1949).

Santa Maria: My Crusade for Portugal (Cleveland/New York: The World Publishing Company, 1961).

Galvão, Henrique and Selvagem, Carlos, *Império ultramarino português: monografia do império, Vol. III: Angola* (Lisbon: Empresa Nacional de Publicidade, 1952).

Gama, Eduardo Diniz da, 'Missão volante de assistência aos indígenas do planalto de Benguela', *Boletim da Assistência Médica aos Indígenas e da Luta contra a Moléstia do Sono* 2.1–8 (1928), 59–66.

'Um ano de chefia no sector Ambaca-Encoje', *Boletim da Assistência Médica aos Indígenas e da Luta contra a Moléstia do Sono* 3.7–12 (1929), 536–41.

Gamble, Mercier, 'An English Translation of Questions asked by General Faria Leal, Administrator of San Salvador do Congo, of Dr. Gamble re Sleeping Sickness', *Journal of Tropical Medicine and Hygiene* 15 (1912), 62–3.

'Sleeping Sickness in the Portuguese Congo: Apparent Cures', *Journal of Tropical Medicine and Hygiene* 16 (1913), 81–4.

'A List of Blood-Sucking Arthropods from the Lower Congo, with a Vocabulary', *Journal of Tropical Medicine and Hygiene* 17 (1914), 148–50.

Garcia, Francisco da Silva, *O vinho do Porto: história, composição, analyse chimica, applicações therapeuticas, falsificações e inconvenientes do seu abuso* (Porto: Imprensa Nacional, 1891).

'Contribuição para o tratamento da doença do somno', *A Medicina Contemporânea* 22 (1904), 271–3.

'Apontamentos sobre a etiologia e tratamento da doença do somno', *A Medicina Moderna* 12 (1905), 288–90.

Garrett, António de Almeida, *Como organizar a luta contra a mortalidade infantil* (Lisbon: Imprensa Nacional, 1928).

Gemmil, William, 'The Growing Reservoir of Native Labour for the Mines', *Optima* 2 (1952), 15–9.

Giraúl, Visconde de, *Ideas geraes sobre a colonização europeia da província de Angola: memória apresentada ao 1. Congresso Colonial Nacional* (Lisbon: Imprensa Nacional, 1901).

'A prophylaxia do paludismo nas nossas colonias', *Revista Portuguesa de Medicina e Cirurgia Práticas* 6.127 (1902), 193–207.

Gleim, Otto, 'Berichte über die Schlafkrankheit der Neger im Kongogebiete', *Archiv für Schiffs- und Tropenhygiene* 4.11 (1900), 358–63.

Gomes, Manuel Gonzaga, 'Reconhecimentos sanitários nas margens dos grandes rios', *Boletim da Assistência Médica aos Indígenas e da Luta contra a Moléstia do Sono* 3.4–6 (1929), 443–56.

Governo Geral de Angola, *Regulamento do recenseamento e cobrança do imposto indígena, aprovado por portaria provincial 30-A de 22 de Janeiro de 1920* (Luanda: Imprensa Nacional, 1920).

Estatutos da Instituição de Assistência às Crianças Indígenas (IACI) (Luanda: Imprensa Nacional, 1936).

Harris, John, *Dawn in Darkest Africa* (London: Smith, Elder & Co, 1912).

Heckenroth, F., Leger, Marcel and Nogue, Maurice, 'L'Afrique Occidentale Française au congrès de médecine tropicale de Saint Paul de Loanda (Juillet 1923)', *Annales de Médecine et de Pharmacie Coloniales* 22 (1924), 5–76.

Hegh, Émile, *Notice sur les glossines ou tsétsés* (London: Hutchinson, 1915).

Heisel, Donald, '*The Indigenous Populations of the Portuguese African Territories*', Unpublished PhD thesis, University of Wisconsin, 1966.

'The Demography of the Portuguese Territories: Angola, Mozambique and Portuguese Guinea', in William Brass (ed.), *The Demography of Tropical Africa* (Princeton: Princeton University Press, 1968), 440–65.

J. S. A., 'Hygiene colonial – doença do somno', *Portugal em África* 10 (1903), 687–91.

Jojot, Ch., 'Le secteur de la prophylaxie de la maladie du sommeil du Haut-Nyong (Cameroun)', *Annales de Médecine et de Pharmacie Coloniales* 19 (1921), 423–42.

Jorge, Ricardo, 'A propósito de Pasteur: crítica da sanidade e da mentalidade portuguesas', in *Sermões dum leigo: discursos e alocuções*, 2nd ed. (Lisbon: Instituto de Alta Cultura, 1974), 181–230.

Junior, Augusto Antonio dos Santos, *Acclimação dos Portuguezes na Provincia de Angola: dissertação inaugural apresentada e defendida perante a Escola Medico-Cirurgica do Porto* (Porto: Typographia do Commercio do Porto, 1883).

Junior, João Cardoso, *Subsídios para a matéria médica e therapeutica das possessões ultramarinas portuguezas*, 2 vols. (Lisbon: Typographia da Academia Real das Sciencias, 1902–5).

Junqueira, Daniel, 'Pelo sul de Angola', *Missões de Angola e Congo* 20 (1940), 5–9, 41–4, 73–7 and 103–8.

Junqueira, Manuel, *As missões católicas e a assistência social aos nossos irmãos africanos* (Coimbra: Livraria Académica, 1943).

Kingsley, Mary, *West African Studies* (London: Macmillan, 1899).

Koch, Robert, 'Schlussbericht über die Tätigkeit der deutschen Expedition zur Erforschung der Schlafkrankheit', *Deutsche Medizinische Wochenschrift* 33.46 (1907), 1889–95.

Kopke, Ayres, 'Escola portugueza de medicina tropical', *A Medicina Contemporânea* 20 (1902), 278–80.

'Investigações sobre a doença do somno', *Archivos de Hygiene e Pathologia Exoticas* 1.1 (1905), 1–65.

'Trypanosomiasis humaine: rapport présenté à la XVII section do XV Congrès International de Médecine, à Lisbonne', *Archivos de Hygiene e Pathologia Exoticas* 1.2 (1906), 159–88.

'Trypanosomiasis humaine', in Sociedade de Geografia de Lisboa (ed.), *XV Congrès International de Médecine (Lisbonne, 19–26 Avril 1906)* (Lisbon: Adolpho de Mendonça, 1906), Vol. 17, 233–59.

'Traitement de la maladie du sommeil: rapport présenté au XIVe Congrès International d'Hygiène et Démographie, Berlin, Septembre 1907', *Archivos de Hygiene e Pathologia Exoticas* 1.3 (1907), 299–347.

'Tratamento da doença do somno pelo atoxyl, verde brilhante e diamido-diphenylurea+ACH', *Jornal da Sociedade das Sciências Médicas de Lisboa* (1907), 3–11.

'Traitement de la trypanosomiase humaine: rapport présenté au XVIe Congrès International de Médecine (à Budapest)', *Archivos de Hygiene e Pathologia Exoticas* 2 (1909), 219–70.

'Trypanosomiase gambiense: sur la résistance du trypanosome gambiense à l'atoxyl et le traitement de la trypanosomiase humaine par l'acide p aminophényl-stibinique', *A Medicina Contemporânea* 27 (1909), 232–4.

'Sobre a doença do somno: progressos na etiologia, tratamento e prophylaxia', *A Medicina Contemporânea* 29 (1911), 225–30.

'Traitement de quelques cas de trypanosomiase humaine par le salvarsan et le neosalvarsan', *A Medicina Contemporânea* 31 (1913), 289–92.

'Escola de Medicina Tropical de Hamburgo', *A Medicina Contemporânea* 32 (1914), 141–5.

Estudo da doença do sono: memória premiada no concurso de 1915 e apresentada sob a divisa Therapia Sterilisans Magna pelo autor à Comissão de Protecção aos Indígenas das Colónias Portuguesas (Lisbon: Typografia da Cooperativa Militar, 1916).

'Ensaios com o galil de Beurmann, Mouneyrat e Tanon, no tratamento da doença do somno', *Portugal Médico* 3 (1917), 23–7.

'Les troubles oculaires dans la maladie du sommeil', *Bulletin de la Société de Pathologie Exotique* 15 (1922), 139–46.

'Tratamento da doença do sono', *Revista Médica de Angola* 4.4 (1923), 49–61.

'A Conferência Internacional sôbre a doença do sôno, Maio de 1925: relatório apresentado a Sua Ex.a o Ministro das Colónias pelo delegado do governo português', *Archivos de Hygiene e Pathologia Exoticas* 7 (1925), 501–66.

'Estudos executados pela missão médica em Moçambique', *Jornal da Sociedade das Sciências Médicas de Lisboa* 92 (1928), 233–73.

Kuczynski, Robert René, *Colonial Population* (Oxford: Oxford University Press, 1937).

The Cameroons and Togoland: A Demographic Study (London: Oxford University Press, 1939).

Külz, Ludwig, 'Zur Pathologie des Hinterlandes von Südkamerun', *Archiv für Schiffs- und Tropenhygiene* 14 (1910), Beiheft, 1–35.

Lapa, Albino, *Conselheiro Ramada Curto* (Lisbon: Agência Geral das Colónias, 1940).

Lapa, J. Pereira and Sousa, Joaquim Morais de, *Serviço de defesa contra a doença do sono nos distritos de Tete e Quelimane (1913)* (Lourenço Marques: Imprensa Nacional, 1915).

Laveran, A. and Mesnil, F., *Trypanosomes et trypanosomiases*, 2nd edn. (Paris: Masson, 1912).

Le Dantec, A., 'L'hygiène sociale à Dakar', *Revista Médica de Angola* 4.2 (1923), 309–48.

Leal, Francisco Cunha, *Oliveira Salazar, Filomeno da Câmara e o Império Colonial Português* (Edição Própria: Lisbon, 1930).

Leal, José Heliodoro de Faria, 'Memórias d'África', *Boletim da Sociedade de Geografia de Lisboa* 32 (1914), 299–330, 343–62, 383–410 and 33 (1915), 15–30, 64–79, 113–28, 162–73, 214–31 and 357–80.

League of Nations Health Organisation (ed.), *Report of the Second International Conference on Sleeping-Sickness (Paris, 5–7 Nov. 1928) (= C.H. 743)* (Geneva, 1928).

Lefrou, G., *Le Noir d'Afrique: anthropo-biologie et raciologie* (Paris: Payot, 1943).
Leitão, Alberto de Souza Maia, *Relatório da visita sanitaria aos concelhos da léste de Loanda mais victimados pela doença do somno* (Porto: Typ. A Vapor, 1901).
'A prophylaxia da doença do somno em Angola', *A Medicina Moderna* 14 (1907), 165–7.
Serviço de saúde colonial: sua reforma (Porto: Imprensa Moderna, 1910).
Lemos, Alberto, 'Introdução ao primeiro censo geral da população de Angola', in Repartição de Estatística Geral da Colónia de Angola (ed.), *Censo geral da população, 1940*, 12 vols. (Luanda: Imprensa Nacional, 1941–7), Vol. I, 1–76.
'Censo da população de 1950: nota introdutória', in Repartição Técnica de Estatística Geral da Província de Angola (ed.), *II Recenseamento geral da população, 1950*, 5 vols. (Luanda: Imprensa Nacional, 1953–6), Vol. 1, 7–65.
Lencastre, António de, 'Ensino da medicina colonial', *Archivos de Hygiene e Pathologia Exoticas* 1.1 (1905), i–xiii.
Letonturier, Charles, Tanon, Louis and Jamot, Eugène, 'La maladie du sommeil au Cameroun et sa prophylaxie', *Revista Médica de Angola* 4.4 (1923), 141–7.
Levy, Izaac, 'Plano de assistência à criança indígena e à mulher grávida', *Boletim Sanitário de Angola* (1943), 169–75.
Lima, José Joaquim Lopes de, *De Angola e Benguella e suas dependencias* (Lisbon: Imprensa Nacional, 1846).
Liverpool School of Tropical Medicine, *Historical Record, 1898–1920* (Liverpool: Liverpool University Press, 1920).
Lopes, Alfredo Luiz, 'Chronica – doença do somno', *Revista Portuguesa de Medicina e Cirurgia Práticas* 6.121 (1901), 1–4.
Lorimer, Frank, 'Introduction', in William Brass (ed.), *The Demography of Tropical Africa* (Princeton: Princeton University Press, 1968), 3–11.
Lugard, Frederick, *The Dual Mandate in British Tropical Africa* (Edinburgh: Blackwood, 1922).
Machado [de Faria e Maia], Carlos Roma, 'Zonas colonisáveis, estudo de adaptação de europeus', in *II Congresso Colonial Nacional de 6 a 10 de Maio de 1924: Teses e Actas das Sessões* (Lisbon, 1924).
'O trabalho dos indígenas portugueses nas colónias visinhas: seu engajamento e emigração clandestinos – modos de os evitar – seu controle oficial', in *III Congresso Colonial Nacional de 8 a 15 de Maio de 1930: Actas das Sessões e Teses* (Lisbon: Tip. Carmona, 1934).
Na fronteira sul de Angola (Lisbon, 1941).
Machado, Ernesto, *No sul de Angola* (Lisbon: Agência Geral do Ultramar, 1956).
Maio, Padre Augusto Teixeira, 'As missões protestantes em Angola e os médicos católicos portugueses', *Acção Médica* 12 (1948), 458–61.
Maldonado, Angelo de Bulhões, 'Doença do somno', *A Medicina Contemporânea* 19 (1901), 96–7.
Manson, Patrick, 'A Clinical Lecture on Sleeping Sickness', *Journal of Tropical Medicine* 1 (1898), 121–8.
Tropical Diseases: A Manual of the Diseases of Warm Climates (New York: William Wood, 1898).
Tropical Diseases: A Manual of the Diseases of Warm Climates, 3rd edn. (London: Cassell, 1903).

et al., 'Discussion on Trypanosomiasis', *The British Medical Journal* 2229 (1903), 645–54.

Martin, Gustave, Leboeuf, Alexis and Roubaud, Émile, *Rapport de la mission d'études de la maladie du sommeil au Congo français, 1906–1908* (Paris: Masson, 1909).

Martin, Louis and Darré, Henri, 'Résultats éloignés du traitement dans la trypanosomiase humaine', *Bulletin de la Société de Pathologie Exotique* 3 (1910), 333–41.

Martins, António Rita, 'A doença do sono: oração de sapiência', *Anuário da Escola Superior Colonial* 19–20 (1938–9), 33–63.

Martins, Manuel Eduardo, 'Relatório da inspecção extraordinária à administração do Hospital Central de Luanda, 31 December 1929', *BOA Série II* (1930), 168–84.

Matos, José Norton de, *Regulamento das circunscrições administrativas da Província de Angola* (Luanda: Imprensa Nacional de Angola, 1913).

A Província de Angola (Porto: Edição de Maranus, 1926).

'Síntese das medidas aconselháveis para impulsionar o povoamento indígena de Angola', in Comissão Executiva dos Centenários (ed.), *Memórias e comunicações apresentadas ao Congresso Colonial (IX Congresso)* (Lisbon, 1940), 479–525.

Memórias e trabalhos da minha vida, 4 vols. (Lisbon: Ed. Marítimo-Colonial, 1944–6).

McCowen, 'A Note on Sleeping Sickness in Principe Island and Angola, West Coast of Africa', *Proceedings of the Royal Society of Medicine* 6 (Section of Epidemiology and State Medicine) (1913), 191–4.

Medical Mission Auxiliary of the Baptist Missionary Society, *The Challenge of Pain: Report for the Year Ended March 31st, 1925* (London: Baptist Missionary Society [1925]).

Melo, A. Brandão de, *Angola: monographie historique, géographique et économique de la colonie destinée à l'Exposition Coloniale Internationale de Paris de 1931* (Luanda: Imprimerie Nationale, 1931).

Mendes, Annibal Correia, 'Glossinas de Angola', *Archivos de Hygiene e Pathologia Exoticas* 1.1 (1905), 66–71.

'Subsídio para a prophylaxia da doença do somno em Angola: distribuição geographica das glossinas no districto de Loanda', *Archivos de Hygiene e Pathologia Exoticas* 1.3 (1907), 392–401.

Mendes, Annibal Correia, Monteiro, Alfredo Silva, Mora, António Damas and Costa, Bernardo Francisco Bruto da, 'Relatório preliminar da missão de estudo da doença do somno na Ilha do Príncipe (1908)', *Archivos de Hygiene e Pathologia Exoticas* 2.1 (1909), 1–45.

'La maladie du sommeil à L'Île du Prince: rapport présenté au Ministère de la Marine et des Colonies', *Archivos de Hygiene e Pathologia Exoticas* 2 (1909), 271–350.

Mense, Carl, *Rapport sur l'état sanitaire de Léopoldville de novembre 1885 à mars 1887* (Brussels: Vanderauwera, 1890).

'Bemerkungen und Beobachtungen über die Schlafsucht der Neger', *Archiv für Schiffs- und Tropenhygiene* 4 (1900), 364–8.

'Deutscher Kolonialkongress 1902', *Archiv für Schiffs- und Tropenhygiene* 7 (1903), 53–6.

'Die menschliche Trypanosomenkrankheit und afrikanische Schlafkrankheit', in Carl Mense (ed.), *Handbuch der Tropenkrankheiten*, vol. 3 (Leipzig: Barth, 1906), 617–67.

(ed.), *Handbuch der Tropenkrankheiten*, 3 vols. (Leipzig: Barth, 1906).

Millman, Edith R. and Millman, William, *Manual a arte de ser mãe: traduzido do inglês por Alfredo Rezende* (London: Carey Press, 1932).

Ministério da Marinha e Ultramar (ed.), *Doença do somno: relatorios enviados ao Ministerio da Marinha pela missão scientifica nomeada por portaria de 21 de Fevereiro de 1901* (Lisbon: Imprensa de Libanio da Silva, 1901).

Ministério do Ultramar – Junta de Investigações do Ultramar (ed.), *Contribuição para o estudo da fertilidade da mulher indígena no Ultramar português* (Lisbon: Junta de Investigações do Ultramar, 1957).

Monteiro, Joachim John, *Angola and the River Congo*, 2 vols. (London: Macmillan, 1875).

Moorshead, Robert Fletcher, *The Appeal of Medical Missions* (New York: Revell, 1913).

The Way of the Doctor: A Study in Medical Missions (London: Carey Press, 1926).

Heal the Sick: The Story of the Medical Mission Auxiliary of the Baptist Missionary Society (London: Carey Press, 1929).

Mora, António Damas, *O serviço de saúde em Timor nos anos de 1914, 1915 e 1916: relatório* (Dili: Imprensa Nacional de Timor, 1917).

'La raison d'être des Congrès de Médecine dans l'Ouest Africain: Allocution', *Revista Médica de Angola* 4.1 (1923), 47–59.

'Les organisations sanitaires en général: organisation sanitaire de l'Angola', *Revista Médica de Angola* 4.1 (1923), 173–83.

'Assistência Médica ao Indígena em África', *A Medicina Contemporânea* 43 (1926), 353–7 and 393–6.

'A Assistência Médica aos Indígenas e a luta contra a propagação da moléstia do sono, em 1927', *Boletim Mensal da Luta contra a Propagação da Moléstia do Sono e da Assistência Médica ao Indígena* 1 (1927), 1–13.

'Dos serviços de assistência aos indígenas durante o primeiro semestre de 1928', *Boletim da Assistência Médica aos Indígenas e da Luta contra a Moléstia do Sono* 2.1–8 (1928), 23–35.

'L'Assistance Médicale Indigène', *Bruxelles-Médical* 8.41 (1928), 1328–37.

'Les services de l'Assistance Médicale Indigène en Angola, pendant 1927', *Revista Médica de Angola* 6 (1928), 9–17.

'Notas sobre um estatuto de "aldeias indigenas"', *Boletim da Assistência Médica aos Indígenas e da Luta contra a Moléstia do Sono* 2.11 (1928), 235–9.

'Os serviços de saúde em Angola e a obra da Assistência Médica aos Indígenas', *Boletim da Assistência Médica aos Indígenas e da Luta contra a Moléstia do Sono* 2.9 (1928), 87–94.

A luta contra a moléstia do sono em Angola (1921–1934) (Luanda, 1934).

'O estado actual da Assistência Médica aos Indígenas na colónia de Angola e outras colónias estrangeiras do grupo da África inter-tropical', in *III Congresso Colonial Nacional de 8 a 15 de Maio de 1930: Actas das Sessões e Teses* (Lisbon: Tip. Carmona, 1934).

'Prefácio', in Bruno de Mesquita, *Considerações sobre a profilaxia da doença do sono em Angola (Tese de Licenciatura, Universidade de Coimbra)* (1934), 13–29.

Publicações médicas e legislação sanitária (Luanda, 1934).

'A mortalidade infantil de brancos e indígenas nas Colónias de Angola e Moçambique, suas causas principais e remédios possíveis: métodos para a organização de estatística da mortalidade infantil', in Comissão Executiva dos Centenários (ed.), *Memórias e comunicações apresentadas ao Congresso Colonial (IX Congresso)* (Lisbon, 1940), 557–625.

Morgado, Nuno Alves, 'Estimativas da populacão das colónias portuguesas para os períodos intercensuários', *Revista do Centro de Estudos Demográficos* 6 (1949), 79–91.

'A demografia do Ultramar português', *Revista do Centro de Estudos Demográficos* 9 (1954–5), 71–283.

'Da razão dos sexos e da distribuição etária nos censos da população de Cabo Verde, Angola (não civilizada) e Moçambique (não civilizada)', *Revista do Centro de Estudos Demográficos* 10 (1956–7), 201–14.

Aspectos da evolução demográfica da população da antiga província do Congo (1949–1956) (Lisbon: CEPS, 1959).

'O crescimento da população do distrito do Congo', *Boletim Geral do Ultramar* 413–14 (1959), 355–60.

'Povoamento em África', *Estudos Ultramarinos* 2 (1960), 101–18.

Morna, Álvaro de Freitas, *Angola: um ano no Governo Geral (1942–1943)*, Vol. 1 (Lisbon: Livraria Popular de Francisco Franco, 1944).

Mouchet, René, 'La natalité et la mortalité infantile dans la Province Orientale', *Annales de la Société Belge de Médecine Tropicale* 6 (1926), 165–74.

Muralha, Pedro, *Terras de África: S. Tomé e Angola* (Lisbon: Publicitas, 1925).

Nascimento, José Pereira do, *O districto de Mossamedes: primeira parte – colonisação europeia* (Lisbon: Typographia de Jornal, 1892).

Nascimento, José Pereira do and Mattos, A. Alexandre de, *A colonização de Angola* (Lisbon: Mendonça, 1912).

Negreiros, António Lobo de Almada, *Angola: brève notice* (Paris: Imprimerie Alcan-Lévy, 1901).

Neves, José da Silva, 'Relatório sobre o serviço de saúde no distrito do Congo, durante o ano de 1919', *Revista Médica de Angola* 1 (1921), 167–80.

Neves, José da Silva and Sousa, Jacinto de, 'Assistência Médica aos Indígenas: relatório apresentado a Sua Ex.a o Ministro das Colónias quando da sua visita a Angola', *Boletim da Assistência Médica aos Indígenas e da Luta contra a Moléstia do Sono* 3.4–6 (1929), 433–42.

Nevinson, Henry W., *A Modern Slavery* (New York: Schocken, 1906).

Nightingale, Consul, *Report on the Trade and Commerce of Angola for the Year 1899* (London: HMSO, 1901).

Nogueira, António Francisco, *A raça negra sob o ponto de vista da civilização da África: usos e costumes de alguns povos gentílicos do interior de Mossamedes e as colónias portuguezas* (Lisbon: Tipografia Nova Minerva, 1880).

Noronha, António da P., 'Algumas plantas medicinais do Zaire, do emprêgo empírico', *Boletim Sanitário de Angola* 2 (1939), 127–36.

Novaes, João, 'Doença do somno em Angola', *A Medicina Contemporânea* 19 (1901), 16–8.

Nunes, José António Pereira, 'A alimentação na Baixa de Cassange: inquéritos de consumo e nutricionais, campanhas alimentares e obras de fomento', *Anais do Instituto de Medicina Tropical* 17.1–2 (1960), 283–435.

Nunes, Silva, 'Aspectos da assistência médica às crianças em Angola e Moçambique', *Anais do Instituto de Medicina Tropical* 10.4.1 (1953), 2595–608.

Ornelas, Augusto, 'Nós e a última conferência internacional da doença do sono', *Boletim da Agência Geral das Colónias* 8 (1926), 86–101.

'A obra de protecção á criança negra', *Boletim da Assistência Médica aos Indígenas e da Luta contra a Moléstia do Sono* 3.7–12 (1929), 523–6.

Primeiro viver: luz e vitaminas (Benguela: Gráfica de Benguela, 1933).

'A assistência maternal e os meios de luta contra a mortalidade infantil em Moçambique', *Moçambique – Documentário trimestral* 27 (1941), 33–48.

Ornelas, Augusto and Mesquita, Bruno Pereira de, *Relatório da missão médica de assistência aos indígenas do Cuanza, 1929* (Lisbon: Agência Geral das Colónias, 1935).

Padua, António de and Lepierre, Charles, *A doença do somno: revista crítica* (Coimbra: Imprensa da Universidade, 1904).

Passos, José, 'Contribuição para o estudo da assistência à criança em Angola: breves notas sobre a actividade e acção social do dispensário de puericultura de Benguela (1935–46)', *Anais do Instituto de Medicina Tropical* 5 (1948), 401–5.

Peiper, Otto, *Geburtenhäufigkeit, Säuglings- und Kindersterblichkeit und Säuglingsernährung im früheren Deutsch-Ostafrika* (Berlin: Schoetz, 1920).

Pélissier, René, 'Conséquences démographiques des révoltes en Afrique portuguaise (1961–1970): essai d'interprétation', *Revue Française d'Histoire d'Outre-Mer* 61.222 (1974), 34–73.

Piot, A., 'Sur le fonctionnement d'un secteur de prophylaxie contre la trypanosomiase au Congo français (1919)', *Bulletin de la Société de Pathologie Exotique* 13 (1920), 376–84.

Primeiro Congresso de Medicina Tropical da África Ocidental, 'Acta da segunda sessão', *Revista Médica de Angola* 4.2 (1923), 7–43.

'Acta da sexta sessão (doença do sono)', *Revista Médica de Angola* 4.4 (1923), 7–46.

Prum, T., 'Observations concernant la natalité et la mortalité infantile de la région de Leverville', *Annales de la Société Belge de Médecine Tropicale* 7 (1927), 15–22.

Rebêlo, António, *A doença do sono no distrito do Tete* (Lourenço Marques: Imprensa Nacional de Moçambique, 1938).

Rebêlo, Frederico Leopoldino, *O Atoxil no tratamento da doença do sono* (Porto: Enciclopédia Portuguesa, 1921).

'Relatório do Chefe da Missão do Zaire referentes ao periodo Agôsto de 1923 a Setembro de 1924', *Revista Médica de Angola* 5 (1927), 80–91.

Reis, Carlos dos Santos and Sarmento, Alexandre, *Manual de estatística médica* (Lisbon: Instituto de Medicina Tropical, 1960).

Rela, José Manuel Zenha, 'Angola: o 'factor população' e o processo de desenvolvimento', *Trabalho. Boletim do Instituto do Trabalho, Previdência e Acção Social de Angola* 29–35 (1970–2), passim.

Repartição de Estatística Geral da Colónia de Angola (ed.), *Censo geral da população, 1940*, 12 vols. (Luanda: Imprensa Nacional, 1941–7).

Repartição Técnica de Estatística Geral da Província de Angola (ed.), *II recenseamento geral da população, 1950*, 5 vols. (Luanda: Imprensa Nacional, 1953–6).

Repartição Técnica de Estatística Geral do Governo Geral de Angola, *Bases para a execução do censo da população da Colónia em 1940* (Luanda: Imprensa Nacional, 1940).

Ribeiro, Aires Pinto, *Apontamentos para o estudo da vitalidade das populações cafreais de Angoche: Assistência Médica ao Indígena durante o ano de 1932* (Lourenço Marques: Imprensa Nacional, 1933).

Ribeiro, Lavrador, 'Notas sobre aspectos nosográficos das endemias de Angola', *Boletim Sanitário de Angola* 5.2 (1942), 45–66 and 6 (1943), 177–98.

'A investigação ciêntífica e o nível sanitário de Angola', *Anais do Instituto de Medicina Tropical* 10.4,1 (1953), 2809–19.

Ribeiro, Manuel Ferreira, 'Molestia de diagnóstico obscuro: communicação lida na sessão de 13 de Maio de 1871', *Jornal da Sociedade das Sciências Médicas de Lisboa* 36 (1871), 204–9.

A colonisação luso-africana: zona occidental (Lisbon: Lallemant Frères, 1884).

Estudos médico-tropicaes durante os trabalhos de campo para o caminho de ferro de Ambaca na Província de Angola, 1877–1878 (Lisbon: Imprensa Nacional, 1886).

Lições práticas de hygiene colonial, Vol. 1 (Lisbon: Typ. do Comercio, 1904).

Rivers, W. H. R., 'The Psychological Factor', in W. H. R. Rivers (ed.), *Essays on the Depopulation of Melanesia* (Cambridge: Cambridge University Press, 1922), 84–113.

Rodenwaldt, Ernst, 'Ein Beitrag zu der Frage des Bevölkerungsrückgangs in den afrikanischen Schutzgebieten', *Mitteilungen aus den deutschen Schutzgebieten* 28.3 (1915), 145–60.

Rodhain, Jerôme, *La mortinatalité et la mortalité infantile au point de vue pathologique – Afrique Centrale* (Genève: UISE, 1931).

Romaniuk, Anatole, 'Infertility in Tropical Africa', in John C. Caldwell and C. Okonjo (eds.), *The Population of Tropical Africa* (New York: Population Council, 1968), 214–24.

Roque, Antonio Bernardino, 'Doença do somno e beri-beri', *A Medicina Contemporânea* 22 (1904), 285–6.

'Sur la prophylaxie du paludisme dans les pays chauds', *Archivos de Hygiene e Pathologia Exoticas* 1.2 (1906), 153–8.

Ross, Edward Alsworth, *Report on Employment of Native Labor in Portuguese Africa* (New York: The Abbot Press, 1925).

Ryckmans, Pierre, 'Démographie congolaise', *Africa. Journal of the International African Institute* 6.3 (1933), 241–58.

Sambon, Louis W., 'Sleeping Sickness in the Light of Recent Knowledge', *Journal of Tropical Medicine* 6 (1903), 201–9.

'The Elucidation of Sleeping Sickness', *Journal of Tropical Medicine* 7 (1904), 61–3, 68–74, 87–91.

Sant'Anna, José Firmino, *Relatório de uma missão de estudo na Zambezia motivada pela doença do sono* (Lourenço Marques: Imprensa Nacional, 1911).

'A tripanosomíase humana da Rhodésia: crónica e particularidades da epidemia, no que interesse ao território português da África Oriental', *Archivos de Hygiene e Pathologia Exoticas* 4 (1913), 3–50.

'O problema da assistência médico-sanitária ao indígena em Africa', *Revista Médica de Angola* 4.2 (1923), 73–178.

Santos, Afonso Costa Valdez Thomaz dos, *Perspectivas económicas de Angola* (Lisbon: Agência Geral das Colónias, 1949).

Santos, Eduardo dos, *Sobre a 'medicina' e a magia dos Quiocos* (Lisbon: Junta de Investigação do Ultramar, 1960).

Santos, Francisco Ferreira dos, 'Assistência Médica aos Indígenas e processos práticos da sua hospitalisação', *Revista Médica de Angola* 4.2 (1923), 51–71.

Santos, Joaquim Pires dos, 'Relatório do Chefe do Sector Sanitário do Congo-Oeste (São Salvador), Junho–Dezembro de 1927', *Revista Médica de Angola* 6 (1928), 147–217.

Sarmento, Alexandre, 'O estudo da população de Angola', *Ocidente. Revista Portuguesa de Cultura* 19.60 (1943), 419–24.

Aspectos da natalidade e mortalidade infantil em Angola: separata do Jornal do Médico (Porto: Costa Carregal, 1944).

'População infantil de Angola', *A Criança Portuguesa* 6 (1946–7), 229–40.

'População indígena de Angola (sondagens e perspectivas demográficas)', *Boletim da Sociedade de Geografia de Lisboa* 66 (1948), 635–49.

'O dispensário de puericultura de Nova Lisboa', *O Médico* 2.24 (1951), 336.

'História breve de uma grande obra: o combate à doença do sono em Angola', *Boletim Clínico e Estatístico do Hospital do Ultramar, 2ª série* 7.3 (1953), 23–38.

'Subsídios para o estudo demográfico da população indígena de Angola', *Anais do Instituto de Medicina Tropical* 14.3–4 (1957), 509–26.

Sarmento, Alexandre and Henriques, Fernando Figueira, 'Alguns aspectos demográficos dos Bochimanes do sul de Angola', *O Médico* 5.149 (1954), 567–72.

Sarraut, Albert, *La mise en valeur des colonies françaises* (Paris: Payot, 1923).

Save the Children International Union, *Proceedings of the International Conference on African Children, Geneva, June 22–25, 1931* (Geneva: Save the Children International Union, 1932).

Saxton, Jack, 'Baby Day at San Salvador', *The Missionary Herald of the Baptist Missionary Society* (1937), 165–6.

'A Medical Missionary's Experience in San Salvador, Portuguese Congo', *Edinburgh Medical Missionary Society – Quarterly Paper* (February 1938), 200–3.

Schwetz, Jacques, 'Compte-rendu succint des travaux de la mission médicale antitrypanosique du Kwango-Kasai (Congo Belge) en 1920–1923', *Revista Médica de Angola* 4.4 (1923), 149–55.

Recherches sur les glossines (Brussels: Hayez, 1919).

'Contribution à l'étude de la démographie congolaise', *Congo. Revue Générale de la Colonie Belge* 4.1 (1923), 297–340.

Secretaria de Colonização e Negócios Indígenas (Província de Angola), *Legislação Provincial* (Luanda: Imprensa Nacional de Angola, 1921).

Sharp, Evelyn, *The African Child: An Account of the International Conference on African Children, Geneva* (London/New York/Toronto: Longmans, Green and Co., 1931).

Sicé, Alphonse, *La Trypanosomiase humaine en Afrique intertropicale* (Paris: Vigot, 1937).

Silva, António Bártolo da, 'Sobre as possibilidades de redução da mortalidade na primeira infância', *Boletim de Assistência Social* 7 (1943), 282–5.

Silva, Avelino Manuel da, *Serviço de Assistência aos Indígenas no distrito do Congo, 1930* (Lisbon: Agência Geral das Colónias [193–]).

Serviço de Assistência aos Indígenas no distrito do Congo, 1° semestre de 1931 (Lisbon: Agência Geral das Colónias, 1931).

Silva, Francisco Venâncio da, 'Relatório do chefe da missão volante do distrito de Malange, Setembro–Novembro de 1927', *Revista Médica de Angola* 6 (1928), 219–43.

'O pian', *Boletim da Assistência Médica aos Indígenas e da Luta contra a Moléstia do Sono* 3.1 (1929), 1–16.

Relatório do serviço permanente de prevenção e combate à peste bubónica no sul de Angola, 1933 (Lisbon: Agência Geral das Colónias, 1936).

Silva, João de Mattos e, 'Doença do somno em Angola', *A Medicina Contemporânea* 18 (1900), 422–3.

Contribuição para o estudo da região de Cabinda: memória para o Congresso Colonial Nacional (Lisbon: Typographia Universal, 1904).

Singer, H. W., 'Demographic Factors in Subsaharan Economic Development', in Melville J. Herskovits and Mitchell Harwitz (eds.), *Economic Transition in Africa* (London: Routledge, 1964), 241–61.

Sleeping Sickness Committee, *Minutes of Evidence taken by the Inter-Departmental Committee on Sleeping Sickness: Presented to Both Houses of Parliament by Command of his Majesty* [= Cd. 7350] (London: HMSO, 1914).

Sociedade das Sciências Médicas, 'Acta da sessão ordinária de 15 de Julho de 1871', *Jornal da Sociedade das Sciências Médicas de Lisboa* 36 (1871), 294–302.

'Relatorio da commissão encarregada de dar um parecer sobre a communicação do sr. Ribeiro acerca da doença do somno', *Jornal da Sociedade das Sciências Médicas de Lisboa* 36 (1871), 251–3, 264–72.

'Representação dirigida ao Governo', *Jornal da Sociedade das Sciências Médicas de Lisboa* (1900), 167–9.

Sousa, Carlos Salazar de, 'Necessidades e deficiências da assistência infantil', *Revista Portuguesa de Pediatria e Puericultura* 2.5 (1939), 221–42.

Sousa, Jacinto de, *Relatório da missão médica volante de Assistência aos Indígenas do Dande, 1928* (Lisbon: Agência Geral das Colónias, [193–]).

'O capital humano', *Boletim da Assistência Médica aos Indígenas e da Luta contra a Moléstia do Sono* 3.2 (1929), 160–2.

Souto, A. Meyrelles do, 'Auxílio médico às missões', *Acção Médica* 12 (1948), 446–55.

Statistical Office of the United Nations (ed.), *Demographic Yearbook for 1948* (New York, 1949).

Demographic Yearbook for 1949–1950 (New York, 1950).

Demographic Yearbook for 1961 (New York, 1961).

Telles, Francisco Xavier da Silva, 'Assistência aos indígenas: these', in *I Congresso Colonial Nacional: Actas das Sessões* (Lisbon: A Liberal, 1902), 25–6.

A transportação penal e a colonização (Lisbon: Typ. Liv. Ferin, 1903).

Thiroux, A., 'La natalité et la mortalité infantile dans les colonies françaises', *Revue Philantropique* 51.408 (1931), 561–9.

Torday, Émil, *La mortinatalité et la mortalité infantile au point de vue économique et social – Afrique Centrale* (Genève: UISE, 1931).

Treille, Georges, 'Mesures propres à assurer la conservation de la race, à prévenir sa dégénérescence physique, à améliorer ses conditions d'existence', in Exposition Universelle Internationale de 1900 (ed.), *Congrès International de Sociologie Coloniale (Paris, 1900)* (Paris: Arthur Rousseau, 1901), Vol. 1, 87–123.

Trolli, Giovanni, 'Le traitement de la trypanose humaine par la Tryparsamide', *Annales de la Société Belge de Médecine Tropicale* 7 (1927), 319–36.

'Impression sur l'organisation du service médical de l'Angola', *Bruxelles-Médical* 9.14 (1929), 401–6.

Rapport sur l'hygiène publique au Congo Belge pendant l'année 1928 (Brussels: Dewit, 1930).

Rapport sur l'hygiène publique au Congo Belge pendant l'année 1929 (Brussels: Dewit, 1931).

'Contribution à l'étude de la démographie des Bakongo', *Bulletin des Séances de l'Institut Royal Colonial Belge* 5.2 (1934), 239–316.

L'Assistance Médicale aux Indigènes du Congo Belge et notre dynastie: historique et nouvelle méthode adoptée par FORÉAMI (Antwerp, 1935).

Trolli, Giovanni and Dupuy, L., *Contribution à l'étude de la démographie des Bakongo au Congo Belge 1933* (Brussels: M. Cock, 1934).

Union of South Africa, *Report to the Council of the League of Nations Concerning the Administration of South West Africa for the Year 1930* (Pretoria: The Government Printer, 1931).

Report to the Council of the League of Nations Concerning the Administration of South West Africa for the Year 1934 (Pretoria: The Government Printer, 1935).

United Nations Population Division, 'Framework for Future Population Estimates, 1950–1980, by World Regions', in *Proceedings of the World Population Conference, Rome, 31 August–10 September 1954* (New York, 1955), Vol. 3, 283–328.

van de Walle, Étienne, 'Characteristics of African Demographic Data', in William Brass (ed.), *The Demography of Tropical Africa* (Princeton: Princeton University Press, 1968), 12–87.

van Hoof, L., 'Thérapeutique de la maladie du sommeil et des trypanosomiases animales africaines', *Revista Médica de Angola* 4.4 (1923), 85–128.

Rapport sur l'hygiène publique au Congo Belge pendant l'année 1939 (Brussels, [1940]).

van Nitsen, René, *Contribution à l'étude de l'enfance noire au Congo Belge* (Brussel: van Campenhout, 1941).

Vasconcelos, Ernesto Júlio de Carvalho, *As colonias portuguezas: geographia physica, política e economica* (Lisbon: Typographia da Companhia Nacional Editora, 1896).

Vassal, Gabrielle, 'Natalité et protection de l'enfance', *Revista Médica de Angola* 4.2 (1923), 45–9.

Vassal, Gabrielle and Vassal, Joseph, *Français, Belges et Portugais en Afrique équatoriale: Pointe-Noire, Matadi, Lobito* (Paris: Éditions Pierre Roger, 1931).

Velho, Luís Baptista de Assunção, 'A tripanossomose humana em Angola (relatórios etc.)', *Revista Médica de Angola* 2 (1921), 7–196.

Villela, Fernandes, 'Rapport sur l'Aide Médicale aux Missions de Belgique', *Acção Médica* 12 (1948), 473–92.

Virchow, Rudolf, 'L'acclimatement', *Revue Scientifique* 22.24 (1885), 737–47.

Warrington, W. B., 'A Note on the Condition of the Central Nervous System in a Case of African Lethargy', *The British Medical Journal* 2178 (1902), 929–31.

Weeks, John, *Among the Primitive Bakongo: A Record of Thirty Years' Close Intercourse with the Bakongo and other Tribes of Equatorial Africa* (London: Seeley, Service & Co., 1914).

Xavier, Ignacio Caetano, 'Relatório do serviço de saúde no Dondo', in *Estatistica Medica dos Hospitaes das Provincias Ultramarinas (1881)* (Lisbon: Imprensa Nacional, 1883), 103–16.

Ziemann, Hans, 'Ist die Schlafkrankheit der Neger eine Intoxikations- oder
    Infektionskrankheit?', *Centralblatt für Bakteriologie, Parasitenkunde und
    Infektionskrankheiten* 32 (1902), 413–24.
'Bericht über das Vorkommen des Aussatzes Lepra, der Schlafkrankheit, der Beri-
    Beri etc. in Kamerun', *Deutsche Medizinische Wochenschrift* 29.14 (1903), 250–2.

Secondary Sources

Adams, Mark B. (ed.), *The Wellborn Science: Eugenics in Germany, France, Brazil,
    and Russia* (New York/Oxford: Oxford University Press, 1990).
Agadjanian, Victor and Prata, Ndola, 'Trends in Angola's Fertility: Paper presented at
    "Workshop on Prospects for Fertility Decline in High Fertility Countries", United
    Nations Population Division, New York (9–11 July 2001)'. www.un.org/en/
    development/desa/population/events/pdf/expert/3/agadjani.pdf (last accessed
    12 February 2021).
Aksoy, Serap et al., 'Human African Trypanosomiasis Control: Achievements and
    Challenges', *PLoS Neglected Tropical Diseases* 11.4 (2017). https://doi.org/10
    .1371/journal.pntd.0005454
Alexandre, Valentim, *Origens do colonialismo português moderno (1822–1891)*
    (Lisbon: Sá da Costa, 1979).
'A política colonial em finais de Oitocentos: Portugal e a sacralização do Império', in
    Valentim Alexandre, *Velho Brasil, novas Áfricas: Portugal e o Império
    (1808–1975)* (Porto: Ed. Afrontamento, 2000), 148–62.
'Nação e Império', in Francisco Bethencourt and Kirti Chaudhuri (eds.), *Do Brasil
    para África (1808–1930)* (Lisbon: Temas e Debates, 2000), 90–142.
Velho Brasil, novas Áfricas: Portugal e o Império (1808–1975) (Porto: Ed.
    Afrontamento, 2000).
'The Portuguese Empire, 1825–1890: Ideology and Economics', in Olivier Pétré-
    Grenouilleau (ed.), *From Slave Trade to Empire: Europe and the Colonisation of
    Black Africa 1780s–1880s* (London: Routledge, 2004), 110–32.
Contra o vento: Portugal, o Império e a maré anticolonial (1945–1960) (Lisbon:
    Temas e Debates, 2017).
Alencastro, Luiz Felipe de, *O trato dos viventes: formação do Brasil no Atlântico Sul,
    séculos XVI e XVII* (São Paulo: Companhia das Letras, 2000).
'Mulattos in Brazil and Angola: A Comparative Approach, Seventeenth to Twenty-
    First Centuries', in Francisco Bethencourt and Adrian Pearce (eds.), *Racism and
    Ethnic Relations in the Portuguese-Speaking World* (Oxford/New York: Oxford
    University Press, 2012), 71–98.
Allina, Eric, *Slavery by Any Other Name: African Life under Company Rule in Colonial
    Mozambique* (Charlottesville: University of Virginia Press, 2012).
Allman, Jean, 'Making Mothers: Missionaries, Medical Officers and Women's Work in
    Colonial Asante, 1924–1945', *History Workshop* 38.1 (1994), 23–47.
'Between the Present and History: African Nationalism and Decolonization', in John
    Parker and Richard Reid (eds.), *The Oxford Handbook of Modern African History*
    (Oxford: Oxford University Press, 2013), 224–42.

Alves, Jorge Fernandes, 'Saúde e Fraternidade: a saúde pública na I República', in
   Comissão Nacional para as Comemorações do Centenário da República (ed.),
   Corpo: estado, medicina e sociedade no tempo da I^a República (Lisbon: Imprensa
   Nacional/Casa da Moeda, 2010), 111–29.
Amaral, Isabel, 'The Emergence of Tropical Medicine in Portugal: The School of
   Tropical Medicine and the Colonial Hospital of Lisbon (1902–1935)', *Dynamis* 28
   (2008), 301–28.
   'Bacteria or Parasite? The Controversy over the Etiology of Sleeping Sickness and
   the Portuguese Participation, 1898–1904', *História, Ciências, Saúde –
   Manguinhos* 19.4 (2012), 1275–300.
Aminoff, Michael Jeffrey, *Brown-Séquard: An Improbable Genius Who Transformed
   Medicine* (Oxford: Oxford University Press, 2011).
Anderson, Benedict, *Imagined Communities: Reflections on the Origin and Spread of
   Nationalism*, Revised Edition (London/New York: Verso, 1991).
Anderson, Warwick, 'Immunities of Empire: Race, Disease, and the New Tropical
   Medicine, 1900–1920', *Bulletin of the History of Medicine* 70.1 (1996), 94–118.
   'Where is the Postcolonial History of Medicine?', *Bulletin of the History of Medicine*
   72.3 (1998), 522–30.
   'The Natures of Culture: Environment and Race in the Colonial Tropics', in Paul
   Greenough and Anna Lowenhaupt Tsing (eds.), *Nature in the Global South*
   (Durham, NC: Duke University Press, 2003), 29–46.
   *Colonial Pathologies: American Tropical Medicine, Race, and Hygiene in the
   Philippines* (Durham, NC: Duke University Press, 2006).
Anderson, Warwick, Roque, Ricardo and Santos, Ricardo Ventura (eds.), *Luso-
   Tropicalism and Its Discontents: The Making and Unmaking of Racial
   Exceptionalism* (New York: Berghahn Books, 2019).
Appadurai, Arjun, 'Number in the Colonial Imagination', in Carol Appadurai
   Breckenridge and Peter van der Veer (eds.), *Orientalism and the Postcolonial
   Predicament: Perspectives on South Asia* (Philadelphia: University of
   Pennsylvania Press, 1993), 314–39.
Araújo, Paulo, *Miguel Bombarda: médico e político* (Casal de Cambra: Caleidoscópio,
   2007).
Arnold, David (ed.), *Imperial Medicine and Indigenous Societies* (Oxford: Oxford
   University Press, 1988).
   *Colonizing the Body: State Medicine and Epidemic Disease in Nineteenth-Century
   India* (Berkeley: University of California Press, 1993).
   'Introduction: Tropical Medicine Before Manson', in David Arnold (ed.), *Warm
   Climates and Western Medicine: The Emergence of Tropical Medicine,
   1500–1900* (Amsterdam: Rodopi, 1996), 1–19.
   (ed.), *Warm Climates and Western Medicine: The Emergence of Tropical Medicine,
   1500–1900* (Amsterdam: Rodopi, 1996).
   The Tropics and the Travelling Gaze: India, Landscape and Science, 1800–1856
   (Seattle/London: University of Washington Press, 2006).
Asiwaju, A. I., 'Migrations as Revolt: The Example of the Ivory Coast and Upper Volta
   before 1945', *Journal of African History* 17.4 (1976), 577–94.
Au, Sokhieng, *Mixed Medicines: Health and Culture in French Colonial Cambodia*
   (Chicago: University of Chicago Press, 2011).

'Medical Orders: Catholic and Protestant Missionary Medicine in the Belgian Congo, 1880–1940', *Low Countries Historical Review* 132.1 (2017), 62–82.

Axelson, Eric, *Portugal and the Scramble for Africa, 1875–1891* (Johannesburg: Witwatersrand University Press, 1967).

Bado, Jean-Paul, *Médecine coloniale et grandes endémies en Afrique, 1900–1960: lèpre, trypanosomiase humaine et onchocercose* (Paris: Karthala, 1996).

Eugène Jamot, 1879–1937: le médecin de la maladie du sommeil ou trypanosomiase (Paris: Karthala, 2011).

Ball, Jeremy, *'The Colossal Lie': The Sociedade Agrícola do Cassequel and Portuguese Colonial Labor Policy in Angola, 1899–1977*. Unpublished PhD thesis, University of California, 2003.

'"Alma Negra" (Black Soul): The Campaign for Free Labor in Angola and São Tomé, 1909–1916', *Portuguese Studies Review* 18.2 (2011), 51–72.

Angola's Colossal Lie: Forced Labor on a Sugar Plantation, 1913–1977 (Leiden/ Boston: Brill, 2015).

Bandeira, Filomena, 'Camoesas, João José da Conceição', in António Nóvoa (ed.), *Dicionário de educadores portugueses* (Porto: Edições Asa, 2003), 237–41.

Baptista, Maria Isabel Rodrigues, 'A demografia em Portugal: um percurso bibliográfico', *Análise Social* 42.183 (2007), 539–79.

Barbieri, Magali, 'De l'utilité des statistiques démographiques de l'Indochine française (1862–1954)', *Annales de Démographie Historique* 113 (2007), 85–126.

Barreto, José, 'Censura', in António Barreto and Joel Serrão (eds.), *Dicionário de história de Portugal, Vol. VII, Supl. A/E* (Porto: Figueirinhas, 1999), 275–84.

Barthélémy, Pascale, 'Sages-femmes africaines diplômées en AOF des années 1920 aux années 1960: une redéfinition des rapports sociaux de sexe en contexte colonial', in Anne Hugon (ed.), *Histoire des femmes en situation coloniale: Afrique et Asie, XXe siècle* (Paris: Karthala, 2004), 119–44.

Africaines et diplômées à l'époque coloniale (1918–1957) (Rennes: Presses Universitaires de Rennes, 2010).

Bashford, Alison, *Imperial Hygiene: A Critical History of Colonialism, Nationalism and Public Health* (Basingstoke/New York: Palgrave Macmillan, 2004).

'Nation, Empire, Globe: The Spaces of Population Debate in the Interwar Years', *Comparative Studies in Society and History* 49.1 (2007), 170–201.

'Population, Geopolitics, and International Organizations in the Mid-Twentieth Century', *Journal of World History* 19.3 (2008), 327–48.

Global Population: History, Geopolitics, and Life on Earth (New York: Columbia University Press, 2014).

Bastos, Cristiana, 'Doctors for the Empire: The Medical School of Goa and Its Narratives', *Identities. Global Studies in Culture and Power* 8.4 (2001), 517–48.

'O ensino da medicina na Índia colonial portuguesa: fundação e primeiras décadas da Escola Médico-cirúrgica de Nova Goa', *História, Ciências, Saúde – Manguinhos* 11 (2004), Supl. 1, 11–39.

'Medical Hybridisms and Social Boundaries: Aspects of Portuguese Colonialism in Africa and India in the Nineteenth Century', *Journal of Southern African Studies* 33.4 (2007), 767–82.

'Migrants, Settlers and Colonists: The Biopolitics of Displaced Bodies', *International Migration* 46.5 (2008), 27–54.

'Corpos, climas, ares e lugares: autores e anónimos nas ciências da colonização', in Cristiana Bastos and Renilda Barreto (eds.), *A circulação do conhecimento: medicina, redes e impérios* (Lisbon: Instituto de Ciências Sociais on-line, 2011), 25–58.

Bastos, Cristiana and Barreto, Renilda (eds.), *A circulação do conhecimento: medicina, redes e impérios* (Lisbon: Instituto de Ciências Sociais on-line, 2011).

Bäumler, Ernst, *Paul Ehrlich: Forscher für das Leben*, 2nd edn. (Frankfurt: Societäts-Verlag, 1980).

Bell, Heather, *Frontiers of Medicine in the Anglo-Egyptian Sudan, 1899–1940* (Oxford: Clarendon Press, 1999).

Bender, Gerald J., *Angola under the Portuguese: The Myth and the Reality* (Berkeley: University of California Press, 1978).

Berman, Bruce J., 'The Perils of Bula Matari: Constraint and Power in the Colonial State', *Canadian Journal of African Studies* 31.3 (1997), 556–70.

Bethencourt, Francisco and Curto, Diogo Ramada (eds.), *Portuguese Oceanic Expansion, 1400–1800* (Cambridge: Cambridge University Press, 2007).

Bethencourt, Francisco and Pearce, Adrian (eds.), *Racism and Ethnic Relations in the Portuguese-Speaking World* (Oxford/New York: Oxford University Press, 2012).

Birmingham, David, *Trade and Conflict in Angola: The Mbundu and Their Neighbours under the Influence of the Portuguese 1483–1790* (Oxford: Clarendon Press, 1966).

'The Coffee Barons of Cazengo', *Journal of African History* 19.4 (1978), 523–38.

Borowy, Iris, 'International Social Medicine between the Wars: Positioning a Volatile Concept', *Hygeia Internationalis* 6.2 (2007), 13–35.

Coming to Terms with World Health: The League of Nations Health Organisation, 1921–1946 (Frankfurt: Peter Lang, 2009).

Borowy, Iris and Gruner, Wolf D., 'Introduction', in Iris Borowy and Wolf D. Gruner (eds.), *Facing Illness in Troubled Times: Health in Europe in the Interwar Years* (Frankfurt: Peter Lang, 2005), 1–16.

Bossard, Eric, *La médecine traditionelle au centre et à l'ouest de l'Angola* (Lisbon: IICT, 1996).

Boyd, John, 'Sleeping Sickness: The Castellani-Bruce Controversy', *Notes and Records of the Royal Society of London* 28 (1973), 93–100.

Brantlinger, Patrick, *Dark Vanishings: Discourse on the Extinction of Primitive Races, 1800–1930* (Ithaca, NY: Cornell University Press, 2003).

Briggs, Laura, *Reproducing Empire: Race, Sex, Science, and U.S. Imperialism in Puerto Rico* (Berkeley: University of California Press, 2002).

Bruchhausen, Walter, 'Medical Pluralism as a Historical Phenomenon: A Regional and Multi-Level Approach to Health Care in German, British and Independent East Africa', in Anne Digby, Waltraud Ernst and Projit B. Muhkarji (eds.), *Crossing Colonial Historiographies: Histories of Colonial and Indigenous Medicines in Transnational Perspective* (Newcastle: Cambridge Scholars, 2010), 99–114.

Burke, Timothy, *Lifebuoy Men, Lux Women: Commodification, Consumption, and Cleanliness in Modern Zimbabwe* (Durham, NC: Duke University Press, 1996).

Burroughs, Robert, *Travel Writing and Atrocities: Eyewitness Accounts of Colonialism in the Congo, Angola and the Putumayo* (London: Routledge, 2010).

Bush, Barbara, 'Motherhood, Morality, and Social Order: Gender and Development Discourse and Practice in Late Colonial Africa', in Joseph Morgan Hodge, Gerald

Hödl and Martina Kopf (eds.), *Developing Africa: Concepts and Practices in Twentieth-Century Colonialism* (Manchester: Manchester University Press, 2014), 270–92.

Caldeira, Maria de Fátima, *Assistência infantil em Lisboa na 1ª República* (Casal de Cambra: Caleidoscópio, 2004).

Caldwell, John C. and Caldwell, Pat, 'The Demographic Evidence for the Incidence and Cause of Abnormally Low Fertility in Tropical Africa', *World Health Statistics Quarterly* 36 (1983), 2–34.

Caldwell, John C. and Schindlmayr, Thomas, 'Historical Population Estimates: Unravelling the Consensus', *Population and Development Review* 28.2 (2002), 183–204.

Callahan, Michael D., *Mandates and Empires: The League of Nations and Africa, 1914–1931* (Brighton: Sussex Academic Press, 2008).

Campbell, Chloe, *Race and Empire: Eugenics in Colonial Kenya* (Manchester: Manchester University Press, 2007).

Campos, Rafael Coca de, *Ocupação, violência e negociação: relações econômicas, políticas e sociais entre as populações africanas pastoris e a sociedade colonial portuguesa no Sudoeste Angolano.* Unpublished MA thesis, Universidade Estadual de Campinas, 2017.

Candido, Mariana Pinho, *An African Slaving Port and the Atlantic World: Benguela and its Hinterland* (Cambridge: Cambridge University Press, 2013).

Castelo, Cláudia, *'O modo português de estar no mundo': o luso-tropicalismo e a ideologia colonial portuguesa (1933–1961)* (Porto: Edições Afrontamento, 1998).

Passagens para África: o povoamento de Angola e Moçambique com naturais da metrópole (1920–1974) (Porto: Edições Afrontamento, 2007).

'Investigação científica e política colonial portuguesa: evolução e articulações, 1936–1974', *História, Ciências, Saúde – Manguinhos* 19.2 (2012), 391–408.

'Reproducing Portuguese Villages in Africa: Agricultural Science, Ideology and Empire', *Journal of Southern African Studies* 42.2 (2016), 267–81.

Castro, Ricardo Themudo de, *A Escola de Medicina Tropical de Lisboa e a afirmação do Estado Português nas colónias africanas (1902–1935).* Unpublished PhD thesis, Universidade Nova de Lisboa, 2013.

Christopher, A. J., '" To Define the Indefinable": Population Classification and the Census in South Africa', *Area* 34.4 (2002), 401–8.

Cinnamon, John M., 'Counting and Recounting: Dislocation, Colonial Demography, and Historical Memory in Northern Gabon', in Karl Ittmann, Dennis D. Cordell and Gregory H. Maddox (eds.), *The Demographics of Empire: The Colonial Order and the Creation of Knowledge* (Ohio: Ohio University Press, 2010), 130–56.

Clarence-Smith, William Gervase, 'The Myth of Uneconomic Imperialism, 1836–1926', *Journal of Southern African Studies* 5.2 (1979), 165–80.

'The Impact of the Spanish Civil War and the Second World War on Portuguese and Spanish Africa', *Journal of African History* 26 (1985), 309–26.

The Third Portuguese Empire, 1825–1975: A Study in Economic Imperialism (Manchester: Manchester University Press, 1985).

'The Effects of the Great Depression of the 1930s on Industrialisation in Equatorial and Central Africa', in Ian Brown (ed.), *The Economies of Africa and Asia in the Inter-war Depression* (London: Routledge, 1989), 170–202.

'The Hidden Costs of Labour on the Cocoa Plantations of São Tomé and Príncipe, 1875–1914', *Portuguese Studies* 6 (1990), 152–72.

'Cocoa Plantations and Coerced Labor in the Gulf of Guinea', in Martin A. Klein (ed.), *Breaking the Chains: Slavery, Bondage, and Emancipation in Modern Africa and Asia* (Madison: University of Wisconsin Press, 1993), 150–70.

'The Redemption of Child Slaves by Christian Missionaries in Central Africa, 1878–1914', in Gwyn Campbell, Suzanne Miers and Joseph C. Miller (eds.), *Child Slaves in the Modern World* (Athens: Ohio University Press, 2011), 173–92.

Cleminson, Richard, *Catholicism, Race and Empire: Eugenics in Portugal, 1900–1950* (Budapest: Central European University Press, 2014).

Cleveland, Todd, *Diamonds in the Rough: Corporate Paternalism and African Professionalism on the Mines of Colonial Angola, 1917–1975* (Athens: Ohio University Press, 2015).

Coale, Ansley J. (ed.), *The Decline of Fertility in Europe* (Princeton: Princeton University Press, 1986).

Coates, Timothy J., *Convict Labor in the Portuguese Empire, 1740–1932: Redefining the Empire with Forced Labor and New Imperialism* (Leiden/Boston: Brill, 2014).

Coghe, Samuël, *Population Politics in the Tropics: Demography, Health and Colonial Rule in Portuguese Angola, 1890s–1940s*. Unpublished PhD thesis, European University Institute, Florence, 2014.

'Inter-imperial Learning and African Health Care in Portuguese Angola in the Interwar Period', *Social History of Medicine* 28.1 (2015), 134–54.

'Reordering Colonial Society: Model Villages and Social Planning in Rural Angola, 1920–1945', *Journal of Contemporary History* 52.1 (2017), 16–44.

'Sleeping Sickness Control and the Transnational Politics of Mass Chemoprophylaxis in Portuguese Colonial Africa', *Portuguese Studies Review* 25.1 (2017), 57–89.

'Reassessing Portuguese Exceptionalism: Racial Concepts and Colonial Policies toward the "Bushmen" in Southern Angola, 1880s–1970s', in Warwick Anderson, Ricardo Roque and Ricardo Ventura Santos (eds.), *Luso-Tropicalism and Its Discontents: The Making and Unmaking of Racial Exceptionalism* (New York: Berghahn Books, 2019), 184–214.

'Disease Control and Public Health in Colonial Africa', *Oxford Research Encyclopedia of African History* (2020), https://doi.org/10.1093/acrefore/9780190277734.013.620.

'Between Colonial Medicine and Global Health: Protein Malnutrition and UNICEF Milk in the Belgian Congo', *Medical History* 65.4 (forthcoming).

Coghe, Samuël and Widmer, Alexandra, 'Colonial Demography: Discourses, Rationalities, Methods', in Population Knowledge Network (ed.), *Twentieth Century Population Thinking: A Critical Reader of Primary Sources* (London/New York: Routledge, 2016), 37–64.

Cohn, Bernard S, 'The Census, Social Structure and Objectification in South Asia', in *An Anthropologist among the Historians and Other Essays* (Delhi: Oxford University Press, 1987), 224–54.

Cole, Joshua, *The Power of Large Numbers: Population, Politics, and Gender in Nineteenth-Century France* (Ithaca: Cornell University Press, 2000).

Comaroff, Jean, 'The Diseased Heart of Africa: Medicine, Colonialism, and the Black Body', in Shirley Lindenbaum and Margaret Lock (eds.), *Knowledge, Power, and Practice: The Anthropology of Medicine and Everyday Life* (Berkeley: University of California Press, 1993), 305–29.

Connelly, Matthew, 'To Inherit the Earth: Imagining World Population, from the Yellow Peril to the Population Bomb', *Journal of Global History* 1.3 (2006), 299–319.

  Fatal Misconception: The Struggle to Control World Population (Cambridge, MA/ London: Belknap Press of Harvard University Press, 2008).

Conrad, Sebastian and Stange, Marion, 'Governance and Colonial Rule', in Thomas Risse (ed.), *Governance Without a State: Policies and Politics of Limited Statehood* (New York: Columbia University Press, 2011), 39–64.

Cook, Harold John, Bhattacharya, Sanjoy and Hardy, Anne (eds.), *History of the Social Determinants of Health: Global Histories, Contemporary Debates* (Hyderabad: Orient BlackSwan, 2009).

Cooper, Ann Clare, *Public Health, the Native Medical Service, and the Colonial Administration in French West Africa, 1900–1944*. Unpublished PhD thesis, University of Texas at Austin, 2010.

Cooper, Barbara, 'Chronic Malnutrition and the Trope of the Bad Mother', in Xavier Crombé and Jean-Hervé Jézéquel (eds.), *A Not-So Natural Disaster: Niger 2005* (New York: Columbia University Press, 2009), 147–68.

Cooper, Frederick, 'Modernizing Bureaucrats, Backward Africans, and the Development Concept', in Frederick Cooper and Randall Packard (eds.), *International Development and the Social Sciences: Essays on the History and Politics of Knowledge* (Berkeley: University of California Press, 1997), 64–92.

  Colonialism in Question: Theory, Knowledge, History (Berkeley: University of California Press, 2005).

Cooter, Roger, 'Introduction', in Roger Cooter (ed.), *In the Name of the Child: Health and Welfare, 1880–1940* (London, New York: Routledge, 1992), 1–17.

Cordell, Dennis D. and Gregory, Joel W. (eds.), *African Population and Capitalism: Historical Perspectives* (Boulder, CO: Westview Press, 1987).

Cordell, Dennis D., Gregory, Joel W. and Piché, Victor, *Hoe and Wage: A Social History of a Circular Migration System in West Africa* (Boulder, CO: Westview Press, 1996).

Cordell, Dennis D., Ittmann, Karl and Maddox, Gregory H., 'Counting Subjects: Demography and Empire', in Karl Ittmann, Dennis D. Cordell and Gregory H. Maddox (eds.), *The Demographics of Empire: The Colonial Order and the Creation of Knowledge* (Athens, OH: Ohio University Press, 2010), 1–21.

Corrado, Jacopo, 'The Fall of a Creole Elite? Angola at the Turn of the Twentieth Century: The Decline of the Euro-African Urban Community', *Luso-Brazilian Review* 47.2 (2010), 100–19.

Corral-Corral, Iñigo and Quereda Rodríguez-Navarro, Carmen, 'Gustavo Pittaluga y la expedición para el estudio de la enfermedad del sueño en los territorios españoles del golfo de Guinea (1909)', *Revista de Neurología* 54.1 (2012), 49–58.

Costa, Cândido Ferreira da, *Cem anos dos missionários do Espírito Santo em Angola, 1866–1966* (Nova Lisboa: Livr. Sampedro Ed., 1970).

Costa, João Paulo Oliveira e, Rodrigues, José Damião and Oliveira, Pedro Aires (eds.), *História da Expansão e do Império Português* (Lisbon: A Esfera dos Livros, 2014).

Costa, Sara, 'Inaugurada a Maternidade Alfredo da Costa', in António Simões do Paço (ed.), *Os anos de Salazar: Vol. I: 1926–1932* (Lisbon: Centro Editor PDA, 2008), 136–47.

Cova, Anne, 'Où en est l'histoire de la maternité', *CLIO. Histoire, femmes et sociétés* 21 (2005), 189–211.

Crozier, Anna, 'What Was Tropical about Tropical Neurasthenia? The Utility of the Diagnosis in the Management of British East Africa', *Journal of the History of Medicine and the Allied Sciences* 64.4 (2009), 518–48.

Crush, Jonathan, Jeeves, Alan and Yudelman, David, *South Africa's Labor Empire: A History of Black Migrancy to the Gold Mines* (Boulder, CO: Westview Press, 1991).

Cruz, Elizabeth Ceita Vera, *O estatuto do indigenato – Angola: a legalização da discriminação na colonização portuguesa* (Lisbon: Novo Imbondeiro, 2005).

Cueto, Marcos, Brown, Theodore M. and Fee, Elizabeth, *The World Health Organization: A History* (Cambridge: Cambridge University Press, 2019).

Curtin, Philip D., *Disease and Empire: The Health of European Troops in the Conquest of Africa* (Cambridge: Cambridge University Press, 1998).

Curto, José C., *Enslaving Spirits: The Portuguese-Brazilian Alcohol Trade at Luanda and its Hinterland, c. 1550–1830* (Leiden/Boston: Brill, 2004).

'Sources for the pre-1900 Population History of Sub-Saharan Africa: The Case of Angola, 1773–1845', *Annales de Démographie Historique* (1994), 319–38.

De Koning, Harry P., 'The Drugs of Sleeping Sickness: Their Mechanisms of Action and Resistance, and a Brief History', *Tropical Medicine and Infectious Diseases* 5.14 (2020), https://doi:10.3390/tropicalmed5010014.

De Roo, Bas, 'Customs in the Two Congos: A Connected History of Colonial Taxation in Africa (1885–1914)', *Journal of Colonialism and Colonial History* 19.1 (2018).

Dias, Jill Rosemary, 'Black Chiefs, White Traders and Colonial Policy near the Kwanza: Kabuku Kambilo and the Portuguese, 1873–1896', *Journal of African History* 17.2 (1976), 245–65.

'Famine and Disease in the History of Angola, c. 1830–1930', *Journal of African History* 22.3 (1981), 349–78.

'Changing Patterns of Power in the Luanda Hinterland', *Paideuma* 32 (1986), 285–318.

Digby, Anne, Ernst, Waltraud and Muhkarji, Projit B. (eds.), *Crossing Colonial Historiographies: Histories of Colonial and Indigenous Medicines in Transnational Perspective* (Newcastle: Cambridge Scholars, 2010).

Direito, Bárbara, '"O terror dos homens e o flagelo dos animais": A doença do sono animal como problema em Moçambique'. Paper presented at the International Conference 'Saber Tropical em Moçambique: História, Memória e Ciência', Lisbon, 25 October 2012.

Domingos, Nuno and Pereira, Victor, 'Introdução', in Nuno Domingos and Victor Pereira (eds.), *O Estado Novo em questão* (Lisbon: Edições 70, 2010), 7–39.

Dores, Hugo Gonçalves, 'La séparation de l'Église et de l'État dans l'Empire portugais: Des limitations d'un principe essentiel de la Première République (1911–1919)', *Histoire, Monde & Cultures Religieuses* 31 (2014), 93–112.

A missão da República: política, religião e o Império Colonial Português (1910–1926) (Lisbon: Edições 70, 2015).

Dörnemann, Maria, *Plan Your Family – Plan Your Nation: Bevölkerungspolitik als internationales Entwicklungshandeln in Kenia (1932–1993)* (Berlin/Boston: De Gruyter Oldenbourg, 2019).

Dörnemann, Maria and Huhle, Teresa, 'Population Problems in Modernization and Development', in Population Knowledge Network (ed.), *Twentieth Century Population Thinking: A Critical Reader of Primary Sources* (London/New York: Routledge, 2016), 142–71.

Dörnemann, Maria, Overath, Petra and Reinecke, Christiane (eds), 'Competing Numbers: Uses of Population Statistics in the Nineteenth and Twentieth Centuries', *Contemporanea. Rivista di Storia dell'800 e del '900* 18.3 (2015), 469–88.

Doyle, Shane, *Crisis and Decline in Bunyoro: Population and Environment in Western Uganda, 1860–1955* (Oxford: Currey, 2006).

Before HIV: Sexuality, Fertility and Mortality in East Africa, 1900–1980 (Oxford: Oxford University Press, 2013).

'Demography and Disease', in John Parker and Richard Reid (eds.), *The Oxford Handbook of Modern African History* (Oxford: Oxford University Press, 2013), 38–55.

Duffy, James, *A Question of Slavery: Labour Politics in Portuguese Africa and the British Protest, 1850–1920* (Oxford: Clarendon Press, 1967).

Duncan, James S., *In the Shadows of the Tropics: Climate, Race and Biopower in Nineteenth Century Ceylon* (Aldershot: Ashgate, 2007).

Eckart, Wolfgang U., 'Malariaprävention und Rassentrennung: Die ärztliche Vorbereitung und Rechtfertigung der Duala-Enteignung 1912–1914', *History and Philosophy of the Life Sciences* 10.2 (1988), 363–78.

'The Colony as Laboratory: German Sleeping Sickness Campaigns in German East Africa and in Togo, 1900–1914', *History and Philosophy of the Life Sciences* 24.1 (2002), 69–89.

'From Questionnaires to Microscopes: Founding and Early Years of the Hamburg Institute of Nautical and Tropical Diseases', in Benedikt Stuchtey (ed.), *Science across the European Empires, 1800–1950* (Oxford: Oxford University Press, 2005), 309–27.

Eckert, Andreas, 'Vom Segen der (Staats-)Gewalt? Staat, Verwaltung und koloniale Herrschaftspraxis in Afrika', in Alf Lüdtke, Michael Wildt and Gadi Algazi (eds.), *Staats-Gewalt: Ausnahmezustand und Sicherheitsregimes: Historische Perspektiven* (Göttingen: Wallstein-Verlag, 2008), 145–65.

'"We Are All Planners Now": Planung und Dekolonisation in Afrika', *Geschichte und Gesellschaft* 34 (2008), 375–97.

Eckl, Andreas E., *Herrschaft, Macht und Einfluß: Koloniale Interaktionen am Kavango (Nord-Namibia) von 1891 bis 1921* (Cologne: Köppe, 2004).

Ehlers, Sarah, *Europa und die Schlafkrankheit: Koloniale Seuchenbekämpfung, europäische Identitäten und moderne Medizin 1890–1950* (Göttingen: Vandenhoeck & Ruprecht, 2019).

Eltis, David and Richardson, David, 'A New Assesment of the Transatlantic Slave Trade', in David Eltis and David Richardson (eds.), *Extending the Frontiers: Essays on the New Atlantic Slave Trade Database* (New Haven/London: Yale University Press, 2008), 1–60.

Atlas of the Transatlantic Slave Trade (New Haven: Yale University Press, 2010).

Esteves, João, 'Adelaide Cabete', in António Nóvoa (ed.), *Dicionário de educadores portugueses* (Porto: Edições Asa, 2003), 203–6.

Farinha, Luís, *O Reviralho: revoltas republicanas contra a Ditadura e o Estado Novo, 1926–1940* (Lisbon: Ed. Estampa, 1998).

'Do Império Português à descolonização: Henrique Galvão e o Império', *História* 21 (2000), 18–28.

Farley, John, *To Cast Out Disease: A History of the International Health Division of the Rockefeller Foundation (1913–1951)* (Oxford: Oxford University Press, 2004).

Feierman, Steven, *The Shambaa Kingdom: A History* (Madison: University of Wisconsin Press, 1974).

Feierman, Steven and Janzen, John M. (eds.), *The Social Basis of Health and Healing in Africa* (Berkeley: University of California Press, 1992).

Ferguson, Angus H., Weaver, Lawrence T. and Nicolson, Malcolm, 'The Glasgow Corporation Milk Depot 1904–1910 and its Role in Infant Welfare: An End or a Means', *Social History of Medicine* 19.3 (2006), 443–60.

Ferreira, Roquinaldo, *Cross-Cultural Exchange in the Atlantic World: Angola and Brazil during the Era of the Slave Trade* (Cambridge: Cambridge University Press, 2012).

'Agricultural Enterprise and Unfree Labour in Nineteenth-Century Angola', in Robin Law, Suzanne Schwarz and Silke Strickrodt (eds.), *Commercial Agriculture, the Slave Trade and Slavery in Atlantic Africa* (Woodbridge: Currey, 2013), 225–43.

Fetter, Bruce (ed.), *Demography from Scanty Evidence: Central Africa in the Colonial Era* (Boulder, CO: Lynne Rienner Publishers, 1990).

'Demography in the Reconstruction of African Colonial History', in Bruce Fetter (ed.), *Demography from Scanty Evidence: Central Africa in the Colonial Era* (Boulder, CO: Lynne Rienner Publishers, 1990), 1–22.

Fischer-Tiné, Harald, *Pidgin-Knowledge: Wissen und Kolonialismus* (Zürich/Berlin: Diaphanes, 2013).

(ed.), *Anxieties, Fear and Panic in Colonial Settings: Empires on the Verge of a Nervous Breakdown* (Basingstoke: Palgrave Macmillan, 2016).

Fisch, Maria, *Die südafrikanische Militärverwaltung (1915–1920) und die frühe Mandatszeit (1920–1936) in der Kavango-Region/Namibia* (Cologne: Köppe, 2004).

Flint, Karen, 'Competition, Race and Professionalisation: African Healers and White Medical Practitioners in Natal, South Africa in the Early Twentieth Century', *Social History of Medicine* 14.2 (2001), 199–221.

Forclaz, Amalia Ribi, *Humanitarian Imperialism: The Politics of Anti-Slavery Activism, 1880–1940* (Oxford: Oxford University Press, 2015).

Ford, John, *The Role of the Trypanosomiases in African Ecology* (Oxford: Clarendon Press, 1971).

Foucault, Michel, *La volonté de savoir* (Paris: Gallimard, 1976).

'Cours du 17 mars 1976', in Mauro Bertani and Alessandro Fontana (eds.), *"Il faut défendre la société": Cours au Collège de France, 1975–1976* (Paris: Gallimard, 1997), 213–35.

Frankema, Ewout and Jerven, Morten, 'Writing History Backwards or Sideways: Towards a Consensus on African Population, 1850–2010', *Economic History Review* 67.4 (2014), 907–31.

Frankema, Ewout and van Waijenburg, Marlous, 'Metropolitan Blueprints of Colonial Taxation? Lessons from Fiscal Capacity Building in British and French Africa, c. 1880–1940', *Journal of African History* 55.3 (2014), 371–400.

Freeland, Alan, '"The Sick Man of the West": A Late Nineteenth-Century Diagnosis of Portugal', in T. F. Earle and Nigel Griffin (eds.), *Portuguese, Brazilian, and African Studies* (Warminster: Aris & Phillips, 1995), 205–16.

Freudenthal, Aida, 'Angola', in A. H. de Oliveira Marques (ed.), *O Império Africano, 1890–1930* (Lisbon: Estampa, 2001), 259–467.

Arimos e fazendas: a transição agrária em Angola 1850–1880 (Luanda: Chá de Caxinde, 2005).

Frey, Marc, 'Experten, Stiftungen und Politik: Zur Genese des globalen Diskurses über Bevölkerung seit 1945', *Zeithistorische Forschungen/Studies in Contemporary History* 4.1–2 (2007), 137–59.

'Neo-Malthusianism and Development: Shifting Interpretations of a Contested Paradigm', *Journal of Global History* 6 (2011), 75–97.

Gabriel, Manuel Nunes, *Angola, cinco séculos de cristianismo* (Queluz: Literal, 1978).

Gardner, Leigh, *Taxing Colonial Africa: The Political Economy of British Imperialism* (Oxford: Oxford University Press, 2012).

Garnel, Rita, 'A consolidação do poder médico: a medicina social nas teses da Escola Médico-cirúrgica de Lisboa (1900–1910)', in Ana Leonor Pereira and João Rui Pita (eds.), *Miguel Bombarda (1851–1910) e as singularidades de uma época* (Coimbra: Universidade de Coimbra, 2007), 77–88.

'Médicos e saúde pública no parlamento republicano', in Fernando Catroga and Pedro Tavares de Almeida (eds.), *Res publica: cidadania e representação política em Portugal, 1820–1926* (Lisbon: Assembleia da República, 2010), 230–57.

'Da Régia Escola de Cirurgia à Faculdade de Medicina de Lisboa: o ensino médico, 1825–1950', in Sérgio Campos Matos and Jorge Ramos do Ó (eds.), *A Universidade de Lisboa, séculos XIX–XX* (Lisbon: Tinta-da-China, 2013), Vol. 2, 538–650.

Garner, Raymond, *Watchdogs of Empire: The French Colonial Inspection Service in Action, 1815–1913*. Unpublished PhD thesis, University of Rochester, 1970.

Gervais, Raymond R. and Mandé, Issiaka, 'Comment compter les sujets de l'Empire? Les étapes d'une démographie impériale en AOF avant 1946', *Vingtième Siècle. Revue d'Histoire* 95 (2007), 63–74.

Giblin, James, 'Trypanosomiasis Control in African History: An Evaded Issue?', *Journal of African History* 31.1 (1990), 59–80.

Gibson, W., Stevens, J. and Truc, P., 'Identification of Trypanosomes: From Morphology to Molecular Biology', in Michel Dumas, Bernard Bouteille and Alain Buguet (eds.), *Progress in Human African Trypanosomiasis, Sleeping Sickness* (Berlin/Heidelberg/New York: Springer, 1999), 7–29.

Glasman, Joël, 'Penser les intermédiaires coloniaux: note sur les dossiers de carrière de la police du Togo', *History in Africa* 37 (2010), 51–81.

Goerg, Odile, 'From Hill Station (Free Town) to Downtown Conakry (First Ward): Comparing French and British Approaches to Segregation in Colonial Cities at the Beginning of the Twentieth Century', *Canadian Journal of African Studies* 32.1 (1998), 1–31.

Gomes, Joaquim Cardoso, *Os militares e a censura: a censura à imprensa na Ditadura Militar e Estado Novo (1926–1945)* (Lisbon: Livros Horizonte, 2006).

Gradmann, Christoph, 'It Seemed about Time to Try One of Those Modern Medicines: Animal and Human Experimentation in the Chemotherapy of Sleeping Sickness 1905–1908', in Volker Roelcke and Giovanni Maio (eds.), *Twentieth Century Ethics of Human Subjects Research: Historial Perspectives on Values, Practices, and Regulations* (Stuttgart: Franz Steiner, 2004), 83–97.

Gradmann, Christoph and Simon, Jonathan (eds.), *Evaluating and Standardizing Therapeutic Agents, 1890–1950* (Basingstoke: Palgrave Macmillan, 2010).

Greenalgh, Susanne, 'The Social Construction of Population Science: An Intellectual, Institutional, and Political History of Twentieth-Century Demography', *Comparative Studies in Society and History* 38.1 (1996), 26–66.

Grenfell, Frederick James, *The History of the Baptist Church in Angola and its Influence on the Life and Culture of the Kongo and Zombo People, 1879–1940.* Unpublished MA thesis, University of Leeds, 1995.

Grosse, Pascal, *Kolonialismus, Eugenik und bürgerliche Gesellschaft in Deutschland, 1850–1918* (Frankfurt: Campus-Verlag, 2000).

Guimarães, Ângela, *Uma corrente do colonialismo português: a Sociedade de Geografia de Lisboa, 1875–1895* (Lisbon: Livros Horizonte, 1984).

Hammond, Richard, *Portugal and Africa, 1815–1910: A Study in Uneconomic Imperialism* (Stanford: Stanford University Press, 1966).

Hardiman, David (ed.), *Healing Bodies, Saving Souls: Medical Missions in Asia and Africa* (Amsterdam: Rodopi, 2006).

'Introduction', in David Hardiman (ed.), *Healing Bodies, Saving Souls: Medical Missions in Asia and Africa* (Amsterdam: Rodopi, 2006), 1–57.

Harries, Patrick, *Work, Culture and Identity: Migrant Laborers in Mozambique and South Africa, c. 1860–1910* (Johannesburg: Witwatersrand University Press, 1994).

Harrison, Mark, *Climates and Constitutions: Health, Race, Environment and British Imperialism in India, 1600–1850* (New York: Oxford University Press, 1999).

Hartmann, Heinrich and Unger, Corinna R. (eds.), *A World of Populations: Transnational Perspectives on Demography in the Twentieth Century* (New York/Oxford: Berghahn Books, 2014).

Havik, Philip J., 'Bóticas e beberagens: a criação dos serviços de saúde e a colonização da Guiné', *Africana Studia* 10 (2007), 235–70.

'Ilhas desertas: impostos, comércio, trabalho forçado e o êxodo das Ilhas Bijagós (1925–1935)', in Centro de Estudos Africanos da Universidade do Porto (ed.), *Trabalho forçado africano: articulações com o poder político* (Porto: Campo das Letras, 2007), 171–89.

'Tributos e impostos: a crise mundial, o Estado Novo e a política fiscal na Guiné', *Economia e Sociologia* 85 (2008), 29–55.

'"Direct" or "indirect" rule? Reconsidering the Roles of Appointed Chiefs and Native Employees in Portuguese West Africa', *Africana Studia* 15 (2010), 29–56.

'Colonial Administration, Public Accounts and Fiscal Extraction: Policies and Revenues in Portuguese Africa', *African Economic History* 41 (2013), 159–221.

'Public Health and Tropical Modernity: The Combat against Sleeping Sickness in Portuguese Guinea, 1945-1974', *História, Ciências, Saúde – Manguinhos* 21.2 (2014), 641–66.

'O IHMT numa perspetiva histórica: trajetórias institucionais desde 1950', *Anais do Instituto de Higiene e Medicina Tropical* 14 (2015), 85–100.

'Hybridising Medicine: Illness, Healing and the Dynamics of Reciprocal Exchange on the Upper Guinea Coast (West Africa)', *Medical History* 60.2 (2016), 181–205.

'Administration, Economy, and Society in the Portuguese African Empire (1900–1975)', in M. S. Shanguhyia and Toyin Falola (eds.), *The Palgrave Handbook of African Colonial and Postcolonial History* (2018), 213–38.

'Public Health and Disease Control in Former Portuguese Africa: Negotiating Health System Management and Strategies, 1945–1965', in Poonam Bala (ed.), *Learning from Empire: Medicine, Knowledge and Transfers under Portuguese Rule* (Newcastle: Cambridge Scholars, 2018), 141–73.

'Public Health, Social Medicine and Disease Control: Medical Services, Maternal Care and Sexually Transmitted Diseases in Former Portuguese West Africa (1920–63)', *Medical History* 62.4 (2018), 485–506.

'Regional Cooperation and Health Diplomacy in Africa: From Intra-colonial Exchanges to Multilateral Health Institutions', *História, Ciências, Saúde – Manguinhos* 27 (2020), Supl. Setembro, 123–44.

Havik, Philip J., Keese, Alexander and Santos, Maciel (eds.), *Administration and Taxation in Former Portuguese Africa, 1900–1945* (Newcastle: Cambridge Scholars, 2015).

Havik, Philip J. and Newitt, Malyn (eds.), *Creole Societies in the Portuguese Colonial Empire* (Bristol: Bristol University Press, 2007).

Hayes, Patricia, 'The "Famine of the Dams": Gender, Labour and Politics in Colonial Ovamboland, 1929–1930', in Patricia Hayes, Jeremy Sylvester, Marion Wallace and Wolfram Hartmann (eds.), *Namibia under South African Rule: Mobility and Containment, 1915–46* (Oxford: James Currey, 1998), 117–46.

Haynes, Douglas Melvin, 'Framing Tropical Disease in London: Patrick Manson, Filaria Perstans, and the Uganda Sleeping Sickness Epidemic, 1891–1902', *Social History of Medicine* 13.3 (2000), 467–93.

Imperial Medicine: Patrick Manson and the Conquest of Tropical Disease (Philadelphia: University of Pennsylvania Press, 2001).

Headrick, Daniel R., *The Tools of Empire: Technology and European Imperialism in the 19th Century* (New York: Oxford University Press, 1981).

'Sleeping Sickness Epidemics and Colonial Responses in East and Central Africa, 1900–1940', *PLoS Neglected Tropical Diseases* 8.4 (2014), https://doi:10.1371/journal.pntd.0002772.

Headrick, Rita, *Colonialism, Health and Illness in French Equatorial Africa, 1885–1935* (Atlanta: African Studies Association Press, 1994).

Hedinger, Daniel and Heé, Nadin, 'Transimperial History: Connectivity, Cooperation and Competition', *Journal of Modern European History* 16.4 (2018), 429–52.

Heintze, Beatrix, *Studien zur Geschichte Angolas im 16. und 17. Jahrhundert: Ein Lesebuch* (Cologne: Köppe, 1996).

Heintze, Beatrix and Oppen, Achim von (eds.), *Angola on the Move: Transport Routes, Communications and History* (Frankfurt: Lembeck, 2008).

Heywood, Linda and Thornton, John, 'Demography, Production, and Labor: Central Angola, 1890–1950', in Dennis D. Cordell and Joel W. Gregory (eds.), *African Population and Capitalism: Historical Perspectives* (Boulder, CO: Westview Press, 1987), 241–54.

'African Fiscal Systems as Sources for Demographic History: The Case of Central Angola, 1799–1920', *Journal of African History* 29.2 (1988), 213–28.

Higgs, Catherine, *Chocolate Islands: Cocoa, Slavery, and Colonial Africa* (Athens: Ohio University Press, 2012).

Hochschild, Adam, *King Leopold's Ghost: A Story of Greed, Terror, and Heroism in Colonial Africa* (Boston: Houghton Mifflin, 1998).

Hodge, Joseph Morgan, *Triumph of the Expert: Agrarian Doctrines of Development and the Legacies of British Colonialism* (Athens: Ohio University Press, 2007).

Hodgson, Dennis, 'Demography as Social Science and Policy Science', *Population and Development Review* 9.1 (1983), 1–34.

Hodgson, Dorothy L., 'Taking Stock: State Control, Ethnic Identity and Pastoralist Development in Tanganyika, 1948–1958', *Journal of African History* 41.1 (2000), 55–78.

Hokkanen, Markku, 'Contestation, Redefinition and Healers' Tactics in Colonial Southern Africa', in Markku Hokkanen and Kalle Kananoja (eds.), *Healers and Empires in Global History: Healing as Hybrid and Contested Knowledge* (Basingstoke: Palgrave Macmillan, 2019), 115–48.

Hoppe, Kirk Arden, *Lords of the Fly: Sleeping Sickness Control in British East Africa, 1900–1960* (Westport, CT: Praeger, 2003).

Hugon, Anne, 'La redéfinition de la maternité en Gold Coast, des années 1920 aux années 1950: Projet colonial et réalités locales', in Anne Hugon (ed.), *Histoire des femmes en situation coloniale: Afrique et Asie, XXe siècle* (Paris: Karthala, 2004), 145–72.

Huhle, Teresa, *Bevölkerung, Fertilität und Familienplanung in Kolumbien: Eine transnationale Wissensgeschichte im Kalten Krieg* (Bielefeld: Transcript, 2017).

Hüntelmann, Axel C., *Paul Ehrlich: Leben, Forschung, Ökonomien, Netzwerke* (Göttingen: Wallstein-Verlag, 2011).

Hunt, Nancy Rose, '"Le Bébé en Brousse": European Women, African Birth Spacing and Colonial Intervention in Breast Feeding in the Belgian Congo', *International Journal of African Historical Studies* 21.3 (1988), 401–32.

'Noise over Camouflaged Polygamy, Colonial Morality Taxation, and a Woman-Naming Crisis in Belgian Africa', *Journal of African History* 32.3 (1991), 471–94.

A Colonial Lexicon of Birth Ritual, Medicalization, and Mobility in the Congo (Durham, NC: Duke University Press, 1999).

'Fertility's Fires and Empty Wombs in Recent Africanist Writing', *Africa. Journal of the International African Institute* 75.3 (2005), 421–35.

'Colonial Medical Anthropology and the Making of the Central African Infertility Belt', in Helen Tilley and Robert J. Gordon (eds.), *Ordering Africa: Anthropology, European Imperialism and the Politics of Knowledge* (Manchester: Manchester University Press, 2007), 252–81.

'Rewriting the Soul in a Flemish Congo', *Past and Present* 198 (2008), 185–215.

A Nervous State: Violence, Remedies, and Reverie in Colonial Congo (Durham, NC: Duke University Press, 2016).

Ikede, B., Ehlassan, E. and Akpavie, S., 'Reproductive Disorders in African Trypanosomiasis: A Review', *Acta Tropica* 45 (1988), 5–10.

Iliffe, John, *East African Doctors: A History of the Modern Profession* (Cambridge: Cambridge University Press, 1998).

Inda, Jonathan Xavier, 'Analytics of the Modern: An Introduction', in Jonathan Xavier Inda (ed.), *Anthropologies of Modernity: Foucault, Governmentality and Life Politics* (Malden, MA: Blackwell, 2005), 1–20.

Isobe, Hiroyuki, *Medizin und Kolonialgesellschaft: Die Bekämpfung der Schlafkrankheit in den deutschen "Schutzgebieten" vor dem Ersten Weltkrieg* (Münster: LIT, 2009).

Ittmann, Karl, 'The Colonial Office and the Population Question in the British Empire, 1918–1962', *Journal of Imperial and Commonwealth History* 27.3 (1999), 55–81.

'"Where Nature Dominates Man": Demographic Ideas and Policy in British Colonial Africa, 1890–1970', in Karl Ittmann, Dennis D. Cordell and Gregory H. Maddox (eds.), *The Demographics of Empire: The Colonial Order and the Creation of Knowledge* (Athens, OH: Ohio University Press, 2010), 59–88.

A Problem of Great Importance: Population, Race, and Power in the British Empire, 1918–1973 (Berkeley: University of California Press, 2013).

Janeiro, Helena Pinto, 'La Primera República portuguesa y las missiones católicas y laicas en Angola: financiación y poder', *Historia y Política* 29.1 (2013), 161–91.

Janzen, John M., *The Quest for Therapy: Medical Pluralism in Lower Zaire* (Berkeley: University of California Press, 1978).

Janzen, John M. and Feierman, Steven, 'Preface', in Steven Feierman and John M. Janzen (eds.), *The Social Basis of Health and Healing in Africa* (Berkeley: University of California Press, 1992), xv–viii.

Jennings, Eric Thomas, *Curing the Colonizers: Hydrotherapy, Climatology, and French Colonial Spas* (Durham, NC: Duke University Press, 2006).

Jennings, Michael, '"A Matter of Vital Importance": The Place of the Medical Mission in Maternal and Child Healthcare in Tanganyika, 1919–1939', in David Hardiman (ed.), *Healing Bodies, Saving Souls: Medical Missions in Asia and Africa* (Amsterdam: Rodopi, 2006), 227–50.

'"Healing of Bodies, Salvation of Souls": Missionary Medicine in Colonial Tanganyika, 1870s–1939', *Journal of Religion in Africa* 38.1 (2008), 27–56.

Jerónimo, Miguel Bandeira, *The 'Civilising Mission' of Portuguese Colonialism, 1870–1930* (Basingstoke: Palgrave Macmillan, 2015).

'"A Battle in the Field of Human Relations": The Official Minds of Repressive Development in Portuguese Angola', in Martin Thomas and Gareth Curless (eds.), *Decolonization and Conflict: Colonial Comparisons and Legacies* (London: Bloomsbury Academic, 2017), 115–36.

Jerónimo, Miguel Bandeira and Monteiro, José Pedro, 'Internationalism and Empire: The Question of Native Labour in the Portuguese Empire (1919–1962)', in Simon Jackson and Alanna O'Malley (eds.), *The Institution of International Order: From the League of Nations to the United Nations* (London/New York: Routledge, 2018), 206–33.

Jerónimo, Miguel Bandeira and Pinto, António Costa (eds.), *Portugal e o fim do colonialismo* (Lisbon: Edições 70, 2014).

The Ends of European Colonial Empires: Cases and Comparisons (Basingstoke: Palgrave Macmillan, 2015).

Jeurissen, Lissia, 'Les ambitions du colonialisme belge pour la "race mulâtre" (1918–1940)', *Belgisch Tijdschrift voor Nieuwste Geschiedenis* 32.3–4 (2002), 497–535.

Kalter, Christoph, *The Discovery of the Third World* (Cambridge: Cambridge University Press, 2016).

Kalusa, Walima T., 'Language, Medical Auxiliaries, and the Re-Interpretation of Missionary Medicine in Colonial Mwinilunga, Zambia, 1922–51', *Journal of Eastern African Studies* 1.1 (2007), 57–78.

Kananoja, Kalle, *Healing Knowledge in Atlantic Africa: Medical Encounters, 1500–1850* (Cambridge: Cambridge University Press, 2021).

Katzenellenbogen, Simon Ellis, *Railways and the Copper Mines of Katanga* (Oxford: Clarendon Press, 1973).

South Africa and Southern Mozambique: Labour, Railways and Trade in the Making of a Relationship (Manchester: Manchester University Press, 1982).

Keese, Alexander, '"Proteger os pretos": havia uma mentalidade reformista na administração portuguesa na África tropical (1926–1961)?', *Africana Studia* 6 (2003), 97–125.

Living with Ambiguity: Integrating an African Elite in French and Portuguese Africa, 1930–61 (Stuttgart: Steiner, 2007).

'Searching for the Reluctant Hands: Obsession, Ambivalence and the Practice of Organising Involuntary Labour in Colonial Cuanza-Sul and Malange Districts, Angola, 1926–1945', *Journal of Imperial and Commonwealth History* 41.2 (2013), 238–58.

'Forced Labour in the "Gorgulho Years": Understanding Reform and Repression in Rural São Tomé e Príncipe, 1945–1953', *Itinerario* 38.1 (2014), 103–24.

'Taxation, Evasion, and Compulsory Measures in Angola', in Philip J. Havik, Alexander Keese and Maciel Santos (eds.), *Administration and Taxation in Former Portuguese Africa, 1900–1945* (Newcastle: Cambridge Scholars, 2015), 98–137.

'Why Stay? Forced Labor, the Correia Report, and Portuguese-South African Competition at the Angola-Namibia Border, 1917–1939', *History in Africa* 42 (2015), 75–108.

Kreike, Emmanuel, *Re-creating Eden: Land Use, Environment, and Society in Southern Angola and Northern Namibia* (Portsmouth, NH: Heinemann, 2004).

Kucklick, Henrika, 'Personal Equations: Reflections on the History of Fieldwork, with Special Reference to Sociocultural Anthropology', *Isis* 102.1 (2011), 1–33.

Kwaschik, Anne, 'Die Verwissenschaftlichung des Kolonialen als kultureller Code und internationale Praxis um 1900', *Historische Anthropologie* 28.3 (2020), 399–423.

Lachenal, Guillaume, 'Le médecin qui voulut être roi: médecine coloniale et utopie au Cameroun', *Annales. Histoire, Sciences Sociales* 65.1 (2010), 121–56.

'A Genealogy of Treatment as Prevention (TasP): Prevention, Therapy, and the Tensions of Public Health in African History', in Tamara Giles-Vernick and James L. A. Webb Jr. (eds.), *Global Health in Africa: Historical Perspectives on Disease Control* (Athens: Ohio University Press, 2013), 70–91.

'Médecine, comparaisons et échanges inter-impériaux dans le mandat camerounais: une histoire croisée franco-allemande de la mission Jamot', *Canadian Bulletin of Medical History* 30.2 (2013), 23–45.

Le médicament qui devait sauver l'Afrique: un scandale pharmaceutique aux colonies (Paris: La Découverte, 2014).

Lains, Pedro, 'Causas do colonialismo português em África, 1822–1975', *Análise Social* 33 (1998), 463–96.

Landau, Paul S., 'Explaining Surgical Evangelism in Colonial Southern Africa: Teeth, Pain and Faith', *Journal of African History* 37.2 (1996), 261–81.

Latour, Bruno, *The Pasteurization of France* (Cambridge, MA: Harvard University Press, 1988).

Lawrance, Benjamin N., Osborn, Emily Lynn and Roberts, Richard L. (eds.), *Intermediaries, Interpreters, and Clerks* (Madison, WI: University of Wisconsin Press, 2006).

Lindner, Ulrike, 'Transnational Movements between Colonial Empires: Migrant Workers from the British Cape Colony in the German Diamond Town of Luderitzbucht', *European Review of History* 16.5 (2009), 679–95.

'The Transfer of European Social Policy Concepts to Tropical Africa, 1900–50: The Example of Maternal and Child Welfare', *Journal of Global History* 9.2 (2014), 208–31.

Livi Bacci, Massimo, *A Century of Portuguese Fertility* (Princeton: Princeton University Press, 1971).

Livingstone, David N., 'Tropical Climate and Moral Hygiene: The Anatomy of a Victorian Debate', *British Journal for the History of Science* 32.1 (1999), 93–110.

Lousada, Isabel, *Adelaide Cabete (1867–1935)* (Lisbon: Presidência do Conselho de Ministros, 2010).

Lyons, Maryinez, 'From "Death Camps" to Cordon Sanitaire: The Development of Sleeping Sickness Policy in the Uele District of the Belgian Congo, 1903–1914', *Journal of African History* 26.1 (1985), 69–91.

The Colonial Disease: A Social History of Sleeping Sickness in Northern Zaire, 1900–1940 (Cambridge: Cambridge University Press, 1992).

'The Power to Heal: African Auxiliaries in Colonial Belgian Congo and Uganda', in Dagmar Engels and Shula Marks (eds.), *Contesting Colonial Hegemony: State and Society in Africa and India* (London: I.B. Tauris & Co, 1994), 202–23.

MacLeod, Roy (ed.), *Disease, Medicine, and Empire: Perspectives on Western Medicine and the Experience of European Expansion* (London: Routledge, 1988).

'Introduction', in Roy MacLeod (ed.), *Disease, Medicine, and Empire: Perspectives on Western Medicine and the Experience of European Expansion* (London: Routledge, 1988), 1–18.

Macola, Giacomo, *The Kingdom of Kazembe: History and Politics in North-Eastern Zambia and Katanga to 1950* (Münster: LIT, 2002).

Madeira, Ana Isabel, 'Popular Education and Republican Ideals: The Portuguese Lay Missions in Colonial Africa, 1917–1927', *Paedagogica Historica* 47.1–2 (2011), 123–38.

Mann, Gregory, 'What Was the Indigénat? The "Empire of Law" in French West Africa', *Journal of African History* 50 (2009), 331–53.

Manning, Patrick, 'African Population: Projections, 1850–1960', in Karl Ittmann, Dennis D. Cordell and Gregory H. Maddox (eds.), *The Demographics of Empire: The Colonial Order and the Creation of Knowledge* (Athens: Ohio University Press, 2010), 245–75.

Mannweiler, Erich, *Geschichte des Instituts für Schiffs- und Tropenkrankheiten in Hamburg, 1900–1945* (Keltern-Weiler: Goecke & Evers, 1998).

Marques, A. H. de Oliveira, 'Introdução: aspectos de política geral', in A. H. de Oliveira Marques (ed.), *O Império Africano, 1890–1930* (Lisbon: Estampa, 2001), 21–30.

Marques, João Pedro, *The Sounds of Silence: Nineteenth-Century Portugal and the Abolition of the Slave Trade* (New York: Berghahn Books, 2006).

Marshall, Dominique, 'Children's Rights in Imperial Political Cultures: Missionary and Humanitarian Contributions to the Conference on the African Child of 1931', *International Journal of Children's Rights* 12.3 (2004), 273–318.

Masuy-Stroobant, Godelieve and Humblet, Perrine C. (eds.), *Mères et nourissons: de la bienfaisance à la protection médico-sociale (1830–1945)* (Brussels: Éditions Labor, 2004).

Matos, Patrícia Ferraz de, *As côres do Império: representações raciais no Império Colonial Português* (Lisbon: Imprensa de Ciências Sociais, 2006).

'Aperfeiçoar a "raça", salvar a nação: eugenia, teorias nacionalistas e situação colonial em Portugal', *Trabalhos de Antropologia e Etnologia* 50 (2010), 89–111.

Matos, Paulo Teodoro de, 'Counting Portuguese Colonial Populations, 1776–1875: A Research Note', *The History of the Family* 21.2 (2016), 267–80.

McIntosh, Tania, *A Social History of Maternity and Childbirth: Key Themes in Maternity Care* (London: Routledge, 2012).

McKelvey, John Jay, *Man against Tsetse: Struggle for Africa* (Ithaca: Cornell University Press, 1973).

Meneses, Filipe Ribeiro de, *Salazar: A Political Biography* (New York: Enigma Books, 2010).

Mertens, Myriam, *Chemical Compounds in the Congo: Pharmaceuticals and the 'Crossed History' of Public Health in Belgian Africa (ca. 1905–1939)*. Unpublished PhD thesis, Universiteit Gent, 2014.

Mertens, Myriam and Lachenal, Guillaume, 'The History of "Belgian" Tropical Medicine from a Cross-Border Perspective', *Belgisch Tijdschrift voor Filologie en Geschiedenis* 90.4 (2012), 1249–72.

Messiant, Christine, *L'Angola colonial, histoire et société: 1961 – les prémisses du mouvement nationaliste* (Basel: Schlettwein, 2006).

Miers, Suzanne, *Slavery in the Twentieth Century: The Evolution of a Global Problem* (Walnut Creek, CA: Altamira Press, 2003).

Miller, Joseph C., *Way of Death: Merchant Capitalism and the Angolan Slave Trade, 1730–1830* (Madison: University of Wisconsin Press, 1988).

Monteiro, José Pedro, *Portugal e a questão do trabalho forçado: um império sob escrutínio (1944–1962)* (Lisbon: Edições 70, 2018).

Montoito, Eugénio, *Henrique Galvão: ou a dissidência de um cadete do 28 de Maio (1927–1952)* (Lisbon: Centro de História da Universidade de Lisboa, 2005).

Mora, Luiz Damas, *António Damas Mora: um médico português entre os trópicos* (Lisbon: By the Book, 2017).

Morier-Genoud, Eric (ed.), *Sure Road? Nationalisms in Angola, Guinea-Bissau and Mozambique* (Leiden/Boston: Brill, 2012).

Moses, A. Dirk (ed.), *Empire, Colony, Genocide: Conquest, Occupation, and Subaltern Resistance in World History* (New York: Berghahn Books, 2008).

Moura, Maria Lúcia de Brito, *A 'guerra religiosa' na I República*, 2nd revised edn. (Lisbon: Universidade Católica Portuguesa, 2010).

Mudimbe, V. Y., *The Invention of Africa: Gnosis, Philosophy, and the Order of Knowledge* (Bloomington: Indiana University Press, 1988).

Musambachime, M. C., 'Protest Migrations in Mweru-Luapula, 1900–1940', *African Studies* 47.1 (1988), 19–34.

Nascimento, Augusto, 'O recrutamento de serviçais moçambicanos para as roças de São Tomé e Príncipe (1908–1921)', in *Actas do Seminário Moçambique: navegações, comércio e técnicas* (Lisbon: Comissão Nacional para as Comemorações dos Descobrimentos Portugueses, 1998), 173–204.

Neill, Deborah Joy, 'Paul Ehrlich's Colonial Connections: Scientific Networks and Sleeping Sickness Drug Therapy Research, 1900–1914', *Social History of Medicine* 22.1 (2009), 61–77.

Networks in Tropical Medicine: Internationalism, Colonialism, and the Rise of a Medical Specialty, 1890–1930 (Stanford: Stanford University Press, 2012).

Neto, Maria da Conceição, 'Ideologias, contradições e mistificações da colonização de Angola no século XX', *Lusotopie* (1997), 327–59.

Neto, Vitor, 'A questão religiosa: Estado, Igreja e conflitualidade sócio-religiosa', in Fernando Rosas and Maria Fernanda Rollo (eds.), *História da Primeira República Portuguesa* (Lisbon: Tinta-da-China, 2009), 129–48.

Newitt, Malyn, *A History of Mozambique* (London: Hurst, 1995).

'British Travellers' Accounts of Portuguese Africa in the Nineteenth Century', *Revista de Estudos Anglo-Portugueses* 11 (2002), 103–29.

'The Portuguese African Colonies during the Second World War', in Judith A. Byfield, Carolyn A. Brown, Timothy Parsons and Ahmad Alawad Sikainga (eds.), *Africa and World War II* (New York: Cambridge University Press, 2015), 220–37.

Nieto-Andrade, Benjamin et al., 'Women's Limited Choice and Availability of Modern Contraception at Retail Outlets and Public-Sector Facilities in Luanda, Angola, 2012–2015', *Global Health: Science and Practice* 5.1 (2017), 75–89.

Nugent, Paul, *Smugglers, Secessionists and Loyal Citizens on the Ghana-Togo Frontier: The Life of the Borderlands since 1914* (Athens: Ohio University Press, 2002).

Oliveira, Pedro Aires, 'O ciclo africano', in João Paulo Oliveira e Costa, José Damião Rodrigues and Pedro Aires Oliveira (eds.), *História da Expansão e do Império Português* (Lisbon: A Esfera dos Livros, 2014), 341–545.

Olmsted, James, *Charles-Édouard Brown-Séquard: A Nineteenth Century Neurologist and Endocrinologist* (Baltimore: Johns Hopkins Press, 1946).

Osborne, Michael A., 'Acclimatizing the World: A History of the Paradigmatic Colonial Science', in Roy MacLeod (ed.), *Nature and Empire: Science and the Colonial Enterprise* (2000), 135–51.

Osterhammel, Jürgen, '"The Great Work of Uplifting Mankind": Zivilisierungsmission und Moderne', in Boris Barth and Jürgen Osterhammel (eds.), *Zivilisierungsmissionen: Imperiale Weltverbesserung seit dem 18. Jahrhundert* (Konstanz: UVK Verlagsgesellschaft, 2005), 363–425.

Overath, Petra, 'Bevölkerungforschung transnational: Eine Skizze zu Interaktionen zwischen Wissenschaft und Politik am Beispiel der "International Union for the Scientific Study of Population"', in Petra Overath (ed.), *Die vergangene Zukunft Europas: Bevölkerungsforschung und -prognosen im 20. und 21. Jahrhundert* (Cologne: Böhlau, 2011), 57–83.

Pacheco, Carlos, 'Arquivos queimados em Angola!', in Carlos Pacheco, *Repensar Angola* (Lisbon: Vega, 2000), 33–7.

Packard, Randall, 'The History of the Social Determinants of Health in Africa', in Harold John Cook, Sanjoy Bhattacharya and Anne Hardy (eds.), *History of the*

Social Determinants of Health: Global Histories, Contemporary Debates (Hyderabad: Orient BlackSwan, 2009), 42–77.

The Making of a Tropical Disease: A Short History of Malaria (Baltimore: Johns Hopkins University Press, 2007).

A History of Global Health: Interventions into the Lives of Other Peoples (Baltimore: Johns Hopkins University Press, 2016).

Paillard, Yvan-Georges, 'Les recherches démographiques sur Madagascar au début de l'époque coloniale et les documents de "l'AMI"', *Cahiers d'Études Africaines* 27.105–6 (1987), 17–42.

Parascandola, John, 'From Mercury to Miracle Drugs: Syphilis Therapy over the Centuries', *Pharmacy in History* 51.1 (2009), 14–23.

Patton, Adell, *Physicians, Colonial Racism, and Diaspora in West Africa* (Gainesville: University Press of Florida, 1996).

Péclard, Didier, '"Eu sou americano": dynamiques du champ missionnaire dans le planalto central angolais au XXe siècle', *Lusotopie* 5 (1998), 357–76.

Les incertitudes de la nation en Angola: aux racines sociales de l'UNITA (Paris: Karthala, 2015).

Pedersen, Susan, *Family, Dependence, and the Origins of the Welfare State: Britain and France, 1914–1945* (Cambridge: Cambridge University Press, 1995).

Pélissier, René, *História das campanhas de Angola: resistência e revoltas (1845–1941)*, 2 vols. (Lisbon: Editorial Estampa, 1986).

Penvenne, Jeanne Marie, 'Settling Against the Tide: The Layered Contradictions of Twentieth-Century Portuguese Settlement in Mozambique', in Caroline Elkins and Susan Pedersen (eds.), *Settler Colonialism in the Twentieth Century: Projects, Practices, Legacies* (New York: Routledge, 2005), 79–94.

Pereira, Ana Leonor, 'Eugenia em Portugal?', *Revista de História das Ideias* 20 (1999), 531–600.

Pereira, Ana Leonor and Pita, João Rui (eds.), *Miguel Bombarda (1851–1910) e as singularidades de uma época* (Coimbra: Universidade de Coimbra, 2007).

Pereira, Victor, 'La dictature salazariste et le "problème démographique"', *Annales de Démographie Historique* 2 (2014), 159–86.

Perrings, Charles, '"Good Lawyers but Poor Workers": Recruited Angolan Labour in the Copper Mines of Katanga, 1917–1921', *Journal of African History* 18.2 (1977), 237–59.

Black Mineworkers in Central Africa (New York: Africana Publ., 1979).

Pesek, Michael, *Koloniale Herrschaft in Deutsch-Ostafrika: Expeditionen, Militär und Verwaltung seit 1880* (Frankfurt/Main: Campus, 2005).

Pestre, Dominique, 'Pour une histoire sociale et culturelle des sciences', *Annales. Histoire, Sciences Sociales* 50.3 (1995), 487–521.

Pimenta, Fernando Tavares, *Angola, os brancos e a independência* (Porto: Edições Afrontamento, 2008).

Pimentel, Irene Flunser, *História das organizações femininas do Estado Novo* (Lisbon: Temas e Debates, 2001).

A cada um o seu lugar: a política feminina do Estado Novo (Lisbon: Círculo de Leitores, 2011).

Polanah, Paulo S., 'An Imperial Mystique: Colonial Discourse and National Identity in Portugal, 1930–1945', *Portuguese Studies Review* 16.1 (2008), 61–86.

Porter, Dorothy, 'Introduction', in Dorothy Porter (ed.), *Social Medicine and Medical Sociology in the Twentieth Century* (Amsterdam: Rodopi, 1997), 1–31.

Porter, Dorothy and Porter, Roy, 'What was Social Medicine? An Historiographical Essay', *Journal of Historical Sociology* 1.1 (1988), 90–106.

Proctor, Robert N. and Schiebinger, Londa (eds.), *Agnotology: The Making and Unmaking of Ignorance* (Stanford: Stanford University Press, 2008).

Proença, Maria Cândida, 'A questão colonial', in Fernando Rosas and Maria Fernando Rollo (eds.), *História da Primeira República Portuguesa* (Lisbon: Tinta-da-China, 2009), 205–28; 503–21.

Quirke, Viviane and Slinn, Judy, 'Introduction', in Viviane Quirke and Judy Slinn (eds.), *Perspectives on Twentieth-Century Pharmaceuticals* (Oxford: Peter Lang, 2010), 1–34.

Raj, Kapil, 'Beyond Postcolonialism . . . and Postpositivism: Circulation and the Global History of Science', *Isis* 104.2 (2013), 337–47.

Ranger, Terence, 'Godly Medicine: The Ambiguities of Medical Mission in Southeast Tanzania', *Social Science and Medicine* 15B.3 (1981), 261–77.

Reinkowski, Maurus and Thum, Gregor (eds.), *Helpless Imperialists: Imperial Failure, Fear and Radicalization* (Göttingen: Vandenhoeck & Ruprecht, 2013).

Riethmiller, Steven, 'From Atoxyl to Salvarsan: Searching for the Magic Bullet', *Chemotherapy* 51 (2005), 234–342.

Rooke, P. T. and Schnell, R. L., '"Uncramping Child Life": International Children's Organisations, 1914–1939', in Paul Weindling (ed.), *International Health Organisations and Movements, 1918–1939* (Cambridge: Cambridge University Press, 1995), 176–202.

Roque, Ricardo, *Antropologia e Império: Fonseca Cardoso e a expedição à Índia em 1895* (Lisbon: Imprensa de Ciências Sociais, 2001).

'The Razor's Edge: Portuguese Imperial Vulnerability in Colonial Moxico, Angola', *The International Journal of African Historical Studies* 36.1 (2003), 105–24.

Headhunting and Colonialism: Anthropology and the Circulation of Human Skulls in the Portuguese Empire, 1870–1930 (Basingstoke/New York: Palgrave Macmillan, 2010).

Rosas, Fernando and Rollo, Maria Fernando (eds.), *História da Primeira República Portuguesa* (Lisbon: Tinta-da-China, 2009).

Rosental, Paul-André, 'Pour une histoire politique des populations', *Annales. Histoire, Sciences Sociales* 61.1 (2006), 7–29.

'Wissenschaftlicher Internationalismus und Verbreitung der Demographie zwischen den Weltkriegen', in Patrick Krassnitzer and Petra Overath (eds.), *Bevölkerungsfragen: Prozesse des Wissenstransfers in Deutschland und Frankreich (1870–1939)* (Cologne: Böhlau, 2007), 255–91.

Saada, Emmannuelle, *Empire's Children: Race, Filiation, and Citizenship in the French Colonies* (Chicago: Chicago University Press, 2012).

Saavedra, Mónica, *A malária em Portugal: histórias e memórias* (Lisbon: Imprensa de Ciências Sociais, 2014).

Sá, Isabel dos Guimarães and Lopes, Maria Antónia, *História breve das Misericórdias portuguesas, 1498–2000* (Coimbra: Imprensa da Universidade de Coimbra, 2008).

Sanderson, Jean-Paul, 'Le Congo belge entre mythe et réalité: une analyse du discours démographique colonial', *Population* 55.2 (2000), 331–55.

Démographie coloniale congolaise: entre spéculation, idéologie et reconstruction historique (Louvain-la-Neuve: Presses Universitaires de Louvain, 2018).

Santos, Boaventura de Sousa, 'Between Prospero and Caliban: Colonialism, Postcolonialism, and Inter-identity', *Luso-Brasilian Review* 39.2 (2002), 9–43.

Santos, Catarina Madeira, 'Administrative Knowledge in a Colonial Context: Angola in the Eighteenth Century', *The British Journal for the History of Science* 43.4 (2010), 539–56.

Santos, Gonçalo Duro dos, 'The Birth of Physical Anthropology in Late Imperial Portugal', *Current Anthropology* 53.S5 (2012), S33–S55.

Santos, Maciel, 'Peasant Tax and the Funding of the Colonial State in the Portuguese Colonies (1900–1939)', in Philip J. Havik, Alexander Keese and Maciel Santos (eds.), *Administration and Taxation in Former Portuguese Africa, 1900–1945* (Newcastle: Cambridge Scholars, 2015), 28–81.

Sarasin, Philipp, *Michel Foucault zur Einführung*, revised 2nd edn. (Hamburg: Junius Verlag, 2006).

Schiebinger, Londa, 'Feminist History of Colonial Science', *Hypatia* 19.1 (2004), 233–54.

Secret Cures of Slaves: People, Plants, and Medicine in the Eighteenth-Century Atlantic World (Stanford: Stanford University Press, 2017).

Schneider, William H., *Quality and Quantity: The Quest for Biological Regeneration in Twentieth Century France* (Cambridge: Cambridge University Press, 1990).

Sealey, Anne, *The League of Nations Health Organisation and the Evolution of Transnational Public Health*. Unpublished PhD thesis, Ohio State University, 2011.

Seibert, Julia, 'More Continuity than Change? New Forms of Unfree Labor in the Belgian Congo, 1908–1930', in Marcel van der Linden (ed.), *Humanitarian Intervention and Changing Labor Relations: The Long-Term Consequences of the Abolition of the Slave Trade* (Leiden/Boston: Brill, 2011), 369–86.

Shapiro, Martin Frederick, *Medicine in the Service of Colonialism: Medical Care in Portuguese Africa, 1885–1974*. Unpublished PhD thesis, University of California, 1983.

Silva, Cristina Nogueira da, *Constitucionalismo e Império: a cidadania no Ultramar português* (Lisbon: Almedina, 2009).

'Natives who were Citizens and Natives who were Indigenas in the Portuguese Empire (1900–1926)', in Alfred W. McCoy (ed.), *Endless Empire: Spain's Retreat, Europe's Eclipse, America's Decline* (Madison: University of Wisconsin Press, 2012), 295–305.

Silva, Daniel B. Domingues da, 'The Atlantic Slave Trade from Angola: A Port-by-Port Estimate of Slaves Embarked, 1701–1867', *International Journal of African Historical Studies* 46.1 (2013), 105–22.

The Atlantic Slave Trade from West Central Africa, 1780–1867 (Cambridge: Cambridge University Press, 2017).

Silva, Sebastião Nuno de Araújo Barros e, *The Land of Flies, Children and Devils: The Sleeping Sickness Epidemic in the Island of Príncipe (1870s–1914)*. Unpublished PhD thesis, University of Oxford, 2013.

Simarro, Pere P. et al., 'The Human African Trypanosomiasis Control and Surveillance Programme of the World Health Organization 2000–2009: The Way Forward',

PLoS – Neglected Tropical Diseases 5.2 (2011), https://doi.org/10.1371/journal
.pntd.0001007.

Sobral, José Manuel, Lima, Maria Luísa, Sousa, Paulo Silveira e and Castro, Paula,
'Perante a pneumônica: a epidemia e as respostas das autoridades de saúde pública
e dos agentes políticos em Portugal', *Varia História* 25.42 (2009), 377–402.

Soff, Harvey G., 'Sleeping Sickness in the Lake Victoria Region of British East Africa,
1900–1915', *African Historical Studies* 2.2 (1969), 255–68.

Soloway, Richard Allen, *Demography and Degeneration: Eugenics and the Declining
Birthrate in Twentieth Century Britain* (Chapel Hill: University of North Carolina
Press, 1990).

Soremekun, Fola, *A History of the American Board Missions in Angola, 1880–1940*.
Unpublished PhD thesis, Northwestern University, 1965.

Sousa, Fernando Alberto Pereira de, *A história da estatística em Portugal* (Lisbon: INE,
1995).

Spittler, Gerd, *Verwaltung in einem afrikanischen Bauernstaat: Das koloniale
Französisch-Westafrika, 1919–1939* (Freiburg: Steiner, 1981).

Stanghellini, A. and Josenando, T., 'The Situation of Sleeping Sickness in Angola:
A Calamity', *Tropical Medicine and International Health* 6.5 (2001), 330–4.

Stanley, Brian, *The History of the Baptist Missionary Society, 1792–1992* (Edinburgh:
T&T Clark, 1992).

Steinmetz, George, *The Devil's Handwriting: Precoloniality and the German Colonial
State in Qingdao, Samoa, and Southwest Africa* (Chicago: Chicago University
Press, 2007).

Stepan, Nancy Leys, *"The Hour of Eugenics": Race, Gender, and Nation in Latin
America* (Ithaca/London: Cornell University Press, 1991).
    Picturing Tropical Nature (London: Reaktion Books, 2001).
    Eradication: Ridding the World of Diseases Forever? (London: Reaktion Books,
    2011).

Steverding, Dietmar, 'The History of African Trypanosomiasis', *Parasites & Vectors*
1.3 (2008), https://doi.org/10.1186/1756-3305-1-3.

Stoler, Ann Laura, *Race and the Education of Desire: Foucault's History of Sexuality
and the Colonial Order of Things* (Durham, NC: Duke University Press, 1995).
    Carnal Knowledge and Imperial Power: Race and the Intimate in Colonial Rule
    (Berkeley: University of California Press, 2002).
    'On Degrees of Imperial Sovereignty', *Public Culture* 18.1 (2006), 125–46.
    Along the Archival Grain: Epistemic Anxieties and Colonial Common Sense
    (Princeton: Princeton University Press, 2008).

Stoler, Ann Laura and McGranahan, Carole, 'Introduction: Refiguring Imperial
Terrains', in Ann Laura Stoler, Carole McGranahan and Peter C. Perdue (eds.),
Imperial Formations (Santa Fe, NM: School for Advanced Research Press, 2007),
3–42.

Stone, Glyn, 'The Foreign Office and Forced Labour in Portuguese West Africa,
1894–1914', in Keith Hamilton and Patrick Salmon (eds.), *Slavery, Diplomacy
and Empire: Britain and the Suppression of the Slave Trade, 1807–1975* (Sussex
Academic Press, 2009), 165–95.

Stornig, Katharina, 'Promoting Distant Children in Need: Christian Imagery in the Late
Nineteenth and Early Twentieth Centuries', in Johannes Paulmann (ed.),

Humanitarianism and Media: 1900 to the Present (Oxford/New York: Berghahn, 2019), 41–66.

Summers, Carol, 'Intimate Colonialism: The Imperial Production of Reproduction in Uganda, 1907–1925', *Signs* 16.4 (1991), 787–807.

Swanson, Maynard W., 'The Sanitation Syndrome: Bubonic Plague and Urban Native Policy in the Cape Colony, 1900–1909', *Journal of African History* 18.3 (1977), 387–410.

Szreter, Simon, 'The Idea of Demographic Transition and the Study of Fertility Change: A Critical Intellectual History', *Population and Development Review* 19.4 (1993), 659–701.

Tantchou, Josiane, *Épidémie et politique en Afrique: maladie du sommeil et tuberculose au Cameroun* (Paris: L'Harmattan, 2007).

Teitelbaum, Michael S. and Winter, Jay, *The Fear of Population Decline* (Orlando: Academic Press, 1985).

Teixeira, Nuno Severiano, *O Ultimatum inglês: política externa e política interna no Portugal de 1890* (Lisbon: Alfa, 1990).

Thébaud, Françoise, 'Le mouvement nataliste dans la France de l'entre-deux-guerres: L'Alliance nationale pour l'accroissement de la population française', *Revue d'Histoire Moderne et Contemporaine* 32 (1985), 276–301.

Quand nos grand-mères donnaient la vie: la maternité en France dans l'entre-deux-guerres (Lyon: Presses Universitaires de Lyon, 1986).

Thomas, Lynn, *Politics of the Womb: Women, Reproduction and the State in Kenya* (Berkeley: University of California Press, 2003).

Thompson, Estevam C., 'Taking the Graduate Students to Luanda and Benguela: A Brazilian Perspective', *Harriet Tubman Newsletter* 31 (2012), 14–25.

Thornton, John K., 'Early Kongo-Portuguese Relations: A New Interpretation', *History in Africa* 8 (1981), 183–204.

A History of West Central Africa to 1850 (Cambridge: Cambridge University Press, 2020).

Tilley, Helen, 'Ecologies of Complexity: Tropical Environments, African Trypanosomiasis, and the Science of Disease Control in British Colonial Africa, 1900–1940', *Osiris* 19 (2004), 21–38.

Africa as a Living Laboratory: Empire, Development, and the Problem of Scientific Knowledge, 1870–1950 (Chicago: Chicago University Press, 2011).

Tomlinson, Richard Peter, 'The "Disappearance" of France, 1896–1940: French Politics and the Birth Rate', *The Historical Journal* 28 (1985), 405–15.

Tornimbeni, Corrado, 'The State, Labour Migration and the Transnational Discourse: A Historical Perspective from Mozambique', *Stichproben. Wiener Zeitschrift für kritische Afrikastudien* 8 (2005), 307–28.

Torres, Adelino, 'Angola: conflitos políticos e sistema social (1928–1930)', *Revista de Estudos Afro-Asiáticos* 32 (1997), 163–83.

Tousignant, Noémi, 'Trypanosomes, Toxicity and Resistance: The Politics of Mass Therapy in French Colonial Africa', *Social History of Medicine* 25.3 (2012), 625–43.

Trotha, Trutz von, *Koloniale Herrschaft: Zur soziologischen Theorie der Staatsentstehung am Beispiel des 'Schutzgebietes Togo'* (Tübingen: Mohr, 1994).

'Was war Kolonialismus? Einige zusammenfassende Befunde zur Soziologie und Geschichte des Kolonialismus und der Kolonialherrschaft', *Saeculum. Jahrbuch für Universalgeschichte* 55 (2004), 49–95.

Tschapek, Rolf Peter, *Bausteine eines zukünftigen deutschen Mittelafrika: Deutscher Imperialismus und die portugiesischen Kolonien* (Stuttgart: Steiner, 2000).

Tucker, John T. (ed.), *Angola: The Land of the Blacksmith Prince* (London/New York/ Toronto: World Dominion Press, 1933).

Turda, Marius and Gillette, Aaron, *Latin Eugenics in Comparative Perspective* (London: Bloomsbury Academic, 2014).

Turrittin, Jane, 'Colonial Midwives and Modernizing Childbirth in French West Africa', in Jean Marie Allman, Susan Geiger and Nakanyike Musisi (eds.), *Women in African Colonial Histories* (Bloomington: Indiana University Press, 2002), 71–91.

Tworek, Heidi J. S., 'Communicable Disease: Information, Health, and Globalization in the Interwar Period', *American Historical Review* 124.3 (2019), 813–42.

Uvin, Peter, 'On Counting, Categorizing and Violence in Burundi and Rwanda', in David Kertzer and Dominique Arel (eds.), *Census and Identity: The Politics of Race, Ethnicity, and Language in National Censuses* (Cambridge: Cambridge University Press, 2002), 148–75.

Vahekeni, Nina et al., 'Use of Herbal Remedies in the Management of Sleeping Sickness in Four Northern Provinces of Angola', *Journal of Ethnopharmacology* 256 (2020), https://doi.org/10.1016/j.jep.2019.112382.

van Beusekom, Monica M., 'From Underpopulation to Overpopulation: French Perceptions of Population, Environment, and Agricultural Development in French Soudan (Mali), 1900–1960', *Environmental History* 4.2 (1999), 198–219.

van den Bersselaar, Dmitri, 'Establishing the Facts: P. A. Talbot and the 1921 Census of Nigeria', *History in Africa* 31 (2004), 69–102.

van Tol, Deanne, 'Mothers, Babies and the Colonial State: The Introduction of Maternal and Infant Welfare Services in Nigeria, 1925–1945', *Spontaneous Generations* 1.1 (2007), 110–31.

van-Dúnem, Maria Manuela Batalha, *Plantas medicinais de Angola: medicamentos ao alcance de todos* (Luanda: Cooperação Portuguesa, 1994).

Vansina, Jan, *Being Colonized: The Kuba Experience in Rural Congo, 1880–1960* (Madison: University of Wisconsin Press, 2010).

Vanthemsche, Guy, *La Belgique et le Congo: empreintes d'une colonie, 1885–1980* (Brussels: Complexe, 2007).

Varanda, Jorge, '*A Bem da Nação*': Medical Science in a Diamond Company in Portuguese Angola. Unpublished PhD thesis, University College London, 2006.

'Um cavalo de Tróia na colónia? As missões de profilaxia contra a doença do sono da Companhia de Diamantes de Angola (Diamang)', in Luís Silva Pereira and Chiara Pussetti (eds.), *Os saberes da cura: antropologia da doença e práticas terapêuticas* (Lisbon: Instituto Superior de Psicologia Aplicada, 2009), 79–110.

'Crossing Colonies and Empires: The Health Services of the Diamond Company of Angola', in Anne Digby, Waltraud Ernst and Projit B. Muhkarji (eds.), *Crossing Colonial Historiographies: Histories of Colonial and Indigenous Medicines in Transnational Perspective* (Newcastle: Cambridge Scholars, 2010), 165–84.

'Cuidados biomédicos de saúde em Angola e na Companhia de Diamantes de Angola, c. 1910–1970', *História, Ciências, Saúde – Manguinhos* 21.2 (2014), 587–608.

Vaughan, Megan, *Curing Their Ills: Colonial Power and African Illness* (Cambridge: Polity Press, 1991).

'Healing and Curing: Issues in the Social History and Anthropology of Medicine in Africa', *Social History of Medicine* 7.2 (1994), 283–95.

Viegas, Valentino, Frada, João and Miguel, José Pereira, *A Direcção-Geral da Saúde: notas históricas* (2006). www2.insa.pt/sites/INSA/SiteCollectionDocuments/ADGSnotashistoricas.pdf (last accessed 12 March 2021).

Vieira, Benedicta Maria, *O Conde de Penha Garcia e a sua vida pública: ensaio biográfico* (Castelo Branco: Estudos de Castelo Branco, 1972).

Vigne, Randolphe, 'The Moveable Frontier: The Namibia-Angola Boundary Demarcation, 1926–1928', in Patricia Hayes, Jeremy Sylvester, Marion Wallace and Wolfram Hartmann (eds.), *Namibia under South African Rule: Mobility and Containment, 1915–46* (Oxford: James Currey, 1998), 289–304.

Vos, Jelmer, 'Of Stocks and Barter: John Holt and the Kongo Rubber Trade, 1906–1910', *Portuguese Studies Review* 19.1–2 (2011), 153–75.

Kongo in the Age of Empire, 1860–1913: The Breakdown of a Moral Order (Madison: University of Wisconsin Press, 2015).

Walker, Timothy, 'Acquisition and Circulation of Medical Knowledge within the Early Modern Portuguese Colonial Empire', in Daniela Bleichmar, Paula De Vos, Kristin Huffine and Kevin Sheenan (eds.), *Science in the Spanish and Portuguese Empires, 1500–1800* (Stanford: Stanford University Press, 2009), 247–70.

Wall, Barbra Mann, *Into Africa: A Transnational History of Catholic Medical Missions and Social Change* (New Brunswick: Rutgers University Press, 2015).

Walters, Sarah, 'Counting Souls: Towards an Historical Demography of Africa', *Demographic Research* 34 (2016), 63–108.

Webel, Mari K., 'Medical Auxiliaries and the Negotiation of Public Health in Colonial North-Western Tanzania', *Journal of African History* 54.3 (2013), 393–416.

The Politics of Disease Control: Sleeping Sickness in Eastern Africa, 1890–1920 (Athens, OH: Ohio University Press, 2019).

Weindling, Paul, 'Social Medicine at the League of Nations Health Organisation and the International Labour Office Compared', in Paul Weindling (ed.), *International Health Organisations and Movements, 1918–1939* (Cambridge: Cambridge University Press, 1995), 134–53.

'Philanthropy and World Health: The Rockefeller Foundation and the League of Nations Health Organisation', *Minerva. A Review of Science, Learning and Policy* 35.3 (1997), 269–81.

Wempe, Sean Andrew, *Revenants of the German Empire: Colonial Germans, Imperialism, and the League of Nations* (Oxford: Oxford University Press, 2019).

Wesseling, H. L., *Divide and Rule: The Partition of Africa, 1880–1914* (Westport, CT: Praeger, 1996).

Wheeler, Douglas, 'The Forced Labour "System" in Angola, 1903–1947: Reassessing Origins and Persistence in the Context of Colonial Consolidation, Economic Growth and Reform Failures', in Centro de Estudos Africanos da Universidade do Porto (ed.), *Trabalho forçado africano: experiências coloniais comparadas* (Porto: Campo das Letras, 2006), 367–93.

'The Galvão Report on Forced Labor (1947) in Historical Context and Perspective: The Trouble-Shooter Who Was "Trouble"', *Portuguese Studies Review* 16.1 (2008), 115–52.

White, Joanna and Schouten, Maria Johanna (eds.), *Normal Birth: Experiences from Portugal and Beyond* (Braga: CICS, 2014).

White, Luise, 'Tsetse Visions: Narratives of Blood and Bugs in Colonial Northern Rhodesia, 1931–9', *Journal of African History* 36.2 (1995), 219–45.

White, Owen, *Children of the French Empire: Miscegenation and Colonial Society in French West Africa, 1895–1960* (Oxford: Clarendon Press, 1999).

Widmer, Alexandra, 'Of Field Encounters and Metropolitan Debates: Research and the Making and Meaning of the Melanesian "Race" during Demographic Decline', *Paideuma* 58 (2012), 69–93.

'The Imbalanced Sex Ratio and the High Bride Price: Watermarks of Race in Demography, Census, and the Colonial Regulation of Reproduction', *Science, Technology & Human Values* 39 (2014), 538–60.

Widmer, Alexandra and Lipphardt, Veronika (eds.), *Health and Difference: Rendering Human Variation in Colonial Engagements* (New York/Oxford: Berghahn Books, 2016).

Williams, Rosa, 'Migration and Miscegenation: Maintaining Boundaries of Whiteness in the Narratives of the Angolan State, 1875–1912', in Philip J. Havik and Malyn Newitt (eds.), *Creole Societies in the Portuguese Colonial Empire* (Bristol: Bristol University Press, 2007), 155–70.

Creating a Healthy Colonial State in Mozambique, 1885–1915. Unpublished PhD thesis, University of Chicago, 2013.

Wilson, Francis, *Labour in the South African Gold Mines, 1911–1969* (Cambridge: Cambridge University Press, 1972).

Worboys, Michael, 'The Comparative History of Sleeping Sickness in East and Central Africa, 1900–1914', *History of Science* 32.1 (1994), 89–102.

'Germs, Malaria and the Invention of Mansonian Tropical Medicine: From "Diseases in the Tropics" to "Tropical Diseases"', in David Arnold (ed.), *Warm Climates and Western Medicine: The Emergence of Tropical Medicine, 1500–1900* (Amsterdam: Rodopi, 1996), 181–207.

'Was There a Bacteriological Revolution in Late Nineteenth-Century Medicine?', *Studies in History and Philosophy of Biological & Biomedical Sciences* 38.1 (2007), 20–42.

Young, Crawford, *The African Colonial State in Comparative Perspective* (New Haven: Yale University Press, 1994).

Index

All persons appear as individual entries, and are indexed by their final surname (e.g. Mora, António Damas and so forth). Page numbers in italics refer to figures. Entries in bold indicate substantial entries with sub-headings. Please note that in the entry for Angola, provinces, districts, zones and cities have been combined into a single entry for simplicity. These provinces, districts, zones and cities overlapped with one another in complex and incomplete ways, and therefore towns within these areas appear in their own right, rather than being nested under the subentries for the relevant area.

308

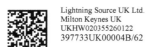

Lightning Source UK Ltd.
Milton Keynes UK
UKHW020355260122
397733UK00004B/62